Value and Quality Innovations in Acute and Emergency Care

Value and Quality Innovations in Acute and Emergency Care

Edited by

Jennifer L. Wiler, MD, MBA, FACEP
Executive Vice Chair and Associate Professor, School of Medicine, Department of Emergency Medicine
Founder and Executive Director, CARE Innovation Center, UCHealth
Associate Professor, Executive Healthcare, School of Business, University of Colorado, Denver, Colorado, USA

Jesse M. Pines, MD, MBA, MSCE
Director, Center for Healthcare Innovation and Policy Research
Professor of Emergency Medicine and Health Policy and Management, George Washington University, Washington, DC, USA

Michael J. Ward, MD, MBA
Assistant Professor, Vanderbilt University Medical Center, Department of Emergency Medicine, Nashville, Tennessee, USA

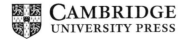

CAMBRIDGE
UNIVERSITY PRESS

CAMBRIDGE
UNIVERSITY PRESS

University Printing House, Cambridge CB2 8BS, United Kingdom

Cambridge University Press is part of the University of Cambridge.

It furthers the University's mission by disseminating knowledge in the pursuit of education, learning and research at the highest international levels of excellence.

www.cambridge.org
Information on this title: www.cambridge.org/9781316625637

© Cambridge University Press 2017

First published 2017

Printed in the United States of America by Sheridan Books, Inc.

A catalogue record for this publication is available from the British Library

Library of Congress Cataloging-in-Publication Data
Names: Wiler, Jennifer L., editor. | Pines, Jesse M., editor. | Ward, Michael J. (Professor of emergency medicine), editor.
Title: Value and quality innovations in acute and emergency care / edited by Jennifer L. Wiler, Jesse M. Pines, Michael J. Ward.
Description: Cambridge, United Kingdom ; New York : Cambridge University Press, 2017. | Includes bibliographical references and index.
Identifiers: LCCN 2016040384 | ISBN 9781316625637 (paperback)
Subjects: | MESH: Emergencies | Emergency Treatment | Acute Disease–therapy | Emergency Medicine–trends | Emergency Medicine–economics | Quality of Health Care | Case Reports
Classification: LCC RC86.7 | NLM WB 105 | DDC 616.02/5–dc23
LC record available at https://lccn.loc.gov/2016040384

ISBN 978-1-316-62563-7 Paperback

....

To my loving family – Dave, Quinn, Reid, and Blake – for their constant support and encouragement. – JLW

To my wife Lori, who gives me the time to let projects like this come together, and to my children, Asher, Molly, and Oren. – JMP

For my family, Marni, Claire, and Evan. You are my reason. Thank you for always keeping me grounded. – MJW

Contents

Contributors

Christopher W. Baugh, MD, MBA, Assistant Professor of Emergency Medicine, Brigham and Women's Hospital, Harvard Medical School, Boston, Massachusetts, USA

Molly Benoit, MPH, Research Assistant, Center for Healthcare Innovation and Policy Research, The George Washington University, Washington, DC, USA

Kelly Bookman, MD, FACEP, Medical Director, Director of EMR, Associate Professor, Department of Emergency Medicine, University of Colorado School of Medicine, Senior Medical Director, ED Service Line, UCHealth, Aurora, Colorado, USA

Roberta Capp, MD, MPH, Assistant Professor, Director of Care Transitions, School of Medicine, Department of Emergency Medicine, University of Colorado Hospital, Aurora, Colorado, USA

Christopher R. Carpenter, MD, MSc, Associate Professor, Division of Emergency Medicine, Washington University in St. Louis School of Medicine, St. Louis, Missouri, USA

Brendan G. Carr, MD, MA, MS, Associate Professor in Department of Emergency Medicine, Vice Chair of Health Care Policy and Delivery, Associate Dean for Healthcare Delivery Innovation, Sidney Kimmel Medical College, Thomas Jefferson University, Director of Emergency Care Coordination Center at US Department of Health and Human Services, Philadelphia, Pennsylvania, USA

Christopher G. Caspers, MD, Assistant Professor of Emergency Medicine, Langone Medical Center, New York University, New York, USA

Jody Crane, MD MBA, Chief Clinical Operations Officer at Sheridan Emergency Medicine, Faculty at University of Tennessee Physician Executive MBA Program, Faculty at Institute for Healthcare Improvement, Cambridge, Massachusetts, USA

T. Eugene Day, DSc, Program Manager for Health Systems, Office of Safety and Medical Operations, Children's Hospital of Philadelphia, Philadelphia, Pennsylvania, USA

M. Kit Delgado, MD, MS, FACEP, Assistant Professor of Emergency Medicine and Epidemiology, Senior Fellow at Leonard Davis Institute of Health Economics, Center for Emergency Care Policy and Research, University of Pennsylvania Perelman School of Medicine, Philadelphia, Pennsylvania, USA

C. Noelle Dietrich, MS, Senior Research Associate, Center for Healthcare Innovation and Policy Research, George Washington University, Washington, DC, USA

Benjamin Easter, MD, Instructor in Emergency Medicine, Administration, Operations and Quality Fellow, University of Colorado School of Medicine, Aurora, Colorado, USA

Wm. Wesley Fields, MD, FACEP, Associate Clinical Professor of Emergency Medicine at University of California, Irvine, Core Faculty in Emergency Medicine at Kaweah Delta Medical Center, Visalia, California, USA

Seth Glickman, MD, MBA, Associate Professor of Emergency Medicine, Director of Office for Population and Value Care, University of North Carolina, Chapel Hill, North Carolina, USA

Eric J. Goldlust, MD, PhD, FACEP, Emergency Physician at Kaiser Permanente Medical Group, Clinical Assistant Professor (Affiliate) in Department of Emergency Medicine, Stanford University School of Medicine, Stanford, California, USA

Joe Guarisco, MD, FAAEM, FACEP, System Chair, Emergency Medicine, Ochsner Health System, Jefferson Parish, Louisiana, USA

Nir J. Harish, MD, MBA, Robert Wood Johnson Foundation Scholar, Department of Emergency Medicine, Yale University School of Medicine, New Haven, Connecticut, USA

Kristi Henderson, DNP, NP-C FAEN, Vice President, Virtual Care and Innovation, Seton Healthcare Family, Austin, Texas, USA

Erik P. Hess, MD, MSc, Associate Professor, Department of Emergency Medicine, Mayo Clinic Medical College, Rochester, Minnesota, USA

Judd E. Hollander, MD, Associate Dean for Strategic Health Initiatives at Sidney Kimmel Medical College, Professor and Vice Chair of Finance and Healthcare Enterprises, Department of Emergency Medicine, Thomas Jefferson University, Philadelphia, Pennsylvania, USA

Nathan R. Hoot, MD, PhD, FACEP, Assistant Professor, Department of Emergency Medicine, University of Texas Health Science Center at Houston, Houston, Texas, USA

Ula Hwang, MD, MPH, Associate Professor in Department of Emergency Medicine and Brookdale Department of Geriatrics and Palliative Medicine, Icahn School of Medicine at Mount Sinai, Geriatric Research, Education and Clinical Center at James J. Peters VAMC, Bronx, New York, USA

Christian Jacobus, MD, FACEP, Medical Director of Bridge Home Health and Hospice, Assistant Professor of Emergency Medicine, University of Toledo College of Medicine and Life Sciences, Findlay, Ohio, USA

Alan E. Jones, MD, Professor and Chairman, Department of Emergency Medicine, University of Mississippi Medical Center, Jackson, Mississippi, USA

James Langabeer II, PhD, MBA, Professor of Emergency Medicine and Informatics, University of Texas Health Science Center, San Antonio, Texas, USA

Fred Lin, MD, Emergency Medicine Resident, Department of Emergency Medicine University of Pennsylvania, Perelman School of Medicine

Suzanne Mason, Professor of Emergency Medicine, School of Health and Related Research, University of Sheffield, Sheffield, South Yorkshire, UK

Christopher McStay, MD, FACEP, FAWM, Chief of Clinical Operations, Associate Professor, University of Colorado School of Medicine, Denver, Colorado, USA

Abhi Mehrotra, MD, MBA, Clinical Associate Professor of Emergency Medicine, Vice-Chair of Strategic Initiatives and Operations, Assistant Medical Director of ED – Chapel Hill, Medical Director of ED – Hillsborough, University of North Carolina, Chapel Hill, North Carolina, USA

Anthony M. Napoli, MD, Associate Professor of Emergency Medicine, Rhode Island Hospital, Warren Alpert Medical School of Brown University, Providence, Rhode Island, USA

Jesse M. Pines, MD, MBA, MSCE, Director, Center for Healthcare Innovation and Policy Research, Professor of Emergency Medicine and Health Policy and Management, George Washington University, Washington, DC, USA

Marc A. Probst, MD, MS, Assistant Professor, Department of Emergency Medicine, Icahn School of Medicine at Mount Sinai, New York, USA

Tammie E. Quest, MD, Professor at Emory University School of Medicine, Director of Emory Palliative Care Center, Department of Veterans Affairs, Atlanta, Georgia, USA

Ali S. Raja, MD, MBA, MPH, Vice Chair, Department of Emergency Medicine, Massachusetts General Hospital, Harvard Medical School, Boston, Massachusetts, USA

Megan Ranney, MD, MPH, Assistant Professor, Director of Emergency Digital Health Innovation Program, Department of Emergency Medicine, Alpert Medical School, Brown University, Providence, Rhode Island, USA

Kristin L. Rising, MD, MS, Assistant Professor, Director of Acute Care Transitions, Department of Emergency Medicine, Thomas Jefferson University, Philadelphia, Pennsylvania, USA

John S. Rozel, MD, MSL, Assistant Professor of Psychiatry and Adjunct Assistant Professor of Law, University of Pittsburgh, Medical Director, re:solve Crisis Network, Pittsburgh, Pennsylvania, USA

Dana R. Sax, MD, MPH, Emergency Physician, Permanente Medical Group, Oakland, California, USA

Tom Scaletta, MD, Chairperson of Department of Emergency Medicine, Medical Director of Patient Experience, Edward-Elmhurst Health, Naperville, Illinois, USA

David J. Schoenwetter, DO, FACEP, Medical Director of Geisinger EMS and Geisinger Life Flight, Attending in Emergency Medicine in Geisinger Health System, Danville, Pennsylvania, USA

Michael J. Schull, MD, MSc, FRCPC, Professor in Department of Medicine, Division of Emergency Medicine, University of Toronto, Sunnybrook Health Sciences Centre, Toronto, Ontario, Canada

Jeffrey S. Selevan, MD, Southern California Permanente Medical Group, Kaiser Permanente Medical Care Program, Pasadena, California, USA

Manish N. Shah, MD, MPH, Associate Professor, John and Tashia Morgridge Vice Chair for Research and Academic Affairs, BerbeeWalsh Department of Emergency Medicine, University of Wisconsin-Madison, Madison, Wisconsin, USA

Olan A. Soremekun, MD, MBA, Associate Professor, Vice Chair for Clinical Operations and New Business Development, Department of Emergency Medicine, Sydney Kimmel Medical College, Thomas Jefferson University and Hospitals, Philadelphia, Pennsylvania, USA

Sarah A. Sterling, MD, Assistant Professor, Department of Emergency Medicine, University of Mississippi Medical Center, Jackson, Mississippi, USA

Michael A. Turturro, MD, FACEP, Associate Professor of Emergency Medicine,

University of Pittsburgh School of Medicine, Chief of Emergency Services, UPMC-Mercy, Pittsburgh, Pennsylvania, USA

Arjun Venkatesh, MD, MBA, MHS, Assistant Professor in Department of Emergency Medicine, Director of ED Quality and Safety Research and Strategy, Co-Director of Emergency Medicine Administration Fellowship, Scientist, Center for Outcomes Research and Evaluation, Yale University School of Medicine, New Haven, Connecticut, USA

Michael J. Ward, MD, MBA, Assistant Professor, Vanderbilt University Medical Center, Department of Emergency Medicine, Nashville, Tennessee, USA

Jody A. Vogel, MD, MSc, Department of Emergency Medicine at Denver Health Medical Center and University of Colorado School of Medicine, Aurora, Colorado, USA

Jennifer L. Wiler, MD, MBA, FACEP, Executive Vice Chair and Associate Professor, School of Medicine, Department of Emergency Medicine; Executive Director, CARE Innovation Center, UCHealth, Aurora, CO; Associate Professor, Executive Healthcare, School of Business, University of Colorado, Denver, Colorado, USA

Dawn Williamson, RN, DNP(c) MSN, PMHCNS-BC, CARN-AP, Clinical Nurse Specialist, Patient Care Services, Emergency Department, Massachusetts General Hospital, Boston Massachusetts, USA

Richard Zane, MD, George B. Boedecker Jr. and Boedecker Foundation Endowed Chair of Emergency Medicine, Professor and Chair of Department of Medicine at University of Colorado School of Medicine, Chief of Emergency Services at University of Colorado Hospital, Executive Director of Emergency and EMS Services, Chief Innovation Officer, University of Colorado Health, Aurora, Colorado, USA

Mark S. Zocchi, MPH, Senior Research Associate, Center for Healthcare Innovation and Policy Research, George Washington University, Washington, DC, USA

Leslie Zun, MD, System Chair in Department of Emergency Medicine at Sinai Health System, Chairman and Professor in Department of Emergency Medicine and Psychiatry, Rosalind Franklin University of Medicine and Science/Chicago Medical School, Chicago, Illinois, USA

Foreword: Delivery System Reform – License to Innovate

Brendan G. Carr

There is no question that we are in the midst of a once in a generation change in the way that healthcare is delivered. The decade started with the passage of a landmark healthcare bill[1] with the lofty goals of increasing the number of Americans with health insurance and fundamentally changing the way that healthcare is delivered in the United States. Though the numbers are always in flux, about 17 million previously uninsured Americans now have coverage, and the uninsured rate is at an all-time low.[1] In January of 2015, the secretary of Health and Human Services outlined ambitious goals for how the Centers for Medicare and Medicaid Services (CMS) would create fundamental changes in payment that would dramatically transform healthcare delivery in the United States.[2] A few months later, Congress passed the Medicare Access and CHIP Reauthorization Act of 2015 (MACRA).[3] MACRA reinforces efforts to pay for care through alternative payment models (APM) (e.g., Accountable Care Organizations) and consolidates the many existing quality reporting structures into a single merit-based incentive payment system (MIPS). One way or another, providers will be motivated to deliver care differently in the future. Expenditures by CMS account for about a third of the $3 trillion spent annually on healthcare in the United States,[1] and the secretary plans for fully half of all spending to use these novel payments and their associated delivery models (e.g., not fee for service) by 2018.

The dramatic shift in how healthcare is paid for has created substantial disruption in the healthcare industry. Many of the efforts to date have been focused on cost reduction through efficient management of high-cost chronic conditions. Health insurance exchanges, Medicaid expansion, hospital readmissions penalties, Accountable Care Organizations, and the precision medicine initiative[4] have dominated headlines over the last 5 years. A central focus moving forward will be on not just how healthcare is paid for but what innovators will do to improve the experience of healthcare. If the future is uncertain in the broader healthcare delivery market, how acute and emergency care will fit into the emerging payment and delivery structures is almost entirely uncharted.[5] With care delivery untethered from payment, market forces, consumer preferences, and lessons learned from industry will allow the United States to translate advances in precision medicine to the population on the whole. This new field – the field of precision delivery – is the next frontier; the delivery system reform initiative sparked by payment change gives healthcare license to innovate.

This book gives us a glimpse into some of the most forward-leaning approaches to date for reinventing acute and emergency care delivery. Americans made over 130 million visits to emergency departments (EDs) and 160 million to urgent care centers in 2012.[6] Retail pharmacies have entered the healthcare space, community paramedics are reinventing the house call, and telemedicine is expected to grow to a $30 billion industry by 2020.[7] In the book's introductory chapters, Easter offers an exceptional review of where emergency care came from, and Harish and Pines paint a vision of the future path toward payment reforms in acute and emergency care. The book offers almost two dozen case-based examples that drive home its central focus: emergency medicine evolved out of the public's need for acute care, and it has never stopped evolving. In some cases, the evolution is about system performance and this is highlighted in chapters examining the United Kingdom's 4-hour rule, the US Veterans Administration's application of discrete event simulation to their access challenges, and the movement of palliative care to the front line. Innovations focused on the ED experience include the elimination of the waiting room at the University of Colorado, the creation of a specialty geriatric ED, and a focus on the patient experience. Still others examine alternatives to acute and emergent care including urgent care centers, telehealth, and the use of community health workers to connect patients to community-based services. The practice of emergency care has always been broad, but the pages that follow are really a glimpse into the future of emergency care practice. Over the last half century, the ED has transformed from a variably staffed "room" where life and limb threats were managed to a safety net for a crumbling health system. The role of the emergency physician continues to evolve to fill the needs of the health system. Practitioners may find themselves staffing the emergency department, the urgent care center, or the observation service; they may be providing on-demand tele-health or medical command support for out of hospital responders to 911 calls; they may be visiting high utilizers or patients recently discharged from the hospital. The next step in the evolution of emergency medicine has recently been referred to as the creation of the "available-ist."

Not all change is readily embraced. Two stories from the recent medical literature come to mind. Despite the fact that Kodak invented digital technology, the company did not readily adopt it as they were concerned that it would erode film sales. Over the course of the next decade, the value of the company plummeted until it declared bankruptcy (after 131 years) in 2012. An editorial in the *New England Journal of Medicine* commented that "Kodak was late to recognize that it was not in the film and camera business: it was in the imaging business." In a second example, a recent editorial offered advice based on the lessons learned from the entry of Uber into the transportation marketplace, explaining that healthcare providers, like taxi drivers have three choices: "ignore innovators and hope for the best; call for increasing regulation to make it harder for innovators to enter the market; or compete on quality and efficiency, disruptive though that might be." Change is here and leaders are emerging. Referencing Kodak's collapse, Asch wrote: "Doctors and hospitals who pay attention to the business they are actually in – defined by the outcomes their 'customers' seek – will leave the doctors and hospitals who don't behind." The pages that follow offer an early lens into the future of emergency care delivery from innovators in the field.

References

1. http://obamacarefacts.com/sign-ups/obamacare-enrollment-numbers/.

2. Burwell SM. Setting value-based payment goals – HHS efforts to improve U.S. health care. *New England Journal of Medicine* 2015;372(10):897–899.

3. Pub. Law 114-10, the Medicare Access and CHIP Reauthorization Act. www.congress.gov/114/bills/hr2/BILLS-114hr2enr.pdf.

4. House TW. The Precision Medicine Initiative. 2015; www.whitehouse.gov/precision-medicine.

5. Brookings Institution. Reimagining emergency medicine: how to integrate care for the acutely ill and injured. 2015; www.brookings.edu/events/2015/05/06-medtalk-emergency-medicine-acute-care.

6. Statistics NCfH. Health, United States, 2014: with special feature on adults aged 55–64. 2014; www.cdc.gov/nchs/data/hus/hus14.pdf-083.

7. Monegain B. Telemedicine market to soar past 30 billion. www.healthcareitnews.com/news/telemedicine-poised-grow-big-time.

Preface

Acute and emergency care plays a critical role in improving population health. These services include diagnostic testing and treatments delivered to people when they are ill and injured. Such care can be delivered in a variety of settings including accident and emergency (A&E) departments in the United Kingdom or emergency departments (EDs) in the United States, hospitals, doctors' offices, urgent care centers, retail clinics, mobile clinics, and by telemedicine. Despite the variety of locations, delivery of this care at the local systems level can be quite challenging. Moreover, while acute and emergency care plays a central role in medicine, its provision comes at considerable cost. In the United States, there has been increased scrutiny on healthcare costs, which are changing the regulations that govern acute and emergency care quality measurement and payment. Exploring how acute and emergency care can become more efficient and cost-effective is an issue of increasing global importance. The critical question is this: "How can acute and emergency care become more efficient, cost-effective, and better designed to meet the needs of patients?"

This book describes the current quality and value movement in acute and emergency care and presents 20 case studies of both US-based and international acute care delivery innovations with expert commentaries. Included in the examples are descriptions of innovations in telehealth, observation medicine, ways to improve patient experience, high utilizer programs, and using informatics to improve clinical decision support. This book is ideal for:

- Stakeholders who are interested in innovation and who want to learn how to improve care while reducing costs and improving quality by following international models that inform global innovation.
- Administrators who want to improve operations and patient flow, particularly in acute and emergency care settings.
- Policymakers who want to better understand the levers for creating positive change in acute and emergency care.

Fifty Years of Transformation of Acute and Emergency Care

Benjamin Easter

In his landmark 1979 piece which defined a specialty, Peter Rosen, MD, called emergency medicine "an unaccountably late development in modern medicine." Rosen strongly argued for a specialty defined not by an organ system or a particular patient population, but by "initial care . . . of life threat[s]."[1] This fundamental notion is now reflected in the American College of Emergency Physicians' (ACEP) definition of emergency medicine as "the medical specialty dedicated to the diagnosis and treatment of unforeseen illness or injury, including the initial evaluation, diagnosis, treatment, coordination of care among multiple providers, and disposition of any patient requiring expeditious medical, surgical, or psychiatric care."[2] Though the framing of a physician's expertise in terms of a phase of care was without precedent 50 years ago, today we understand it implicitly.

The Ancestor to the Emergency Physician

In his book, *Anyone, Anything, Anytime: A History of Emergency Medicine*, Brian Zink, MD, deems the primary care physician (previously, a general practitioner) "the ancestor to the emergency physician."[3] To be sure, an early twentieth-century primary care physician had a similar scope of practice to a modern emergency physician: internal medicine, minor surgical care, obstetrics, pediatrics, and psychiatry. Prior to World War II, fully three-quarters of American physicians identified themselves as primary care physicians. However, this umbrella term belied significant heterogeneity in training. Early 1900s primary care physicians were likely to have gone straight into independent clinical practice after completing medical school, which at the time involved primarily "book" work. Those who trained after the Flexner Report of 1910 (which stands as the foundation of American medical training curricula to this day) were more likely to have had at least 1 year of post-graduate internship.

The standardization and organization called for by the Flexner Report, coupled with the growth in medical knowledge, accelerated a trend toward specialization. Organization of specialty societies and boards – the American College of Surgeons in 1913 and the American Board of Ophthalmology in 1916 – followed, and many hospitals began to require post medical school training and certification prior to credentialing. The diverse group of primary care physicians would not unify into the American Academy of General Practice until 1947.

By this point, the healthcare landscape had changed significantly. Specialists, on account of their training and credentialing, had better access to hospitals and performed more of the medical school teaching, and patients came to expect the standard of care provided by a specialist. By 1966, only 31 percent of physicians were primary care physicians.[3] As their scope of practice narrowed, primary care physicians had to see more patients per day. This made it difficult to maintain the always-available philosophy that had defined them for decades. In addition, the aforementioned explosion of medical knowledge made mastery of a diverse range of subjects increasingly difficult.

The Growing Role of the Hospital and the Crisis of the Emergency Room

A similar transformation was occurring in the location that Americans received healthcare. In the post–World War II era, the United States completed its transition from home care to hospital care. The Hill-Burton Act of 1946 fueled a postwar spending binge on hospital growth with the number of US hospitals increasing 21 percent between 1946 and 1965. In addition, the growth in medical knowledge and technology altered the public's perception of hospitals from a place of convalescence to a place of cure.[3] Sophisticated new technologies, such as radiographs, were expensive, leading to their concentration in hospitals, which had the capital to purchase them and the volume to use them profitably. For similar reasons, specialists concentrated in hospitals as well. Many physicians moved their practice locations to the area around the hospital for their own and their patients' convenience. As Zink argues, these changes catalyzed a paradigm shift from primary care physician-centered healthcare to system-centered healthcare.[3]

Use of the emergency room (ER) became common at this time as well. (N.B. The term "ER," as it was called at the time, is specifically used to contrast it with the more modern "emergency department"). From 1954 to 1965, US ER visits tripled in just over a decade. A number of factors contributed to this sudden growth. Demographic changes in the United States were chief among these. Increased population during the Baby Boom years led to increased demand for medical care overall.[4] In addition, suburban sprawl made it more difficult for a traditional primary care physician to perform house call. As office-based practice became more routine and scheduled, it became more difficult for providers to leave time for acute or unscheduled patients. Primary care physicians also followed the general population emigration from cities, leaving the burden of care to the ERs of public hospitals and urban academic medical centers.[3] In fact, the change was so significant that it was presciently noted in 1957 that "Americans came to '…take for granted that hospitals have emergency service at all hours where any problem, surgical, medical, or psychiatric can be treated. … In time, the hospital emergency service may find its scope extended to meet any general medical and surgical problems, which the patient, at least, will deem urgent.'"[3]

Despite this, the ER remained an afterthought in the priorities of many hospitals. At the time, emergency medicine as a specialty did not yet exist. In many settings, physicians who had been censured or could not meet credentialing requirements were placed there. Former criminals, alcoholics, and foreign medical graduates trying to learn English were common. In academic settings, the most junior of housestaff cared for ED patients, frequently with no supervision. In a 1956 survey of hospitals, 71 percent staffed their ER with house officers.[3] A mere 21 percent used private physicians, typically a rotating call schedule of all of the hospital's practitioners, including even those that did not normally treat medical or surgical patients, such as psychiatrists or pathologists.[5] Greater than half of ambulance transports were provided by funeral directors or morticians because their vehicles allowed for horizontal transport of patients.

However, the pressing needs of ER patients led to calls for improved emergency care. In 1958, the *New England Journal of Medicine* published an article titled "The ER and the

Changing Pattern of Medical Care," which detailed historical data on ER use at Hartford Hospital and called for staffing of ERs with "professional personnel of adequate training and mature judgment."[6] An accompanying editorial boldly declared "the experience and judgment of the physician who directs [emergency] care is the indispensable sine qua non.[7]

Thus, a gap was emerging. Both patients and the system demanded a new age specialty-trained physician with content and technical expertise across multiple fields, but who was also a throwback to the primary care physician's ethical obligation to provide care to whomever and whenever it was needed.

The Alexandria Plan

Into this gap stepped Dr. James Mills. In 1961, Dr. Mills was a primary care physician working in Alexandria, VA. He had an affiliation with Alexandria Hospital, which faced many of the challenges detailed above – rising patient volumes and lack of consistent and appropriately trained staff for its ER. ER nurses would triage patients, and then call on housestaff or private physicians (who frequently, in turn, called housestaff) to see patients. But Alexandria Hospital had many unfilled internship slots, and a pilot to staff the ER with medical students had failed.

Dr. Mills decided that he personally would leave his practice behind and work full time in the ER. He convinced one other primary care physician and two internists to join him. They contracted with the hospital to work 12-hour shifts, 5 days on and 5 days off. Their experiment was incredibly successful. ER volume doubled within 5 years, and both private practice physicians and patients were increasingly satisfied with the care provided.

A similar pattern emerged in Pontiac, MI. There, a group of approximately 30 physicians from various specialties contracted to provide care in the emergency room. Each worked 16–32 hours per month. The Pontiac group was quite successful financially, and the participating providers soon found they could make a higher hourly salary in the ER than in their other practices. This was no doubt a strong impetus for the development of emergency medicine as a specialty.

From Emergency Room to Emergency Department

Dr. Mills's contract with Alexandria Hospital specified work in the "emergency department" as opposed to the "emergency room." This seemingly trivial change in language was suggestive of the organizational transformation that emergency medicine would undergo over the next several decades.

In 1968, eight physicians from Michigan founded the American College of Emergency Physicians. ACEP's logo, which still exists today, was designed by the son of one of the founders.[8] It depicts a large square made of 64 smaller squares, which represented the organization of American medicine. One square, however, is missing, representing the lack of emergency medicine in this framework. Just a year later, the first emergency medicine national meeting, the ACEP Scientific Assembly, was held in Denver, CO. The College had a strong early focus on the finances of emergency medicine. Many practitioners were nervous about leaving their stable practices behind for the ED, and the College fought for reimbursement for EPs as specialists.

Around this time, the University of Cincinnati was also approved by the American Medical Association to start a 2-year emergency medicine training program. Still wary of the young specialty, it was formally approved under family practice with a certification of advanced training in emergency medicine. Nonetheless, in 1972, Bruce Janiak, MD, became the first residency-trained emergency physician in the United States.

From the outset, there was disagreement among the ACEP members about specialty status. Some even advocated for becoming a sub-section of the American Academy of General Practice. However, after rejecting this thought, the College began to pursue a path toward specialty certification. A number of things would be required: codifying the scope of practice, developing initial training and continuing education programs, creating academic departments, writing an exam, and defining a body of research.[3] Formal recognition of the specialty would soon follow.

In 1975, the AMA approved a section on emergency medicine and established training standards for residencies. In 1979, emergency medicine was recognized as the 23rd medical specialty approved by the American Board of Medical Specialties, and the American Board of Emergency Medicine (ABEM) was granted administrative rights to provide board certification. The first test was offered the following year. The format of the ABEM oral examination was unique at the time, and the rigor of the certification process was important for the young specialty. Originally, ABEM was a "conjoint" board with representatives from other so-called "parent" specialties. This led to interesting challenges. In one discussion about how much training emergency medicine residents should have in other specialties, the seven specialties on the board created a training program 13 years in length.[3] However, only a decade later, ABEM would become its own, primary board.

Thus, emergency medicine became a formal part of the house of medicine. Prior to Dr. Janiak, no emergency physician had been trained as such; all were converts who pioneered a new practice. But having learned from the experience of primary care physicians, early emergency physicians quickly recognized the need for and codified a formal structure of training, credentialing, and practice. This was fortunate, as a number of external factors would drastically increase the need for emergency physicians in the years to come.

Outside Influences

Parallel to these developments, there was growing recognition of the importance of acute illness in society. In 1966, the National Academy of Sciences released a landmark report titled "Accidental Death and Disability: The Neglected Disease of Modern Society," which bemoaned this "epidemic" and the relative "public apathy" with which it was being confronted.[9] In particular, the group was concerned about the paucity of attention paid to trauma in comparison to cardiovascular disease or cancer. This report catalyzed the development of a national emergency phone number (911), pre-hospital services, and regional emergency care networks. The year 1965 had seen the inauguration of Medicare and Medicaid, which brought millions of elderly and indigent patients, many of whom had been underserved or completely without medical care, back to the frontlines. This placed additional pressure on generalists and specialists alike, and made it even more difficult to expect them to cover both scheduled and unscheduled care. Furthermore, relatively little attention had been paid at the national level to ensuring there were sufficient providers for this influx of patients. Many turned to the ED.

The Vietnam War also profoundly impacted the development of emergency medicine. In Vietnam, mortality rates plummeted compared to prior wars as a system of rapid triage and evacuation to definitive care was implemented. Advances in intravenous fluids, blood product administration, and antibiotics were also brought back to civilian practice.

Hospitals also continued to grow in size and complexity. Perhaps ironically, the more complex and organizationally detailed they became, the more patients came to the ED for care. As Zink wrote, "Hospitals had become little fiefdoms . . . [and] presenting to the ED at a hospital complex was the simplest and most convenient way to gain entry into a system that could seem imposing and confusing from the outside." The ED became the "default point of contact . . . for millions of urban people."[3] Medicare and Medicaid also allowed hospitals to make money on patients that had previously been charity care. Accordingly, the ED became an increasing point of emphasis, and hospitals desired high-quality emergency physicians. In addition, many private physicians were happy to have less work on nights, weekends, and holidays, and to have a source to refer their acute patients at other times.

Growing a Specialty

The 1980s would see explosive growth in emergency medicine education and training. Following the University of Cincinnati program, dozens of other emergency medicine residencies were started. The American College of Graduate Medical Education approved the requirements for EM residencies in 1982. Originally, a preliminary internship year followed by 24 months of emergency medicine was required, though this was later changed to 36 months of emergency medicine. In 1989, the path to board certification was closed for non-residency trained emergency physicians. Less than 30 years after Dr. Mills started the Alexandria plan, every new board certified emergency physician in the United States would be residency trained.

EM quickly became a competitive choice among American medical students. The educational philosophy was also unique. During the foundational years, leaders in the specialty debated whether training programs in emergency medicine should have 24-hour supervision by faculty.[10] This question was especially pertinent, given the then routine staffing of ERs with housestaff only. The decision was made that EM faculty should always be present, a defining characteristic of EM in American academic medical centers that distinguished it from virtually every other specialty. Peter Rosen, a founding pioneer of the specialty, further defined the educational mission in "The Biology of Emergency Medicine," calling for the need for the right patient pathology, the right faculty, and the right number of residents.[1]

In 1986, Congress formalized the ED's role as the safety net of American healthcare with its passage of the Emergency Medical Treatment and Active Labor Act (EMTALA). EMTALA requires EDs to provide appropriate evaluation and medical stabilizing treatment for any person seeking care with an emergency medical condition. Technically, the law applies only to hospitals accepting federal payer sources, but this pertains to virtually every hospital in the United States. Written to prohibit "dumping" of patients based on payer status, EMTALA guaranteed a rudimentary level of universal access to the ED for all patients in the United States.

Emergency Medicine Internationally

Internationally, emergency medicine has developed most quickly in the British Common-wealth. In the United Kingdom, it is frequently known as Accident and Emergency (A+E), and developed during a similar time period. Maurice Ellis served as the first "casualty consultant" in 1952. The British Association for Accident and Emergency Medicine was founded in 1967, and the first certification exam took place in 1983. A similar path toward specialty certification occurred, as an Intercollegiate Board, analogous to ABEM's conjoint board, was founded in 1991. In 2006, the boards merged to become a joint College of Emergency Medicine, which was designated the Royal College of Emergency Medicine in 2015, of which there are over 5,000 members today.[11] The Canadian Association of Emergency Physicians and the Australasian College for Emergency Medicine were founded several years later. Both serve similar functions in their respective countries.

The above organizations all collaborated in the founding of the International Federation for Emergency Medicine (IFEM) in 1989. IFEM works to promote emergency medicine as a recognized specialty in countries around the world, helping to shepherd them through the above process.

Emergency medicine has been slower to emerge in the developing world. Traditionally, global health has focused on prevention of illness, maternal and child health, and treatment of childhood diseases.[12] This focus, while important, has failed to produce comprehensive and timely healthcare systems that are capable of caring for emergencies. Nevertheless, there is certainly unmet need. In fact, seven of the top fifteen causes of death and six of the top fifteen causes of disability in developing countries have evidence that early intervention improves outcomes.[13] In addition to their primary mission, EDs can also play important roles augmenting public health and primary prevention efforts, including vaccine administration, training of clinical personnel in high volume areas, referral for treatment and secondary prevention, and disaster care.[14]

All emergency medical systems must have certain components, including a need for public education about recognition of illness and accessing the system, communication about patients and a means for transporting them, triage, and training of medical personnel in the principles of emergency medicine. However, while minimum standards must be created, local communities should define the particular illnesses to be targeted and interventions to be offered.[13] By way of example, an economic analysis of a hypothetical emergency medical response system for cardiac arrest in Kuala Lumpur, Malaysia, showed that it would cost approximately $2.5 million to produce four neurologically intact survivors of cardiac arrest.[15] The high cost is principally a result of Kuala Lumpur's young population, illustrating the need for local determination (rather than wholesale import) of the menu of emergency services.

To be sure, international emergency medicine faces stiff challenges: lack of first aid training among the lay public, poorly developed transportation systems, and lack of formal education in emergency medicine all compound already existing financial and infrastructure constraints. As a temporizing measure, IFEM created a curriculum in basic emergency medicine for international medical students, laying out the basic principles of emergency care that physicians of every specialty should know.[16] Success stories do exist, however. Botswana recently recognized emergency medicine as a specialty, and created a residency-style training program and research center.[17]

Acute and Emergency Care: The ED and Beyond

Having evolved from one room "ERs," the modern ED is a sprawling and complex place. The ED is the de facto point of entry into the hospital for virtually all patients. Patients present of their own accord, many are referred by outside providers, and ambulances also transport patients. EDs may incorporate many different areas to help "stream" patients by complaint and acuity. Low-acuity, urgent complaints may be handled in a fast-track area. Specialized rooms exist for the care of specific patient populations, such as gynecology, otolaryngology, or psychiatry. A high acuity or resuscitation area allows for the treatment of the most acute patients, and can provide many of the services of an Intensive Care Unit or Operating Room. In addition, space is needed for the many ancillary services that ED patients need quick access to, including radiology (plain radiographs, computerized tomography (CT), ultrasound, and potentially MRI), laboratory analyses, case management, and security. Easy access to an ambulance bay and helipad are generally needed.

Though it is still the most common, the hospital ED is far from the only location to receive acute and emergency care patients. Urgent care centers and retail clinics have become well-established alternatives for lower acuity, unscheduled care. More recently, freestanding emergency departments and telemedicine have also entered the acute care space.

Urgent care centers developed as a means to provide unscheduled care to lower acuity patients. There are almost 7,000 such centers in the United States.[18] Urgent care represents a niche market – patients generally do not have access to or are unable to get a timely appointment with their primary care physician for an unscheduled illness, but their illnesses are not emergent or they wish to avoid the costs and times associated with an ED. Most urgent care centers perform basic testing, such as a dipstick urinalysis or plain radiographs. They are most frequently staffed by family physicians followed by emergency physicians. Charges seen by the patient are significantly lower than most EDs.[19] While urgent care centers have considerably longer hours than most physicians' offices, most are not open 24 hours per day.

Retail clinics are a variation on the urgent care model. These are clinics located in, and typically affiliated with, stores, pharmacies, or supermarkets. Most are staffed with physician assistants or nurse practitioners. Approximately 2,000 exist in the United States. They treat routine illnesses, such as upper respiratory infections, and also offer health screenings and vaccinations. Unscheduled visits and extended hours are the norm. In contrast to most of the rest of the US healthcare landscape, prices are generally fixed and visible in advance.[20] In addition, for care within the scope of practice of retail clinics, costs tend to be lower than comparable care in a primary care physician's office, urgent care, or ED. Up to 90 percent of patients report that they were very or somewhat satisfied with the quality of their care, and the National Committee for Quality Assurance has found several retail clinics to be among the highest performers in quality metrics pertaining to primary care and urgent care. However, it is unclear if the convenience of retail clinics simply adds additional encounters to the healthcare system rather than replacing them with lower cost substitutes.[20] In addition, care coordination and continuity of care with a patient's physician is very limited.

In the last few years, the United States has seen the proliferation of freestanding emergency departments (FSED). These are physically separate from acute-care hospitals, though they may be affiliated with such. They seek to fill the gap between the traditional ED and urgent care. Generally, FSEDs provide many services that might be available only in an ED, such as CT scans or electrocardiography, and are staffed with emergency physicians, but also provide the proximity and convenience traditionally associated with an urgent care center. There is significant state-to-state variation in the regulations governing FSEDs with respect to credentialing, payment, and accessibility. Of concern though is their concentration in areas with a favorable payer mix, and not in those areas where healthcare resources are scarce.[21]

Telemedicine can take two forms. The first is real-time patient management with collaboration between two providers. High-fidelity video and audio equipment are used to help the provider at a distance obtain information as if he/she were at the bedside. This type of telemedicine is frequently used in rural or remote areas to obtain consultation with higher levels of care or specialists, such as trauma surgeons or a stroke team. Another opportunity is for a virtual patient-provider encounter without an office visit. Fees are generally lower than an in-person visit, but it takes less time and gives the clinician freedom to work from a location of his/her choosing. One study based on this premise examined the laceration treatment decisions of emergency physicians who were given a medical history and four mobile phone pictures of the laceration. The same EP then examined the patient directly. There was agreement about treatment decision in 87 percent of patients.[22] While quite innovative, lack of consistent reimbursement for telemedicine applications remains a challenge, however.

Acute and Emergency Care: Transformed but Still in Need of Innovation

Today, there are approximately 40,000 practicing emergency physicians in the United States, almost 1 in 25 physicians. There are approximately 200 residency programs (allopathic and osteopathic) graduating 2,000 new EPs annually. There are 130 million U.S. ED visits per year. It would seem ironic to the founders of the specialty, so worried that their efforts would be thwarted by private physicians afraid to lose their patients, that 80 percent of patients who called their family physician about a new medical complaint were directed to the ED.[23]

There are clear hallmarks of success over the last three decades. A national 911 program, with sophisticated emergency medical services, places emergency care within minutes of most Americans. Air medical transport, combined with regional care networks, can rapidly move patients to higher levels of care. Morbidity and mortality for devastating acute illnesses – myocardial infarction, stroke, and trauma, to name a few – have plummeted.

This is not to say, however, that improvements are not necessary. In fact, ACEP's 2014 rating of the US emergency care system was a woeful "D+." In categories that included Access to Emergency Care, Quality and Patient Safety Environment, Medical Liability Environment, Public Health and Injury Prevention, and Disaster Preparedness, no category scored better than a "C."[23] Access, operations, quality/safety, and cost issues plague many modern emergency departments, and threaten the substantial progress made over the last 50 years.

In some ways, EDs have been a victim of their own success, with growth in ED visits exceeding twice the growth in the US population.[23] Coupled with a decrease in acute care hospital beds, this growth has led to significant crowding in EDs and boarding of admitted patients. Increasingly, the ED and its patients are understood not to be the source of crowding, but its most recognizable victim as research demonstrates that crowding is a hospital and community-wide problem.[24,25] Nevertheless, crowding has been associated with adverse outcomes, treatment delays, and increased rates of patients leaving prior to seeing a physician, and future innovations must address this vexing problem.[26,27,28]

Simultaneously, the ED handles significant public health roles, and serves as the safety net of the healthcare system. Patients who are under- or uninsured, homeless, struggle with substance abuse, have high risk medical conditions, or even who simply are unable to see a primary care physician in a timely fashion utilize the ED. Because of the broad cross-section of society that uses the ED for some type of care, EDs are increasingly serving surveillance roles for HIV infection and substance abuse in addition to more traditional public health roles such as vaccination, secondary prevention, and diagnosis of chronic illness and referral for treatment. "Although the principal mission of EM is to care for patients with acute illness and injury, this is not its only mission and it is naïve to believe our role is strictly confined to the former. Since its inception as a recognized medical specialty . . . emergency practitioners have consistently provided preventive care services, many of which have become standard of care. We do . . . strongly advocate for performing preventive interventions that make the most sense in the context of available resources."[29]

Compounding these problems, there is renewed focused on the cost of medical care in many countries. In the United States, approximately 17 percent of Gross Domestic Product is spent on healthcare with little to no marginal improvement in outcomes over countries spending half that amount. Government and private payers are actively seeking alternative payment models that simultaneously reduce costs and deliver greater value. Many other countries, including the United Kingdom, have considerably more experience with the healthcare value equation and understand the need for cost-effective, evidence-based solutions. Nonetheless, they still face the perception that emergency care is costly and inefficient. Therefore, there is a need to clearly define the value of acute and emergency care, and describe case studies of innovative solutions that have enhanced this value through improved outcomes and decreased costs.

References

1. Rosen P. The biology of emergency medicine. *Journal of the American College of Emergency Physicians*. 1979;8:280–283.

2. American College of Emergency Physicians. Definition of emergency medicine. Available at www.acep.org/Clinical–Practice–Management/Definition-of-Emergency-Medicine/. Accessed November 30, 2015.

3. Zink B. *Anyone, Anything, Anytime: A History of Emergency Medicine*. Elsevier Health Science, 2006.

4. Southern Illinois University. The history and future of emergency medicine. Available at www.siumed.edu/students/emig/history.pdf. Accessed November 30, 2015.

5. Suter RE. Emergency medicine in the United States: a systematic review. *World Journal of Emergency Medicine*. 2012;3(1): 5–10.

6. Shortliffe EC, Hamilton TS. The emergency room and the changing pattern of medical care. *New England Journal of Medicine*. 1958;258:20–25.

7. Emergency Ward Service. *New England Journal of Medicine*. 1958;258:47–48.

8. American College of Emergency Physicians. The ACEP logo: what it really means. www.acep.org/About-Us/The-ACEP-Logo–What-it-Really-Means/. Accessed December 3, 2015.

9. National Academy of Sciences, Division of Medical Sciences, Committee on Trauma and Committee on Shock. *Accidental Death and Disability: The Neglected Disease of Modern Society*. Washington, DC, 1966.

10. Harkin KE, Cushman JT, eds. *Emergency Medicine: A Comprehensive Guide to the Specialty*. Dallas, TX: Emergency Medicine Residents' Association, 2007.

11. Royal College of Emergency Medicine. Landmarks in the development of

the specialty. Available at http://www.rcem.ac.uk/. Accessed December 3, 2015.

12. Macfarlane S, Racelis M, Muli-Musiime F. Public health in developing countries. *Lancet*. 2000;356:841–846.

13. Razzak JA, Kellerman AL. Emergency medical care in developing countries: is it worthwhile? *Bulletin of the World Health Organization*. 2002;80(11):900–905.

14. Anderson P, Petrino R, Halpern P, et al. The globalization of emergency medicine and its importance for public health. *Bulletin of the World Health Organization*. 2006;84(10):835–839.

15. Hauswald M, Yeoh E. Designing a prehospital system for a developing country: estimated cost and benefits. *American Journal of Emergency Medicine*. 1997;15(6):600–603.

16. Slinger A, Hobgood C, Kilroy D, et al. International federation for emergency medicine model curriculum for medical student education in emergency medicine. *Emergency Medicine Australasia*. 2009;21 (5):367–372.

17. Caruso N, Chandra A, Kestler A. Development of emergency medicine in Botswana. *African Journal of Emergency Medicine*. 2011;1(3):108–112.

18. Urgent Care Association of America. Industry FAQs. Available at www.ucaoa.org/general/custom.asp?page=IndustryFAQs. Accessed December 8, 2015.

19. Weinick RM, Bristol SJ, DesRoches CM. Urgent care centers in the U.S.: findings from a national survey. *BMC Health Services Research*. 2009;9:79.

20. Bachrach D, Frohlich J, Garcimonde A, Nevitt K. Building a culture of health: the value proposition of retail clinics. Robert Wood Johnson Foundation. Available at www.rwjf.org/content/dam/farm/reports/issue_briefs/2015/rwjf419415. Accessed December 8, 2015.

21. Schuur JD, Baker O, Wilson M, Cutler D. Where do freestanding emergency departments choose to locate? A socio-demographic analysis in three states. *Annals of Emergency Medicine*. 2015 Oct;66 (4S):S2.

22. Sikka N, Pirri M, Carlin K, Strauss R, Rahimi F, Pines J. The use of mobile phone cameras in guiding treatment decisions for laceration care. *Telemedicine Journal and e-Health*. 2012;18(70):554–557.

23. American College of Emergency Physicians. America's emergency care environment: a state-by-state report card – 2014. Available at www.emreportcard.org/uploadedFiles/ACEP-ReportCard-10-22-08.pdf.pdf. Accessed December 3, 2015.

24. Schneider SM, Gallery ME, Schafermeyer R, et al. Emergency department crowding: a point in time. *Annals of Emergency Medicine*. 2003;42:167–172.

25. Schull MJ, Lazier K, Vermeulen M, et al. Emergency department contributors to ambulance diversion: a quantitative analysis. *Annals of Emergency Medicine*. 2003;41:467–476.

26. Sun BC, Hsia RY, Weiss RE, et al. Effect of emergency department crowding on outcomes of admitted patients. *Annals of Emergency Medicine*. 2013;61(6):605–611.

27. Liu S, Hobgood C, Brice JH. Impact of critical bed status on emergency department patient flow and overcrowding. *Academic Emergency Medicine*. 2003;10:382–385.

28. Polevoi SK, Quinn JV, Kramer NR. Factors associated with patients who leave without being seen. *Academic Emergency Medicine*. 2005;12:232–236.

29. Bernstein SL, Haukoos JS. Public health, prevention, and emergency medicine: a critical juxtaposition. *Academic Emergency Medicine*. 2008;15(2):190–193.

Chapter

2

Fragmentation in Acute and Emergency Care
Causes, Consequences, and Solutions

Jesse M. Pines, Mark S. Zocchi, C. Noelle Dietrich, and Molly Benoit

Introduction

The landmark Patient Protection and Affordable Care Act (ACA), signed into law in 2010, was enacted with two major objectives: expand access to health insurance and reform the healthcare delivery system.[1] One of the goals of the ACA's delivery system reform is to reduce care fragmentation, where multiple providers and organizations provide care to patients with no single entity coordinating overall aspects of care. Care fragmentation is prominent in acute, unscheduled care, particularly in episodic settings like emergency departments (EDs) and urgent care centers that may not have complete information about patient's prior records and or any connection to patients' longitudinal providers, particularly primary care physicians. The uncoordinated, fragmented care delivery system results in higher costs, sometime conflicting care plans, preventable hospitalizations, and lower quality, along with frustration for both patients and providers.[2,3,4,5,6,7,8]

Driving fragmentation in the acute care system is the fee-for-service (FFS) payment model, where providers are reimbursed separately for each service, where there is no monetary incentive to ensure that care is coordinated across settings. Specifically, there is no direct incentive to reduce unnecessary and duplicative tests and to improve care transitions.[9] This chapter will present some of the shortcomings of the US healthcare system that have resulted in this fragmented acute care system, the consequences of poor coordination between acute care and longitudinal providers, and discuss policy options to encourage the better care, higher quality, and lower cost within acute and emergency care settings.

Fragmentation in Acute and Emergency Care

For many people with the occasional injury or illness, the acute care system works well. The acute care system provides complex services without appointment. EDs are open 24/7 and will see anyone regardless of ability to pay. Treating time-sensitive life-threatening conditions is the hallmark of the acute care system. However, many people who use the acute care system have multiple complex conditions and require care from multiple providers. In the absence of coordinated care, these patients and their families must navigate a complex healthcare system, often in a time of high emotional and financial stress that comes along with acute illness and injury.[10]

The Agency for Healthcare Research and Quality describes care coordination as "deliberately organizing patient care activities and sharing information among all of the participants concerned with a patient's care to achieve safer and more effective care. This means that the patient's needs and preferences are known ahead of time and communicated at the right time to the right people, and that this information is used to provide safe, appropriate, and effective care to the patient."[11] A significant body of research exists on using care coordination to reduce the number of acute exacerbations of chronic conditions, ED visits, and hospitalizations.[12,13,14] Further hindering care coordination efforts in episodic settings is a lack of technology for truly interoperable electronic health record (EHR) systems. In some cases, EHR systems can differ even within a facility. The inability of acute care providers to obtain a complete medical record results in a reliance on patient recall of medical care and may result in the incorrect information being used as the basis for care decision making.

Impact of Care Fragmentation

The process of fragmentation increases healthcare costs, causes preventable hospitalizations, and lowers quality.[15] Acute care providers that do not have access to complete and timely medical information cannot make the most optimal treatment decisions, resulting in preventable medical errors, duplication of tests, and patient frustrations. Many people who visit ED and other episodic settings do not have a primary care physician and arrive at the ED with ongoing medical problems. A recent multistate study found that 1 in 5 patients return to the ED within 30 days and 1 in 12 return within 3 days. Of those who return, almost 1 in 3 go to a different ED.[16] Lack of a primary care physician and visits to multiple EDs make fragmentation a particular challenge for acute care providers. ED providers who do not have the test results from the patient's previous ED encounter sometimes end up redoing tests. One study estimated that a fully standardized health information exchange and interoperability could yield a net benefit of $77.8 billion per year by reducing redundancy in laboratory and diagnostic testing.[17]

Patients who receive fragmented care for their acute care episode sometimes continue to experience the effects of fragmented care after discharge. Discharge instructions provide critical information for patients to manage their care at home. However, as many studies have shown, many patients do not understand these discharge instructions or do not recall the instructions they received. Poor understanding limits a patient's ability to properly take medication, follow treatment plans, recognize complications, and receive follow-up care.[18] One study found that nearly 1 out of every 6 patients experienced a preventable adverse event within 3 weeks of discharge.[19] Even for those who do see a primary care physician after discharge, fragmentation impacts their care as only 12–34 percent of physicians report receiving a hospital discharge summary for their patient's first post-discharge visit.[20]

Continuity of care is especially important for patients with multiple chronic medical conditions. These patients are hospitalized more often, are more likely to need the ED, and receive more outpatient care.[21,22] Opportunity for fragmentation of care in this population is especially high. However, integrated systems with high levels of interoperability have been shown to lower healthcare utilization in this vulnerable patient population.[23]

Reducing Fragmentation and Its Impact in Acute and Emergency Care

With new payment models that move away from FFS to bundled payments and that move toward accountable care organizations and capitated models, there will be a greater incentive to reduce fragmentation and prevent the negative impact of fragmentation on care quality and efficiency. Solutions to fragmentation require the development of systems to improve patient connectedness and information availability for providers. For example, some delivery interventions focus on reducing fragmentation in outpatient care through patient-centered medical home models or broadening the scope of services through social work and case management to coordinate care across settings. The ultimate goal is for providers, particularly in episodic settings, to be connected to patients' longitudinal care providers such that: (1) care is provided in the context of their existing and ongoing medical needs; (2) transitions in care are smooth and seamless where all providers caring for the patient have complete information; and (3) the system actively works to ensure that patients are followed over time through and after an acute care episode. Several system interventions have been implemented over the past decade to try to reduce fragmentation in acute and emergency care.[24]

Connecting to Providers before an Acute Care Visit

When patients become ill or are injured, they need to make decisions about where and if to seek care. These decisions are made based on their knowledge of the expected care needs for their condition, their prior experiences with the healthcare system, and their access to healthcare resources.[25] One intervention that can reduce the fragmentation is for groups to allow patients to connect early in their care decision-making process to help decide on whether they need to get medical care and, if so, the best setting.

An example of this sort of service is telephone triage staffed by nurses who provide online medical advice for patients seeking care. Some medical practices have open lines of communication where patients can call in and speak to an on-call provider, while some call-in lines are run by health insurance companies. A recent systematic review of telephone triage found that while some programs are effective in reducing visits, some actually increase utilization, particularly referrals to EDs.[26] In addition, the review also concluded that telephone triage in general was a safe practice. At the regional level, poison control centers are a good example of a consumer-facing system that can help triage patients before they seek acute care, and also helps providers with guidance on care for poisonings and overdoses.[27]

As described in Case Study 6 in this book, Kaiser Permanente OnCall (KP OnCall) is a program run by an integrated health system that receives capitated payments (i.e., fixed payments from members). KP OnCall is a robust system that is staffed by both nurses and physicians and is a center for clinical advice that patients can call into 24 hours a day, 7 days a week. KP OnCall reduces fragmentation by working with the patient to make the best decision about when and where to seek care in the context of their current medical issues. A recent study of KP OnCall described 850,000 calls in Southern California alone in 2011, 34 percent of which were safely managed by primary care appointments in non-ED settings, 18 percent were sent to the ED, 15 percent were directed to urgent care centers, 10 percent were provided with advice for home care, and 1 percent were told to dial "911" for immediate transfer to the hospital.[28] The remainder of the calls received no specific advice for additional care.

Another patient-facing intervention to help with care-seeking decisions is direct-to-consumer (DTC) telemedicine. In this system, patients can call in and get medical advice from a physician. However, in many models of DTC telemedicine, the provider does not have direct access to the patient's information and is not directly involved in after-care. This results in a fragmented visit where the recommendations may never make it into a patients' longitudinal chart. Some health systems, particularly those that are participating in accountable care organizations, have been starting DTC telemedicine programs that are directly affiliated with a health system where providers have not only patient records but access to longitudinal care providers for after-care. As payment shifts away from FFS, it is likely the more connected, less fragmented approaches will flourish.

Improving Care Transitions after an Acute Care Visit

Fragmentation can also occur after an acute care visit, where sometimes information about the encounter is lost. In many cases, because there is no direct connection between the acute care provider and the "next" provider that will continue managing the patient, there is information that is lost. This is because they may not share the same EHR or because there may be no system in place to communicate while the patient is being treated in the acute care settings. Some EDs have systems in place to send the ED chart and results to the primary care office after an ED visit, while many do not have any such system in place. For the most part, many urgent care centers and retail clinics do not coordinate after-care. In the absence of systems to transmit information, the patient or their family is often left to be the courier of this information across settings.

There have been several innovations that have directly addressed transitions in care after acute care visits, particularly ED visits. These were described in a recent report published by the Agency for Healthcare Research and Quality in 2014.[29] Broadly, the report describes issues that can hamper the discharge process, specifically with respect to the communication and education of patients specifically about what happened during the visit (i.e., diagnoses, tests, and procedures), coordination with other providers and services, reconciling medication lists, communication about the expected course of illness and symptoms to watch for, and, finally, ensuring that treatment plans are implemented as planned. Fragmentation can hamper many of these processes, and several interventions can be implemented to reduce the impact of fragmentation on acute care after-care processes.

Screening tools may be helpful in identifying patients who are at risk for problems after ED care and suffer problems from fragmented care. For example, several validated survey tools exist to screen particularly older adult populations for functional problems (i.e., memory and activities of daily living) that may identify high-risk patients who require closer follow-up after discharge. Once patients are identified as high risk, interventions can be performed in acute care settings to ensure that high-risk patients are provided with the best information on after-care, to ensure that they and their families understand the plan of care, and to keep in contact with the patient in the short term. Call-back programs are a popular way to keep in touch with patients after discharge and have been shown to identify high-risk problems shortly after ED discharge that can be addressed. Other interventions can focus on trying to coordinate care directly with longitudinal care providers, such as not only communicating the care plan but also scheduling a follow-up appointment for the patient. Systems such as Kaiser have 24/7 call-in lines for providers to coordinate care with other providers to reduce fragmentation when Kaiser members use acute care settings outside the Kaiser network. In addition, because social determinants can be an important risk factor for fragmented care, some hospitals have tried interventions to address social determinants directly such as providing assistance with prescriptions, transportation, and housing. Many of these functions can be taken on in the ED by a new class of worker called "ED navigators." These new positions are starting to be tested in EDs to improve care coordination and reduce fragmentation.

Building Systems for Providers to Share and Exchange Information

The concept of the interoperability of health information technology (IT) – specifically defined as the ability of IT systems and software to communicate with one another, exchange data, and display that information in usable ways – is vital to improve fragmentation. Not having complete information about a patients' prior care is associated with fewer informed decisions, more duplication, and even safety risks. Because healthcare is delivered across multiple providers and locations, including acute care settings, getting up to date and comprehensive information to the provider at the point of care is vital.

Improving information availability can also reduce the likelihood of communication-related problems in treatment decisions. Today, many EHR systems are not interoperable, and data are kept in silos that are not shared. However, as a first step, several communities have implemented health information exchanges, which can be useful in gathering information on prior visits. For example, in Maryland and Washington, DC, hospitals the Chesapeake Regional Information System for Our Patients allows data sharing across hospitals and includes such information as radiology testing results, laboratory results, prescriptions, and discharge summaries, which can be very useful particularly for complex patients in an acute care or ED setting.

Another example of an interoperable system is the Veterans Affairs (VA) EHR, which contains data for every VA hospital and clinic across the United States. Similarly, Kaiser's HealthConnect is a resource that provides universal information to Kaiser providers on Kaiser patients across settings. In December 2015, the US Office of the National Coordinator for Health Information Technology released the documents "Connecting Health and Care for the Nation: A 10-Year Vision to Achieve an Interoperable Health IT Infrastructure" and the "Shared Nationwide Interoperability Roadmap," which describe a 10-year vision of integrating interoperability of health IT across US healthcare settings.[30] Solving the issue of interoperability and usability of health IT, improving care coordination across settings, and reimaging payment models will be vital to improving the ability of providers to practice cost-consciously.[31]

References

1. The Patient Protection and Affordable Care Act, P.L. 111–148, March 23, 2010.

2. NPR/Robert Wood Johnson Foundation/Harvard School of Public Health. Poll: Sick in America. May 2012. Available at www.npr.org/documents/2012/may/poll/summary.pdf.

3. Elhauge E, ed. The Fragmentation of U.S. Health Care: Causes and Solutions. New York: Oxford University Press, USA, 2010.

4. Schrag D, Xu F, Hanger M, Elkin E, Bickell NA, Bach PB. Fragmentation of care for frequently hospitalized urban residents. Medical Care. 2006;44:560–567.

5. Bourgeois FC, Olson KL, Mandl KD. Patients treated at multiple acute health care facilities: quantifying information fragmentation. Archives of Internal Medicine. 2010;170:1989–1995.

6. Institute of Medicine. Hospital-Based Emergency Care: At the Breaking Point. Washington, DC: National Academies Press, 2007.

7. Bodenheimer T, Pham HH. Primary care: current problems and proposed solutions. Health Affairs. 2010;29:799–805.

8. Colla CH, Morden NE, Sequist TD, Schpero WL, Rosenthal MB. Choosing Wisely: Prevalence and Correlates of Low-Value Health Care Services in the United States. Springer. Journal of General Internal Medicine. 2015;30(2):221–228.

9. Pines J, George M, McStay F, McClellan M. Successful Acute Care Payment Reform Requires Working with the Emergency Department. Health Affairs blog, May 5,

2015. Available at http://healthaffairs.org/blog/2015/05/05/successful-acute-care-payment-reform-requires-working-with-the-emergency-department/.

10. Mate KS, Compton-Phillips AL. The antidote to fragmented health care. *Harvard Business Review*. December 15, 2014.

11. Care Coordination. Agency for Healthcare Research and Quality. May 2015. Available at www.ahrq.gov/professionals/prevention-chronic-care/improve/coordination/index.html.

12. Fromer L. Implementing chronic care for COPD: planned visits, care coordination, and patient empowerment for improved outcomes. *International Journal of COPD*. 2011;6:605–614.

13. Scruggs B. Chronic health care: it is so much different than acute health care – or it should be. *Home Health Care Management and Practice*. 2009;22:43–48.

14. Boult C, Green AF, Boult LB, Pacala JT, Snyder C, Leff B. Successful models of comprehensive care for older adults with chronic conditions: evidence for the institute of medicine's "retooling for an Aging America" report. *Journal of the American Geriatrics Society*. 2009;57:2328–2337.

15. Elhauge E, ed. *The Fragmentation of U.S. Health Care: Causes and Solutions*. New York: Oxford University Press USA, 2010.

16. Duseja R, Bardach NS, Lin GA, Yazdany J, Dean ML, Clay TH, et al. Revisit rates and associated costs after an emergency department encounter: a multistate analysis. *Annals of Internal Medicine*. 2015;162:750–756.

17. Walker J, Pan E, Johnston D, Adler-Milstein J, Bates DW, Middleton B. The Value of Health Care Information Exchange and Interoperability. *Health Affairs*. January 19, 2005. Available at http://content.healthaffairs.org/content/early/2005/01/19/hlthaff.w5.10.

18. Alberti TL, Nannini A. Patient comprehension of discharge instructions from the emergency department: a literature review. *Journal of the American*

Academy of Nurse Practitioners. 2013;25:186–194.

19. Forster AJ, Murff HJ, Peterson JF, Gandhi TK, Bates DW. The incidence and severity of adverse events affecting patients after discharge from the hospital. *Annals of Internal Medicine*. 2003;138:161–167.

20. "Health Policy Brief: Care Transitions." *Health Affairs*. September 13, 2012. Available at www.healthaffairs.org/healthpolicybriefs/brief.php?brief_id=76.

21. Steiner CA, Friedman B. Hospital utilization, costs, and mortality for adults with multiple chronic conditions, Nationwide Inpatient Sample, 2009. *Preventing Chronic Disease*. 2013;10:E62.

22. Sambamoorthi U, Tan X, Deb A. Multiple chronic conditions and healthcare costs among adults. *Expert Review of Pharmacoeconomics & Outcomes Research*. 2015;15:823–832.

23. Bayliss EA, Ellis JL, Shoup JA, Zeng C, McQuillan DB, Steiner JF. Effect of continuity of care on hospital utilization for seniors with multiple medical conditions in an integrated health care system. *Annals of Family Medicine*. 2015;13:123–129.

24. Katz EB, Carrier ER, Umscheid CA, Pines JM. Comparative effectiveness of care coordination interventions in the emergency department: a systematic review. *Annals of Emergency Medicine*. 2012;60:12–23.

25. Ragin DF, Hwang U, Cydulka RK, et al. Reasons for using the emergency department: results of the EMPATH Study (Emergency Medicine Patients' Access to Healthcare (EMPATH) Study Investigators). *Annals of Emergency Medicine*. 2005;12:1158–1166.

26. Telephone consultation and triage: effects on health care use and patient satisfaction. Available at www.cochrane.org/CD004180/EPOC_telephone-consultation-and-triage-effects-on-health-care-use-and-patient-satisfaction.

27. Mowry JB, Spyker DA, Cantilena LR, McMillan N, Ford M. 2013 Annual Report of the American Association of Poison Control Centers' National Poison Data System

(NPDS): 31st Annual Report. *Clinical Toxicology (Phila).* 2014;52:1032–1283.

28. Pines JM, Seleven J, McStay F, George, M, McClellan M. *Kaiser Permanente – California: A Model for Integrated Care for the Ill and Injured.* Washington, DC: Center for Health Policy at Brookings; May 4, 2015. Available at www.brookings.edu/~/media/Research/Files/Papers/2015/05/04-emergency-medicine/KaiserFormatted_150504RH-with-image.pdf?la=en.

29. Improving the emergency department discharge process: environmental scan report. Johns Hopkins University, Armstrong Institute for Patient Safety and Quality. (Prepared by Johns Hopkins University, Baltimore, MD, under Contract No. HHSA 2902010000271.) Rockville, MD: Agency for Healthcare Research and Quality; December 2014 . AHRQ.

Publication No. 14(15)-0067-EF. Available at www.ahrq.gov/sites/default/files/wysiwyg/professionals/systems/hospital/edenvironmentalscan/edenvironmentalscan.pdf.

30. Connecting Health and Care for the Nation: A Shared Nationwide Interoperability Roadmap (executive summary). Washington, DC: The Office of the National Coordinator for Health Information Technology. Available at www.healthit.gov/sites/default/files/hie-interoperability/Roadmap-Executive%20Summary-100115–4pm.pdf.

31. Katz EB, Carrier ER, Umscheid CA, Pines JM. Comparative effectiveness of care coordination interventions in the emergency department: a systematic review. *Annals of Emergency Medicine.* 2012;60:12–23.

Measuring and Improving Quality of Care

Benjamin Easter and Arjun Venkatesh

In "Crossing the Quality Chasm," the Institute of Medicine's landmark report on American healthcare, substantial shortcomings were identified in Americans receiving the care that they "should" receive, that meets their needs, and that is based on the best scientific evidence. Indeed, the shortcomings were significant enough that the report remarked that, "between the healthcare we have and the care we could have lies not just a gap, but a chasm."[1] To be sure, acute and emergency care has difficulties and complexities that further challenge these efforts – high acuity, significant volume unpredictability, and episodic nature, to name a few.

However, quality gaps have been described across several dimensions of emergency care for various conditions, including delays in the early recognition and application of evidence-based bundles for sepsis,[2,3] the overuse of computed tomography (CT) imaging for minor head trauma,[4] and poor compliance with medication recommendations for treatment of acute myocardial infarction and pneumonia.[5] Taken as a whole, these studies confirm substantial opportunities to improve the quality of acute and emergency care. Many emergency departments (EDs) have identified these gaps locally and successfully developed robust quality improvement programs, particularly for highly visible metrics such as those reported publicly by US federal agencies and nonprofit organizations.

In response to the desire of many emergency care clinicians for newer and better measures of acute care quality, numerous proposals have offered a way forward for emergency care to develop quality measures that target the Triple Aim. The Triple Aim is a framework developed by the Institute for Healthcare Improvement, which describes an approach to optimizing health system performance via (1) improving the patient experience of care, (2) improving the health of populations, and (3) reducing the per capita cost of health care.[6,7,8] However, the path to defining, measuring, and improving quality of care has presented several unique challenges that emergency care leaders must consider. We describe the past, present, and future of emergency care quality measurement so that providers can best design quality improvement to improve patient outcomes and demonstrate success both locally to hospitals as well as nationally through public reporting.

History of Quality Improvement in Acute and Emergency Care

The Hospital Quality Alliance (HQA) played a key role in early efforts at quality measurement. The HQA was a collaboration among the Centers for Medicare and Medicaid Services (CMS), the Joint Commission on Accreditation of Healthcare Organizations (JCAHO), the American Hospital Association, and the American Association for Retired Persons. The HQA served as a national clearinghouse for data on specific medical conditions, namely, acute myocardial infarction, congestive heart failure, and pneumonia. The

HQA focused on 10 measures with varying degrees of relevance to the ED. CMS later reported these measures publicly on its website with attribution at the individual hospital level. Importantly, HQA measures were not designed specifically for acute care; rather, they impacted the ED through its role in delivering hospital-based care.[9]

In contrast, physician groups developed measures specifically targeted to acute and emergency care. In 2006, the American Medical Association's Physician Consortium for Performance Improvement developed its own set of emergency medicine–specific measures. Six of these measures were also incorporated into CMS's Physician Quality Reporting System (PQRS). At the time, CMS's PQRS program was a voluntary quality reporting system offering emergency physicians a payment bonus for submitting quality measure scores on select conditions such as acute myocardial infarction and pneumonia.

The American College of Emergency Physicians (ACEP) also created its own set of quality measurements, some of which were incorporated into PQRS. Both sets, however, were not widely adopted, hampered by a lack of governmental or payer involvement as well as difficulties with abstraction and submission as a result of underdeveloped health information technology.

Nevertheless, 22 of the above measures were later endorsed by the National Quality Forum with an express purpose of "standardizing quality measurement in hospital-based EDs."[10] In addition, they were designed to be attributable at levels from the individual clinician to a multihospital system. Many of these measures quickly became recognizable to front-line emergency physicians, including door-to-electrocardiogram (ECG) time, aspirin for acute myocardial infarction, compliance with sepsis bundles, and lengths of stay for admitted and discharged patients.

Although pioneering, these early attempts at quality improvement had clear limitations. Measurement of emergency care quality was based on performance on select variables of specific diseases and ignored the ED's myriad functions, such as timely access, diagnosis, prognosis, treatment, and disposition. Moreover, no unifying vision of quality existed, and the resulting "patchwork of measures ... neither align[ed] with national quality priorities nor reflect[ed] the full scope of ED care".[11]

Successes and Failures of Quality Improvement Efforts

For those leading EDs and caring for patients on the front lines, these quality improvement efforts have generated mixed reactions as some targets have yielded radical improvements in care while others have resulted in highly visible unintended consequences.

The use of quality measurement, particularly door-to-balloon (D2B) time for patients with ST-elevation myocardial infarction (STEMI), represents a certain success. In 2005, only one-third of patients had a D2B time less than 90 minutes, and the median time was 96 minutes, despite clear evidence of the benefits of rapid intervention.[12] In light of overwhelming data, CMS made D2B time a publicly reported quality measure in 2005. Shortly thereafter, the D2B Alliance was founded, a national effort to improve the diagnosis and treatment of patients with STEMI. The D2B Alliance sought to make extraordinary performance ordinary by providing hospitals with key evidence-based strategies and supporting tools needed to begin reducing their D2B times.[13]

Following the recommendations of the D2B Alliance, D2B time was endorsed by the NQF in 2007 and included in CMS's Value-Based Purchasing Program in 2013. In addition to this powerful process measure, CMS also developed a complementary set of additional acute myocardial infarction process measures and outcome measures, including 30-day mortality and readmissions, to support broad-based quality improvement across the healthcare system. These measures have been tremendously successful in creating improvement in the care of these patients. In 5 years, D2B time fell 32 minutes,[10] driven by multidisciplinary efforts at early identification and treatment of STEMI. Moreover, this decline in D2B time is associated with declines in mortality, resulting in thousands of lives saved.[14]

However, quality measurement in emergency care has also brought unintended consequences. Amid an environment in which few measures existed and many were rapidly developed, CMS promulgated two measures of pneumonia care that would subsequently draw substantial criticism: a process measure seeking to provide antibiotic treatment within 4 hours of ED arrival and another promoting obtaining blood cultures prior to antibiotics. The 4-hour target was based on limited observational data, and to make matters worse, the clock was to start on ED arrival, which posed numerous challenges in collecting clinical data when pneumonia was suspected. To improve measure performance, many EDs developed strategies to ensure early blood culture collection and antibiotic administration in any patient with suspected pneumonia. In short course, national performance on both measures improved; however, many patients with simple upper respiratory infections or altered mental status began to receive unnecessary antibiotics.[15] Moreover, the amount of blood cultures increased significantly, leading to substantial increases in false positive rates and concomitant downstream costs, without affecting clinical management.[16] Ultimately, science has prevailed, and the research demonstrating the unintended consequences of these measures resulted in loss of NQF endorsement and removal from CMS quality reporting programs.

As ED crowding increases and ED directors are increasingly looked to by hospital administrators to improve acute care throughput, a second commonly cited example of ED quality measurement is the National Health Service rule in 2005. This measure called for the elimination of ED stays greater than 4 hours for admitted patients. While this national rule quickly resulted in substantial changes to many hospital operations, resulting in improvements in patient flow, the rigid and universal nature of this metric for all EDs also generated ED and hospital practices consistent with "gaming" of the measure, such as moving patients to a different unit solely to meet regulatory requirements or, even worse, admitting patients just before the 4-hour target who may have otherwise been discharged.[17] Subsequently, the rule was relaxed to 95 percent and a broader set of measures of quality was released.

Current Taxonomy of Quality Measurement

In recent years, the use of quality measures has grown, both locally for quality improvement and nationally for accountability reporting and pay-for-performance. To help organize these efforts, several governmental and nongovernmental initiatives have sought to create overarching strategies for quality. In fact, the Institute of Medicine has identified quality measurement as essential to a learning healthcare system and to changing US healthcare delivery.

Quality measures are defined by CMS as tools that help measure or quantify healthcare processes, outcomes, patient perceptions, and organizational structure and/or systems that are associated with the ability to provide high-quality health care and/or that relate to one or more quality goals for health care.[18]

Chief among efforts to develop quality measures is the US National Quality Strategy (NQS), which resulted from convening a wide range of stakeholders, including providers, purchasers, patients, and others, to identify three aims of high-quality healthcare:

1. Better Care: Improve the overall quality, by making health care more patient-centered, reliable, accessible, and safe.
2. Healthy People/Healthy Communities: Improve the health of the US population by supporting proven interventions to address behavioral, social, and environmental determinants of health in addition to delivering higher-quality care.
3. Affordable Care: Reduce the cost of quality health care for individuals, families, employers, and government.[19]

To achieve these aims, the NQS also identified six priorities that have subsequently been adopted by CMS in the CMS Quality Strategy[20] and are used to guide the development of quality metrics and the use of metrics for performance programs[21]:

1. Making care safer by reducing harm caused in the delivery of care.
2. Ensuring that each person and family is engaged as partners in their care.
3. Promoting effective communication and coordination of care.
4. Promoting the most effective prevention and treatment practices for the leading causes of mortality, starting with cardiovascular disease.
5. Working with communities to promote wide use of best practices to enable healthy living.
6. Making quality care more affordable for individuals, families, employers, and governments by developing and spreading new healthcare delivery models.

From Quality Strategy to Quality Measures

While these strategies outline areas in which quality measures need to be developed, the value of individual quality measures has come under greater scrutiny. Originally, quality measures were targeted at processes of care that were perceived as easy to achieve and with limited linkage to a patient outcome (i.e., checking an oxygen saturation on pneumonia patients). In more recent years, however, an emphasis has been placed on developing more robust outcome measures, focused on patient mortality and morbidity as well as patient-reported outcomes such as functional status.

However, the recent push for measure development has resulted in significant numbers of quality measures with frequent duplicates and overlapping or, at times, competing goals. As a result, the proliferation of measures and classification schemes has led to a new focus on "harmonizing" quality measures based on content area, target populations, exclusions, calculation methodology, and data sources.[19] Moreover, a call has begun to eliminate the volume and total cost of measurement, particularly for older, lower value measures.[22]

As newer measures are developed to fill existing gaps in the NQS, federal agencies such as CMS and even private payers are looking to develop and use measures of acute and emergency care for multiple purposes. Payers and policymakers seek to develop measures that are horizontally and vertically "aligned." Horizontal alignment refers to the development of complementary quality measures for related healthcare settings so that incentives are shared. For example, the development of a back pain imaging appropriateness measure for both primary care physicians as well as the ED can ensure higher quality care without patients simply being shuffled between settings to avoid measurement. Vertical alignment refers to the development of a quality measure that can be applied at several levels of measurement, for example, at the point of care (tobacco cessation counseling) and at the population level (example reduced rate of smoking in a managed population). Developing a quality measure that can be "rolled up" from an individual clinician to a hospital or health system and ultimately to a regional geography like a county or state can ensure that providers have consistent incentives within larger organizations such as hospitals and public health agencies. These vertically aligned measures are essential to the NQS goal of better population health since they enable the development and evaluation of Accountable Care Organizations (ACOs) and other innovative payment models.

Emergency medicine's role in these newer quality measures reflects the position of the ED as the critical interface between outpatient and inpatient care. As the front porch to the hospital, the ED is the primary and sometimes only source of acute, unscheduled hospitalizations – therefore, the ED can often determine a hospital's success in population outcome measures of hospital admission and readmission rates. ED directors seeking to demonstrate the value of the ED to hospital and health system leaders will increasingly need to identify quality improvement targets and interventions that result in improved system-wide performance on these high-profile, publicly reported quality measures, many of which carry substantial financial implications.

Stakeholders in Quality Measurement

Numerous stakeholders participate in the development of quality measures. The Joint Commission (TJC) has long held a role in quality measurement, starting with its participation in the HQA described previously. More recently, TJC has employed Core Measure Sets and accreditation standards to improve quality. While few specifically target ED care, many indirectly apply through emergency medicine's position as a hospital-based specialty (myocardial infarction, pneumonia, stroke, and ED flow).

In addition to the roles already described, CMS also encourages reporting on quality through the Physician Quality Reporting System (PQRS). PQRS originally provided a Medicare payment bonus for those physicians or groups reporting on quality measures and a penalty for those who did not report. As of 2016, a bonus is no longer provided, but a penalty still exists for failure to report. Moving forward, the Medicare Access and CHIP Reauthorization Act (MACRA) legislation of 2015 triggered a more substantial role for CMS's quality measurement programs for individual physicians. PQRS will be retired and a new Merit-Based Incentive System (MIPS) will be introduced. MIPS includes the potential for 20 percent of a physicians' payments from Medicare to be related to quality measures.[23]

Recent federal legislation also encourages groups of physicians, including specialty societies, to develop their own quality measures.[19] ACEP has followed suit with development of the Clinical Emergency Data Registry (CEDR), which was specifically developed by and for the emergency medicine community. This registry carries some similarities to well-known clinical registries in other specialties such as the National Cardiovascular Disease Registry (NCDR) and the National Surgical Quality Improvement Program (NSQIP). As a CMS Qualified Clinical Data Registry (QCDR), the new emergency medicine registry includes all ED patients (not just those over 65 years of age reported to CMS) and newer measures that can be developed by the emergency medicine community, such as pregnancy tests for reproductive age females with abdominal pain, and is based on electronic health record data instead of manual chart abstraction by a coder or a nurse.

The ED Benchmarking Alliance (EDBA) also measures and tracks emergency care in the United States. The EDBA conducts an annual survey that serves as a benchmarking tool that measures structures and processes of care with a primary focus on flow and throughput. Although EDBA has no public reporting or accountability implications, many ED medical directors have found the detailed data available in the survey invaluable to managing their departments and presenting key emergency care concepts to hospital leaders.

Finally, the NQF, while not a developer of quality measures, uses a consensus-based process to vet measures proposed by outside groups. Importantly, NQF is not a governmental agency, but rather convenes stakeholders representing often competing interests to generate consensus about quality measures. While the process to obtain NQF endorsement is lengthy and costly, measures that achieve this status are more likely to be utilized, to have accountability for reporting, and to have monetary implications.

Thus, while a veritable "alphabet soup" of regulatory agencies and organizations measure acute and emergency care quality, the lack of a common framework for emergency care quality measurement makes it likely that numerous and occasionally competing incentives are likely to continue.

Emergency Care Quality Measures of the Future

While the use of quality measures to improve the quality of emergency care has generated mixed results in the past, several notable advances in measurement science, the availability of data through healthcare information technology, and, most important, a cultural acceptance and hunger for better quality measures in the emergency medicine community have generated several proposals with much promise.

Chief Complaint–Based Measures

Because most quality measures have historically identified cohorts of patients for inclusion based on International Classification of Disease (ICD) discharge diagnoses, these metrics have largely been disease specific.[24] Furthermore, because discharge diagnoses often fail to capture the reason patients sought emergency care (e.g., a patient who presents with chest pain but is discharged with gastroesophageal reflux disease), discharge diagnosis–based measures often fail to include many ED patients in assessing quality.[25] A recent proposal to combat this limitation has been to develop chief complaint–based measures of emergency care quality.[26] Such measures would be constructed around the reasons patient seek care, such as chest pain, seizures, or even suspected diseases such as pulmonary embolism – all conditions for which emergency care–specific clinical practice guidelines exist.

Patient-Reported Outcome Measures

Previous emergency care quality measures have largely been focused on care processes and not patient outcomes. The development of outcome measures for emergency care had historically been difficult given the limited and episodic amount of time emergency clinicians spend with patients. As a result, little clinical engagement exists for a traditional outcome measure such as 30-day mortality or readmission to be attributed to an individual emergency care physician or even the ED as a whole. As quality measures move beyond the use of billing data to capture outcomes, however, newer outcome measures offer much potential in identifying gaps in emergency care. For example, newer patient-reported outcomes measures such as a patient-reported angina questionnaire or 6-month functional status have become cornerstones for assessing the effectiveness of procedures such as elective percutaneous coronary intervention and total hip or knee replacement, respectively. In the context of the ED, a patient-reported outcome measure could be created to assess headache improvement or return-to-work for patients with acute migraine or even functional and cosmetic improvement for laceration repair. Ultimately, the development of such patient-reported outcome measures also offers the potential to move away from much-criticized metrics of patient satisfaction toward measures of more meaning to patients that can support ED efforts to deliver more patient-centered care.

Group Measurement

Most of the quality measures initially developed for emergency medicine were designed to quantify the care provided by an individual physician as opposed to a group of physicians working in an ED. These individual measures were an outgrowth of CMS policy that required individual physicians to report quality performance and efforts in other specialties to develop many individual quality measures for office-based care. More recently, CMS has developed mechanisms for group reporting to support both hospital-based providers as well as those working in large healthcare organizations. Group reporting also supports efforts by EDs to move toward team-based care in which high-quality outcomes require not only teamwork between emergency physicians, mid-level providers, and nursing staff, but also safe handoffs and transitions between providers. Group measurement can also support the development of measures that cross specialties and settings. For example, an efficiency measure of risk-adjusted ED admission rates for asthma could be paired with a process measure of primary care follow-up following an ED visit for asthma. If both the ED and local primary care providers were measured under this example, then tremendous incentives would exist to redesign ED operations and communications systems to support effective care coordination. As the ED has evolved into the locus of acute care, many group measures of quality will require engagement between the ED and health systems to ensure high quality.

Electronic Clinical Quality Measures

Within the past decade virtually every ED has adopted the use of an electronic health record. As a result, quality measures no longer need to be based solely on administrative billing data. The use of standardized data elements contained within the EHR allows for patients to be identified for quality measurement using clinical data. For example, a recently developed measure of appropriate CT imaging use for suspected pulmonary embolism has been specified for use in electronic health records using clinical data such as D-dimer testing results to assess ED imaging efficiency. The new ACEP CEDR has been designed to capture these electronic clinical quality measures. Such EHR-based quality measurement tools provide ED directors with access to real-time, benchmarking quality data that can be fed back to clinicians and hospital leadership, and avoid the burden of manual abstraction of charts by nurses to calculate quality scores.

As quality measurement's role in healthcare delivery evolves into its second generation, particularly with regard to acute and emergency care, many risks and opportunities exist for ED leaders. The era of process metrics that required formidable chart abstraction efforts with little impact on patient outcomes will be replaced by better patient- and provider-centered measures designed to support common incentives across a learning healthcare system striving for the Triple Aim. Emergency care leaders should embrace these newer models of care delivery, or they will risk not only large financial penalties but, more important, the opportunity to improve care for millions of ED patients per year.

References

1. Institute of Medicine. *Crossing the Quality Chasm: A New Health System for the 21st Century.* National Academy Press, 2001.

2. Ferrer R, Artigas A, Levy MM, et al. Improvement in process of care and outcome after a multicenter severe sepsis educational program in Spain. *JAMA.* 2008;299(19):2294–2303.

3. Levy MM, Dellinger RP, Townsend SR, et al. The surviving sepsis campaign: results of an international guideline-based performance improvement program targeting severe sepsis. *Journal of Intensive Care Medicine.* 2010;38(2):367–374.

4. Jagoda AS, Bazarian JJ, Bruns JJ Jr, et al. Clinical policy: neuroimaging and decision-making in adult mild traumatic brain injury in the acute setting. *Annals of Emergency Medicine.* 2008 Dec;52(6):714–748.

5. Pham JC, Kelen GD, Pronovost PJ. National study on the quality of emergency department care in the treatment of acute myocardial infarction and pneumonia. *Academic Emergency Medicine.* 2007;14 (10):856–863.

6. Pines J, Venkatesh A. Taking control of quality measurements. *Emergency Physicians Monthly.* Available at http://epmonthly.com/ article/taking-control-of-quality-measurements/. Accessed April 12, 2016.

7. Agrawal S. Aligning emergency care with the triple aim: opportunities and future direction after healthcare reform. *Healthcare.* 2014; 2:184–189.

8. Venkatesh A. Emergency care and the national quality strategy: highlights from the Centers for Medicare and Medicaid Services. *Annals of Emergency Medicine.* 2015;65(4):396–399.

9. Jha AK, Li Z, Orav EJ, et al. Care in U.S. hospitals: the hospital quality alliance program. *New England Journal of Medicine.* 2005;353(3):265–274.

10. National Quality Forum (NQF). National voluntary consensus standards for emergency care: a consensus report. NQF, 2009. Available at www.qualityforum.org/ Publications/2009/09/Emergency_Care_ full.aspx. Accessed April 12, 2016.

11. Schuur JD, Hsia RY, Burstin H, et al. Quality measurement in the emergency department: past and future. *Health Affairs.* 2013;32(12):2129–2138.

12. Krumholz HM, Herrin J, Miller LE, et al. Improvements in door-to-balloon time in the United States: 2005–2010. *Circulation.* 2011;124(9):1038–1045.

13. Krumholz HM, Bradley EH, Nallamothu BK, et al. A campaign to improve the timeliness of primary percutaneous coronary intervention: door-to-balloon: an alliance for quality. *Journal of American College of Cardiology Intervention.* 2008;1 (1):97–104.

14. Rathore SS, Curthi JP, Chen J, et al. Association of door-to-balloon time and mortality in patients admitted to hospital with ST elevation myocardial infarction: national cohort study. *BMJ.* 2009;338; b1807.

15. Kanwar M, Brar N, Khatib R, et al. Misdiagnosis of community-acquired pneumonia and inappropriate utilization of antibiotics: side effects of the 4-h antibiotic administration rule. *Chest.* 2007;131:1865–1869.

16. Ramanujam P, Rathlev NK. Blood cultures do not change management in hospitalized patients with community-acquired pneumonia. *Academic Emergency Medicine*, 2006;13:983–985.

17. Mason S, Weber EJ, Coster J, et al. Time patients spend in the emergency department: England's 4-hour rule – a case of hitting the target but missing the point? *Annals of Emergency Medicine.* 2012;59 (5):341–349.

18. Centers for Medicare and Medicaid Services. Measures management system. Available at www.cms.gov/Medicare/Quality-Initiatives-Patient-Assessment-Instruments/MMS/index.html. Accessed April 10, 2016.

19. Agency for Healthcare Research and Quality. About the national quality strategy. Available at www.ahrq.gov/workingforquality/about.htm#aims. Accessed April 11, 2016.

20. Centers for Medicare and Medicaid Services. A blueprint for the CMS measures management system. Available at www.cms.gov/Medicare/Quality-Initiatives-Patient-Assessment-Instruments/MMS/Downloads/Blueprint112.pdf. Accessed April 13, 2016.

21. AHRQ. About the national quality strategy. Available at www.ahrq.gov/workingforquality/about.htm#aims. Accessed April 11, 2016.

22. Berwick DM. Era 3 for medicine and health care. *JAMA*. 2106;315(13):1329–1330.

23. Wiler JL, Granovsky M, Cantrill SV, et al. Physician quality reporting system updates and the impact on emergency medicine practice. *Western Journal of Emergency Medicine*. 2016;27(2):229–237.

24. Kanzaria HK, Mattke S, Detz AA, et al. Quality measures based on presenting signs and symptoms of patients. *JAMA*. 2015;313(5):520–522.

25. Raven MC, Lowe RA, Maselli J, et al. Comparison of presenting complaint versus discharge diagnosis for identifying "nonemergency" emergency department visits. *JAMA*. 2013;309(11):1145–1153.

26. Griffey RT, Pines JM, Farley HL, et al. Chief complaint based performance measures: a new focus for acute care quality measurement. *Annals of Emergency Medicine*. 2015;65(4):387–395.

Chapter 4

Alternative Payment Models in Acute, Episodic Care
Moving from Volume to Value

Nir J. Harish and Jesse M. Pines

Introduction

One of the defining features of the US health care system is volume-based reimbursement, typified by the traditional fee-for-service (FFS) payment model that still dominates much of American health care. In an FFS system, providers are able to generate more revenue for seeing more patients or performing more services per patient. In this system, providers forfeit revenue when they provide care that results in keeping patients healthy and out of the hospital. As a result, there is a growing consensus that the volume-based payment system has trapped the United States in a tangle of rising costs, fragmented care delivery, and variable care quality.

Since the early 1990s, when "health reform" first became a perennial political buzzword, a parade of alternative reimbursement systems has been proposed to replace volume-based care. Most failed, like the early attempts at capitation by health maintenance organizations (HMOs) that reduced patient choice about which doctors they could see and focused primarily on building up the role of insurers in the practice of medicine. This included negotiating lower prices with networks of doctors, and gatekeeping, in which patients required referrals to see specialists, neither of which were popular with patients or physicians. By contrast, other efforts were more successful. Integrated delivery models, like Kaiser Permanente, have proved popular with patients in a variety of settings. In these systems, members pay premiums to providers and hospitals to manage their care, rather than using an insurance company as an intermediary. In this model, providers have direct incentives to deliver more efficient care and stand to benefit when lower costs are incurred through care delivery.

In 2010, the passage of the ACA established a series of structural, regulatory, and financial changes in the United States that have set in motion a large-scale shift away from volume-based reimbursement and toward a system that aims to keep patients healthy and out of the hospital by reducing cost while maintaining quality and not reducing access to care. The underlying assertion of this shift is that higher quality care and a longer time frame of accountability will result in lower costs and better patient outcomes.

In 2015, the US Department of Health and Human Services announced that 90 percent of all Medicare spending would be "value-based" by 2018. This announcement provided a sense of urgency that has led providers, specialty societies, insurers, state governments, and other stakeholders to develop and test a range of new reimbursement systems, or alternative payment models (APMs), that share the goal of paying providers to deliver higher value care that will reduce downstream costs. Value, in this context, can be thought of as the effectiveness of care for a given cost, or "what you get for your money."

To date, most attempts at value-based alternative payment models have not directly focused on improving acute, episodic care delivered in settings like emergency departments (EDs) and urgent care centers. Instead, models like Accountable Care Organizations and Primary Care Medical Homes are designed with the explicit goal of reducing demand for acute, episodic care but are not designed to engage providers who work in those settings.[1]

Acute care presents a unique set of challenges in the move to value-based payment models. Acute and emergency care, because they are episodic in nature, make FFS an easy fit. This episodic nature creates an obstacle for payment models that are based on holding providers accountable for long-term outcomes. Acute care providers often see a patient only once, so holding them accountable for downstream outcomes is challenging. It is also difficult to hold a single acute care provider group or hospital accountable for longer-term patient outcomes, because patients in need of acute care sometimes have little choice in where to get their care – for example, after a motor vehicle collision – and do not necessarily return to the same group or hospital for care.

Furthermore, acute and emergency care providers often treat patients with incomplete information because there is no prior relationship with the patient and medical records may be incomplete or inaccessible. Combined with the high-risk nature of many acute care complaints, this makes cost-efficient practice a challenge in acute care. For the same reasons, it is often difficult to retrospectively determine the appropriateness of initial care. In the United States, the high volume of uncompensated care that is provided in EDs must also be accounted for in payment models, as the Emergency Treatment and Active Labor Act (EMTALA) mandates the provision of medical screening exams regardless of ability to pay. Finally, any payment system for acute care must take into account the additional costs incurred by providers to maintain excess capacity in case of mass casualty incidents, natural disasters, or other public health emergencies.

As the move to APMs gains momentum, however, new delivery models will need to be developed in ways that include acute, episodic settings. In this chapter, we'll explore what volume and value mean in the context of acute and emergency care. We'll consider system-, facility- and patient-level levers can be used to promote value in acute care within the current system. We will then examine a range of APMs, and how they might be applied in acute and emergency care, ranging from quality performance incentives to fully capitated payments.

What Is Wrong with Volume-Based Acute Care?

The traditional fee-for-service (FFS) reimbursement system pays physicians and facilities separately. Physicians bill most payers using codes based on relative-value units (RVUs), which are determined using the Resource-Based Relative Value Scale (RBRVS), reviewed annually by Medicare. While commercial payers do not need to use the RVU system, most choose to use it, or a version of it, out of convenience. RVUs are meant to account for the "intensity" of work required per unit of time for every service provided by a physician. Emergency physicians bill using one of five "evaluation and management" (E&M) codes, reflecting the overall intensity of the evaluation and management of the patient, as well as separate codes for any discrete procedures performed, such as a laceration repair or tracheal intubation. Facilities bill most payers for each individual service provided – for example, the use of a pulse oximeter, the placement of an intravenous catheter by a nurse, or the administration of a medication.

Healthcare providers are motivated by much more than just profit, but the current FFS system makes it difficult for providers to prioritize anything other than volume – seeing as many patients as possible. Whenever a provider spends extra time addressing a complex social problem, he or she is forfeiting the revenue of seeing another patient. In the long run, however, keeping the patient healthy is better for the patient and less costly for the health system. Yet under FFS, the provider does not benefit financially when patients are healthier. Similarly, in most FFS systems, physicians who engage in shared decision-making – taking into account the patient's values and preferences – risk being doubly penalized if the patient elects not to have a test or procedure: once because the provider spent additional time with the patient instead of seeing a new patient, and again because the provider refrained from performing the billable test or procedure. In this way, FFS can make it hard for providers to focus on delivering care that is in the best interest of the patient.

In addition to the volume incentive, one frequently cited challenge of the current payment system is that the RVRBS is often seen as rewarding procedural services over cognitive or preventive services. In most cases, procedural services are reimbursed more highly than cognitive and preventive services. Some researchers have suggested that a revision of the RVRBS could, in itself, lead to many of the value-oriented changes that payers and policymakers are seeking, for example, by rewarding services that promote long-term outcomes, such as team-based discharge planning or post-ED care coordination. At the present time, however, the relative value of these services remains a moot point, because most payers do not reimburse for these services at all.

What Does High-Value Acute Care Look Like?

An ideal acute care system should utilize the unique skills and services of acute care facilities and providers to help patients get healthy and stay healthy. It is a system that enables acute care providers to deliver the best care they can, more efficiently, with more support for discharge planning, care coordination, and other services that help reduce potentially avoidable hospital admissions. It is a system where providers do not overuse testing because it is easier than taking a good history and making a more informed decision or engaging in shared decision making. It is a system that broadens the role of the acute care provider beyond the "here and now," to include the "there and later." In this system, there is less of "Well, I've taken care of your main complaint" and more of "What else can we address today?" It is a system in which the acute care provider is not an island, but part of a larger continuum of care.

Let's consider some examples:

1. **Better coordination of post-ED services to reduce avoidable admissions**. A 64-year-old patient with congestive heart failure (CHF) presents to the ED with a mild exacerbation. No recent echocardiogram has been done, but after initial treatment, it is determined that there is no pulmonary edema, and the patient is stable despite mild volume overload. Instead of admitting the patient, the ED provider is able to arrange a next-day home visit from a nurse on the patient's primary care team, and an outpatient echocardiogram is scheduled prior to ED discharge.

2. **Acute care visits are seen as opportunities to prevent additional visits**. An elderly patient comes in after a minor mechanical fall, with a skin abrasion. A high-value system would identify this visit as an opportunity to identify fall risks, perhaps arranging a physical therapy evaluation and a home safety assessment, so that the next ED visit is not for a hip fracture.

3. **Proactive care that is patient-centered, not just chief complaint–centered**. A 40-year-old male comes in with gastroenteritis. In a high-value system, the provider might be made aware that the patient had multiple elevated blood pressure readings during unrelated visits to a local retail clinic, and initiate appropriate follow-up to ensure that this patient does not receive follow-up care and treatment.

4. **A more intensive ED workup that can save downstream costs**. A 62-year-old female presents with a headache that is thought to represent a first-time migraine, although she has not had any neuroimaging. Instead of performing a low-yield computed tomography (CT) scan, a high-value system might actually pursue a more intensive initial workup, to eliminate the need for additional downstream appointments. For example, this patient might have magnetic resonance imaging (MRI) in the ED to obviate the need for a follow-up visit.

5. **Willingness to be held accountable for outcomes after the end of the visit**. After a 40-year-old construction worker is discharged from the ED for presumed musculoskeletal back pain, the provider calls him back to see whether the recommended exercises and non-steroidal anti-inflammatory drugs (NSAID) were effective and, if not, offers to set up an appointment for physical therapy or, if his symptoms are worsening, a recheck in the ED at no extra cost.

The goal, as depicted in the scenarios above, is to design a system that enables providers to provide the care that will best serve the patient, not just for the short term but also to ensure that their symptoms are addressed in a way that maximizes efficiency, where outcomes are measured, and positive outcomes rewarded.

What Can We Do within the Current System to Promote Value?

There are a number of system-, facility-, and patient-level levers that can be used to improve the quality and value of care within the existing payment system.

System-Level Levers

1. **Public reporting and transparency of outcomes, quality, and price data**. The theory is that if there were more transparency about quality, price, and outcomes, which capture much of what we consider "high value" care, patients and payers would migrate to the best providers, thus creating a strong but nonmonetary incentive for providers to deliver higher value care. There are challenges with this approach, however. As discussed in other chapters, choosing good, measurable quality and outcome metrics is difficult. In addition, a wave of hospital and physicians' practice mergers has significantly reduced competition in many markets, meaning that patients and payers may have less choice.

2. **Narrow networks.** Narrow networks are the fastest-growing product on the health insurance exchanges created by the ACA.[2] In a narrow network, insurers choose a small number of local providers to include in a plan (less than 30 percent of available providers, by definition). Similar to managed care in the 1990s, this is a business intervention rather than a delivery one, and limits choices. With narrow networks, the insurer is able to negotiate a steep discount with a provider in order to include them in the plan. This reduces the insurer's costs by keeping patients away from more expensive providers. However, there is often no guarantee of high-value care for the patient.

3. **Efforts to reform the RVRBS system to add or revalue nonprocedural services.** As mentioned earlier, it is possible that placing a higher monetary premium on nonprocedural services, such as time spent with a patient, discharge planning, palliative care, and care coordination, could alter incentives significantly. However, while providers might bill for "care coordination," there is still only limited incentive for the provider to ensure that the patient's downstream care is truly optimized. In other words, doing the minimal amount of care coordination required for billing might not add much value to the patient.

Facility-Level Levers

1. **Care pathways and decision-support tools.** Care pathways have been heralded as a way to reduce variation in care. For example, sepsis care pathways have been used successfully in acute care settings to ensure that all patients receive timely antibiotics and appropriate fluid resuscitation by removing the variability among providers.[3] Ensuring high-quality care is a key step toward high-value care. Care pathways and decision-support tools can also be used to promote specific high-value services. For example, a care pathway for an elderly patient who has suffered a fall can trigger a social work evaluation. Similarly, a decision support tool for a young patient with back pain can help the provider determine whether imaging is actually indicated.
2. **Interoperable health information technology.** The ability to rapidly access patient records and to electronically communicate with downstream providers is critical to the provision of high-value care. It reduces the likelihood of unnecessary duplication of testing and improves care planning to ensure appropriate follow-up and execution of a care plan.
3. **Alternative settings of care.** One way to increase value is to provide care at a lower cost. A high-value system can help direct patients to the most efficient care setting for their needs. Kaiser Permanente, for example, has a 24-hour call line that can make next-day appointments for patients with acute complaints who do not require immediate ED evaluation. Retail clinics, urgent care centers, telemedicine, and freestanding EDs can offer similar value.

A Provider-Level Lever

Patient callbacks. A simple intervention is to have providers call certain patients (e.g., high-risk patients) after discharge.[4] This allows the provider to assess whether the recommended treatment is working, and adjust the treatment plan over the phone, avoiding an unnecessary return visit. Alternatively, if the symptoms are worsening, the provider might ask the patient to return to the ED for an early reevaluation, avoiding further deterioration in the patient's condition that could have led to a worse outcome and more expensive course.

Which Alternative Payment Models Can Lead to Higher Value in Acute Care?

The subtitle of this chapter, "Moving from Volume to Value," implies that volume and value are somehow dichotomous, on opposite ends of a spectrum. The reality is that both

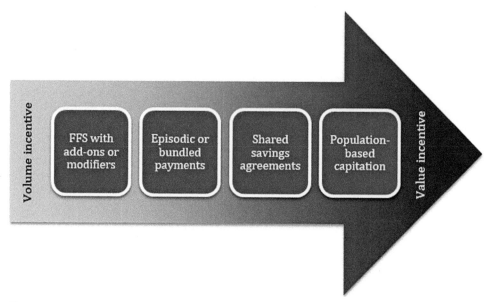

Figure 4.1 Spectrum of alternative payment models.

often coexist along a continuum that begins with minor add-ons to traditional FFS payments and goes all the way to fully capitated population-based payments. In this section, we will consider each of these in turn. Figure 4.1 provides a spectrum of alternative payment models.

FFS with Add-Ons and Modifiers

Public and commercial payers have begun to embrace efforts to counter the disincentives for value that are built into traditional FFS by layering quality- and value-based incentives onto the traditional FFS structure. These can take a number of forms, including the following:

1. **New billable procedure codes**. These codes would cover "high value" services, such as discharge planning, palliative care consultations, or care coordination, and be billed the same as other FFS codes. This model faces the same limitations as any other FFS system, however, including a volume incentive, an incentive to prioritize highly paid codes over lower codes, and a lack of long-term accountability.

2. **Fixed per-person payments**. The ED would bill payers a small per-person charge to fund services such as care coordinators, case managers, etc. This fee would not be directly tied to a particular service, but would likely require the ED to demonstrate downstream benefits in cost and outcomes over time.

Another way to adjust the FFS model to promote value is to adjust existing reimbursement up or down based on quality or performance metrics. A well-known example of this approach is Medicare's Hospital Readmissions Reduction Program (HRRP). Under the HRRP, hospitals that exceed the national average readmission rates for certain conditions face a fixed percentage reduction in their Medicare reimbursement rates. In fact, the Affordable Care Act (ACA) mandated that Medicare phase in a value modifier (VM) for all FFS payments to physicians in large groups by 2017. The VM was recently bundled into a larger initiative, the Merit-Based Incentive Payment System (MIPS), which assigns providers a composite score based on quality, resource utilization, meaningful use of electronic health records, and quality improvement activities. Based on the MIPS score, Medicare will adjust payments to the provider up or down. In the current plan, the maximum adjustment up or down in 2022 will be ±9 percent. MIPS will apply to EM providers in groups larger than 100 providers.

While MIPS will apply only to Medicare payments, similar arrangements have been considered in the commercial market. One could imagine, for example, that payments could be adjusted up or down based on adherence to agreed-on protocols, ED admission rates, ED revisit rates, or other metrics.

Episodic and Bundled Payments

The terms *episodic* and *bundled* are often used interchangeably. In this text we define them as follows:

- *Episodic payment*: Single payment to a single provider triggered by an acute episode and covering a predetermined time period.
- *Bundled payment*: Single payment covering multiple providers triggered by an acute episode and covering a predetermined time period.

The key difference is that *episodic* payments are to a single provider, and *bundled* payments cover multiple providers.[5] With episodic payments, the payer would pay each provider separately and the facility/hospital separately. With a bundled payment, there is one single payment covering the hospital and all providers, who then have to determine how to divide the revenue internally.

Medicare has been using episodic payments for inpatient hospitalizations since 1983 using the diagnosis-related group (DRG) system. In this system, the hospital is reimbursed a predetermined amount per admission based on the discharge diagnosis of the patient. Because these payments are separate from the physician fee payments, we classify them as episodic payments, rather than bundled payments.

Episodic and/or bundled payments are frequently proposed as APMs for acute care. They are appealing because they are triggered by acute episodes, and therefore fit intuitively with the nature of acute and emergency care. Payments would be focused on specific disease entities or chief complaints, such as pneumonia, urinary tract infection, back pain, or headache.

Let's imagine an episodic payment for "low back pain," a common complaint in acute care settings. In the current system, a visit for low back pain may result in bills for a low-acuity E&M code, perhaps administration of a medication or two, possibly some imaging, and recommendations for exercises and NSAIDs. If the patient feels no better in a week and returns to the ED, the provider can bill again for the same services. Arguably, the provider has little incentive to make sure the treatment plan actually works. In an episodic or bundled payment, the provider would bill not for all of the individual services provided, but simply for a "low back pain" visit. That payment would cover a set amount of time – a warranty, of sorts – say, 4 weeks. If the patient returns within 4 weeks for the same complaint, the provider could not bill again. Therefore, there is a greater incentive to come up with a plan that actually works – maybe this would involve physical therapy or a more detailed discussion of the natural course of low back pain. At the same time, any services provided would come out of the single payment. So if the provider elects to perform an expensive test such as MRI, that expense would come out of the payment. At the same time, if the patient truly needed MRI, due to progressive motor weakness, for example, presumably they would return within the 4 weeks, so it is not in the interest of the provider to delay necessary care.

It is important to recognize that both episodic and bundled payments are still fundamentally volume based. The incentive is still to have more episodes or bundles. However, they have a number of key attributes that alter the associated incentives:

1. Providers are accountable for a longer-term outcome. In the ED context, this means accountability for how a patient does after leaving the ED.
2. Providers have no incentive to perform unnecessary tests or services, because there is no additional reimbursement associated with them.

In essence, in an episodic or bundled payment, the provider is placed *at risk* for any expenses above the payment rate that accrue during the visit or in the defined time period after the visit.

Bundled payments function much like episodic payments, but would include additional providers, such as the patient's primary care provider, physical therapist, or radiologist, along with any hospital- or office-based facility fees. The benefit of this system is that it would require providers to coordinate care, including agreeing to a coherent treatment plan and avoiding duplication of services.

Bundled payments present a particular challenge, however, because the revenue needs to be divided among multiple parties. Often, these internal payment allocations become a microcosm of the same problems facing the system as a whole. For example, within a bundled payment, is the radiologist still paid per scan? Are procedures still valued over cognitive services?

Despite these challenges, many policymakers and scholars feel that episodic and bundled payments represent a promising approach to bringing value-based payments to acute and emergency care.

Shared Savings Programs

One of the most widely discussed APMs since the ACA has been the Accountable Care Organization (ACO), established by the ACA as part of the Medicare Shared Savings Program. The idea behind the ACO model, and shared savings programs in general, is simple: a provider that reduces the overall cost of care can receive a payment for some of the savings generated. This should, in theory, align providers with payers.

In general, ACOs are formed by large multispecialty groups and/or hospital-based groups. These groups are assigned a panel of patients, and take accountability for the overall quality and cost of care for those patients. If the ACO generates a minimum of 2 percent savings compared with a predetermined benchmark, it is eligible to recoup some percentage (up to 50 percent) of the savings.

Several criticisms of ACOs have been suggested, such as the following:

1. Shared savings programs do not help defray the up-front costs of redesigning care or hiring necessary staff for care coordination and other services.
2. Shared savings programs are built on top of the existing FFS system; if providers reduce the number of services they provide, they will still lose revenue. The shared savings will reduce the size of the loss, but it will still be a loss of revenue from baseline.

3. Shared savings are based on reducing costs from the original baseline. It is unclear how this model will evolve once costs have been reduced.

At the time of this writing, there are still no major examples of ACOs that include an emergency physician group in the shared savings program. It has been suggested, however, that ACOs might eventually include emergency physicians and other acute care providers, offering a piece of the shared savings, to align incentives across a broader segment of the care continuum.

There are a number of ways that emergency physician groups could work with or within an ACO. A simple relationship could entail contracting with the ACO for FFS payments, with bonuses or adjustments based on providing certain high-value services or meeting specific metrics. Alternatively, to more closely align the group with the ACO, the emergency physicians could be made eligible for a portion of any overall shared savings achieved by the ACO.

Population-Based Capitation

At the far end of the APM spectrum is full, population-based capitation, also known as global payments or comprehensive care payments. In a capitated system, a group of providers and associated facilities receives a fixed payment to provide care for a population of patients over a defined time period. A key component to most capitation models being proposed today, unlike those used in the early 1990s, is that the payments must be risk adjusted, to reduce the incentive for providers to cherry-pick only healthy patients. Integrated payer–provider systems, like Kaiser Permanente, can also be considered as a variant of the capitated model in practice, with each patient's annual premium serving as the capitated payment.

Of the models we have considered, capitation is the only system free of volume incentives. In these systems, the provider is not paid per service, but per person. There is no incentive to overutilize tests or services. There is a strong incentive to reduce the overall cost of care for each patient, because any expenses come out of a predetermined capitated rate. At the same time, there is an incentive to reduce access to services because payments are fixed, so marginal investment in improving service quality does not necessarily lead to higher revenue.

However, integrated systems, like Kaiser Permanente in California, have demonstrated how integrated and capitated systems can create value in the acute care setting, in ways that volume-based systems often cannot. Kaiser Permanente, as mentioned previously, maintains a 24-hour nurse hotline to help direct patients to the right care setting for unscheduled complaints. Kaiser Permanente has also developed effective programs to identify frequent users of the ED with chronic conditions and develop high-touch strategies where patients' treatment is frequently assessed and they are better engaged to reduce their future ED use. Finally, exemplifying the benefits of a non-volume-based system, in Kaiser Permanente hospitals, "ED flow is not prioritized over ensuring that patients receive comprehensive work-ups, so that patients who do not require hospitalization are not admitted, even in favor of a longer ED stay."[2]

Capitation systems are also faced with some of the reverse challenges of volume-based systems. Whereas volume-based systems are criticized for encouraging providers to overtest and overutilize services, capitated systems are criticized for encouraging providers to do the bare minimum. While capitated providers may be held to quality and outcome metrics, it may not be possible to detect more subtle effects of underutilization, such as effects on patient experience and patient-centered goals of care. Similarly, while volume-based providers may be incentivized to see "too many" patients in a day, a capitated provider may be underincentivized to see patients, leading to long waits for appointments.

In the United Kingdom, where the National Health Service operates the single-payer system, there are longstanding issues with access to care, and especially scheduled care. Recently, there have been efforts to promote capitation using capitated outcome-based and incentivized contracts (COBICs) within the mostly volume-based payment system in the National Health Service. The key elements of this new payment model are (1) multiyear instead of annual payments, (2) capitation rather than FFS, and (3) up to 20 percent in additional payments for patient- and population-level outcomes. Notably, even within a single-payer system, this process has been met with challenges.[6]

Where Should We Go from Here?

This chapter has reviewed the broad continuum of APMs that have been proposed primarily in the United States to replace volume-based care, and how they might apply in the acute care setting. So now the question is, which one should we choose? While it would be nice to find a single APM that would perfectly align the incentives of providers and payers with the best interest of the patient, it turns out that the answer is: it depends.

Both episodic payments and global payments offer solutions that enable acute care providers to shift their focus beyond the immediate visit and the next patient waiting to be seen, opening up new possibilities for providing high value acute care. The key difference between them, however, is whether the provider is held accountable for the number of "unnecessary" visits.

For some conditions, especially chronic conditions like congestive heart failure, acute care providers can play a big role in helping patients stay healthy, through careful coordination with other providers. For these conditions, a global payment that encompasses the patient's whole care team might reasonably incentivize all providers to cooperate on keeping the patient healthy and out of the hospital.

There are other conditions, however, where no one can reasonably control the volume of visits. Consider, for example, appendicitis or pregnancy. For these conditions, episodic or bundled payments would be a reasonable way to cover the acute costs of care while ensuring that providers are incentivized to keep downstream costs limited and long-term outcomes optimized.

In reality, it is possible that there is not one single model that will work for all providers, health systems, and patients, and it is likely that more than one payment model will be needed to support a complex health system like that in the United States. However, the cost of increased complexity in payment models is higher spending on low-value administrative costs, which would risk offsetting the benefits of value-based APMs.

While payment models continue to be developed and tested, there remains the possibility that changes within the FFS system, such as payment for care coordination services, greater use of care pathways, and better interoperability of health information technology, will significantly enhance the value of care without radically changing the payment system.

Through the ongoing process of payment reform, it will be critical to remain focused on untangling the web of rising costs, fragmented care delivery, and variable care quality, and ensure that providers are paid for keeping patients healthy and out of the hospital.

References

1. Pines JM, George M, McStay F, McClellan M. Successful acute care payment reform requires working with the emergency department. *Health Affairs* blog. May 5, 2015. Available at http://healthaffairs.org/blog/2015/05/05/successful-acute-care-payment-reform-requires-working-with-the-emergency-department.

2. Haeder SF, Weimer DL, Mukamel DB. Narrow networks and the Affordable Care Act. *JAMA.* 2015;314(7):669–670.

3. Miller RR, Dong L, Nelson NC, et al. Multicenter implementation of a severe sepsis and septic shock treatment bundle. *American Journal of Respiratory and Critical Care Medicine.* 2013;188(1):77–82.

4. Jones JS, Young MS, LaFleur RA, Brown MD. Effectiveness of an organized follow-up system for elder patients released from the emergency department. *Academic Emergency Medicine.* 1997;4 (12):1147–1152.

5. Miller HD. From volume to value: better ways to pay for health care. *Health Affairs.* 2009;28(5):1418–1428.

6. Hicks N and Bell D. English developments in value-based care: the beginnings of a revolution? *Health Affairs* blog. March 16, 2016. Available at http://healthaffairs.org/blog/2016/03/16/english-developments-in-value-based-care-the-beginnings-of-a-revolution.

Chapter

5 Improving Timeliness and Access of Acute and Emergency Care
The Science of Improving Emergency Department Crowding

Olan A. Soremekun

Introduction

Patients routinely face crowded emergency departments (EDs), prolonged wait times, and diminished access to care in the United States and throughout the world.[1] In several studies, ED crowding and prolonged wait times have been associated with delayed diagnosis and treatment of time-sensitive conditions, worse patient outcomes, and diminished patient satisfaction.[2]

In 2001 the Institute of Medicine (IOM) report, in conjunction with the growing body of evidence on the negative impact of ED crowding, led the Center for Medicare and Medicaid Services (CMS) and other payers to adopt ED-specific quality metrics that reflect the timeliness of ED care. In the United States today, many EDs must publicly report their "left without been seen" (LWBS) rates, time-to-provider, and the length of stay for their admitted and discharge patients to CMS and other payers. These metrics also contribute to overall hospital ratings such as the CMS star ratings. These publicly reported hospital metrics and rankings are increasingly used by patients to make decisions about where to obtain emergency care, further incentivizing EDs to improve the timeliness of care.

The increased focus on improving the timeliness of ED care has led ED managers and researchers to enhance their focus on the science of ED operations. By leveraging prior work in the field of operations research and advances in other industries such as manufacturing, ED managers are redesigning the ED care processes to make ED care more responsive to patients seeking emergency care. Early research in ED operations focused on measuring ED crowding, its contributors, and how ED crowding affects patient outcomes. More recently, ED operations research has shifted toward interventions to decrease crowding and increase timeliness of care.

In this chapter we describe how ED crowding is measured, conceptual models to understand ED crowding, and some key concepts from the field of operations management and how these concepts apply to the ED.

Measuring Timeliness of ED Care and ED Crowding

The publicly reported measures for timeliness include median times to evaluation by a qualified medical provider, average time before pain medication for a broken bone, average time spent in the ED before a decision to admit to the hospital, and average length of stay for admitted and discharged patients. These metrics are reported quarterly with the majority of hospitals using sampling to obtain these data. While the use of averages does not fully describe the spectrum of performance for an ED, nor do they quantify crowding. Since these are static metrics that provide a snapshot of ED performance, these timeliness metrics are of limited use to an ED manager who is attempting to develop interventions to reduce crowding.

To quantify levels of crowding, researchers have designed scales that are used by many EDs to assess the current state of the ED and to activate ED and hospital-level interventions (e.g., ED diversion). The National ED Overcrowding Scale (NEDOCS) and the ED Work Index (EDWIN) scores are commonly used for quantifying the level of ED crowding.[3,4] The NEDOCS scale has been validated in multiple peer-reviewed studies and is calculated using five variables: total beds in the ED, total admits in the ED, number of respirators in the ED, longest admit time (in hours), and waiting room time for last patient put in an ED bed.[3] The NEDOCS scale goes from 0 to 200. At scores of 100–140 an ED is considered crowded, 140–180 severely overcrowded, and 180–200 dangerously overcrowded.[3]

The EDWIN score is calculated using distinct variables from NEDOCS and is simpler to compute. The EDWIN score uses the number of patients in the ED, number of attending physicians on duty, total number of ED beds, and number of inpatient holds in the ED to numerically quantify patient crowding. At EDWIN scores of 1.5–2, EDs are considered busy, while at a scores greater than 2, EDs are considered crowded.[4]

Other commonly used, less complex, and easier to derive crowding measurements are the total ED patient hours at the time of arrival and ED occupancy rates.[5,6] Though these scales have been validated in various settings, recent studies have demonstrated limitations at extremely high levels of ED crowding,[7] conditions under which most EDs function. Regardless of the methodology used, crowding measured at the daily level has been shown to mask hourly variation.

Conceptual Model of ED Crowding

The Input-Throughput-Output model is a popular conceptual model commonly used to identify the factors that influence ED crowding.[8] In this model, *input* refers to the demand for emergency services and is divided into patients who require emergency care, unscheduled urgent care in the ED, and safety-net care in the ED. The *throughput* component reflects the ED care processes from the time a patient arrives until the time the practitioner makes a disposition decision to either admit, discharge, or transfer the patient. The last component of the model describes the *output*, or outflow of patients after the disposition decision has been made. For example, output includes the ED boarding of inpatients, representing admitted patients who remain in the ED awaiting an inpatient bed, is an often cited in the literature for causing ED crowding.[1,9] Despite the development and familiarity of this conceptual model focused on the external forces that influence ED care, research is predominantly focused on throughput interventions. This focus is likely a result of ED management's ability to have much more control over these interventions. Interventions changing how patients arrive and leave the ED (i.e., input and output) are far more difficult to control.

Operations Research Concepts and ED Throughput

A substantial advancement in the study of ED operations is the use of systems science methods. These scientific disciplines, which include operations management, operations research, and industrial or systems engineering, apply scientific principles to improve the management of an organization facilitating complex decision-making. For decades, principles and concepts from operations research have been applied to improve the performance of organizations in many industries. Applying key principles from operations research to the ED identifies important drivers of ED throughput, and subsequently potential solutions. Three example concepts from operations research that are particularly relevant to the ED are (1) process capacity and bottleneck, (2) queuing theory and the waiting time formula, and (3) frontier analysis.

The first concept from operations research that applies to the ED flow is process capacity and bottleneck. In a multistep process, the process capacity represents the capacity of the entire process and is based on the capacity of the slowest step in the process: the bottleneck. A capacity of the bottleneck dictates the speed of the overall process, and thus to shorten service time, the capacity of the bottleneck must be increased. Defining the ED process capacity and identifying bottlenecks is complicated due to the number of steps involved in the care process and the different care paths for the different patient complaints. Therefore to identify the bottlenecks, ED managers need detailed process maps and need to identify the capacity of each step in the care process for various patient types. Once bottlenecks are identified, ED managers can account for the possibility that these bottlenecks may shift. As capacity increases, the bottleneck may shift to another step in the process. An ED manager that neglects the entire process may fail to see improvement in overall service time as the bottleneck may shift to another, similarly slow step in the process.

Another concept from operations research that is applicable to ED flow is queuing theory. Queuing theory is a mathematical formula describing the relationship between service time, process capacity, and arrivals in the system, all of which affect how the system performs (i.e., wait time). Service time refers to the time it takes to complete a specific process, for example, the time to triage a new patient arriving at the ED. Capacity, on the other hand, refers to the resources available to perform a task. As service times and variability increase or capacity decreases, wait time increases, sometimes nonlinearly, resulting in a dramatic increase in wait times. The variability in patient arrival and service times leads to some patients having to wait to receive care even when an ED has spare capacity in its overall system.

Finally, frontier analysis allows a standard comparison of multiple EDs based on how they use their resources to achieve performance. Frontier analysis uses the concept of efficiency, or inputs into a system to achieve a level of output. EDs on the frontier maximize their output (i.e., patient satisfaction) for a given input (i.e., number of staff). The efficient frontier identifies facilities that are maximally efficient for a given level of inputs or resources. Eliminating waste in ED processes can result in an ED moving closer to the frontier. The approach to eliminating waste to increase efficiency often referred to as "lean management" has been used in some EDs to improve flow. Besides eliminating waste, reducing variability and increasing flexibility also move EDs closer to the frontier.[10] As there are limited interventions to manage variability in ED demand, there has been an increased focus on ways to increase flexibility of ED capacity to meet variable demand. Examples of areas that increase flexibility in capacity include increasing the flexibility of physical resources (e.g., converting single rooms to double rooms or vertical spaces as needed) or human resources (e.g., on-call systems).

Interventions to Improve ED Flow and Reduce ED Crowding

The peer-reviewed literature provides some examples of interventions to improve ED flow and decrease ED crowding. In addition to interventions published in the peer-reviewed literature, we also describe other operational interventions discussed in the lay press and how they may impact ED flow. We organize these interventions based on the input-throughput-output model described by Asplin et al.[8] These interventions have demonstrated varying effects on timeliness of ED care. The varying effect of interventions on outcomes may be due to the heterogeneity of the environments in which they are implemented, lack of uniformity in the intervention, and how these interventions were implemented across study sites. Multiple sites and differing interventions present a challenge to assess the true impact of these interventions on ED crowding and wait times. Below we describe interventions by the components of the input-throughput-output conceptual model for ED flow.

Input

From the operations management perspective, managing the input, or arrivals at the ED, has to do with the overall demand (volume of patients arriving at the ED) as well as managing variability in the demand or arrival pattern. Given that government regulations in the United States and other countries mandate evaluation of patients presenting to EDs, the following interventions have been targeted to manage inflow.

1. **Triage to other clinical providers**. Some EDs have piloted interventions to send patients with nonemergent conditions to same-day primary care appointments after a brief medical screening examination.[11] In addition to triaging patients from the ED to other clinical providers (e.g., primary care physician), nurse–physician triage lines are being implemented by insurance providers and health systems that are staffed with ED physicians to reduce overall ED visits.

2. **Ambulance diversion**. Some EDs divert ambulance traffic when an ED exceeds capacity to control the inflow. Ambulance diversion has a limited effect given that only a small fraction of ED patients arrive via ambulance.[12] In addition, the systemic effect of ambulance diversion (one hospital going on diversion leads to multiple hospitals in the area receiving the majority of ambulance transports, which then become crowded and thus require diversion) makes diversion an inefficient and largely ineffective method to control ED inflow. In several states in the United States, ambulance diversion for crowding is no longer an option for EDs. In those states where ambulance diversion is still possible, the impact on quality and financial impact (ambulance patients are generally sicker and associated with higher revenue) has led to a decrease in diversion hours.

3. **Scheduled ED visits**. Some EDs now allow patients to schedule their ED visit using online tools. While the scheduling of ED visits may not reduce the overall arrivals at the ED, this intervention helps the ED manage the variability in ED arrivals by smoothing patient arrivals and lowering peak demand time periods. However, limited data exist in the peer-reviewed literature on this intervention.

4. **Expanded options for acute unscheduled care**. In the past, EDs in many communities served as the only option for acute unscheduled care. More recently, urgent care centers are available to provide care for low acuity complaints. In addition, due to changing market incentives, primary care practices also increasingly providing same-day or next-day appointments for their patients with acute complaints. Despite alternative options for acute, unscheduled care, national ED volumes continue to increase.

Throughput

The majority of ED-based interventions in the peer-reviewed literature focus on managing throughput, or processes that occur within the ED. From an operations perspective, these interventions target common principles in process design. Some concepts common in manufacturing plants, such as parallel as opposed to serial processing (first-line orders by triage nurses and physicians), Toyota production systems and identification of bottlenecks (split flow and dedicated fast-tracks), and eliminating wasted time through the application of lean management, are now being applied to patient care. Given the multitude of published interventions on improving throughput, we will focus on the most common interventions.

1. **Physician-in-triage**. Physician-in-triage (PIT) places a physician in triage to expedite care. Due to heterogeneous implementation in EDs, the impact of PIT models on patient care varies. For the majority of these programs, PIT does not replace the nurse who performs triage in the ED. At most study sites, PIT supplements nurse triage and becomes an additional step in the process. When the main objective of a PIT program is to have the physician initiate work-ups, these programs often have a limited impact on ED flow.[13] These programs incorrectly assume that initiating work-ups removes the bottleneck to see the physician. The limited impact on ED flow is likely due to shifting to other bottlenecks (e.g., physician disposition, ED beds) that may impact flow, a so-called hurry-up-and-wait approach that merely shifts where wait time occurs. PIT programs that have shown the largest impact on ED flow are those programs where the physician is responsible for initiating work-ups and managing disposition of certain types of patients.[13,14] These programs both address the bottleneck related to work-ups and perhaps, more importantly, add capacity when arranging for the disposition of a subset of patients.

2. **Split-flow models, dedicated fast-tracks, and streaming**. In split-flow models and streaming, similar patient types are clustered together. Considering they have similar needs, they can potentially reduce provider cognitive load and improve efficiency. For example, in a split-flow model, the traditional lengthy ED nursing triage process is eliminated and replaced with a quick triage process to distinguish patients with higher severity from those with lower severity. The physician in the split-flow model identifies patients who can be kept on the "fast" lane and could be discharged either immediately on arrival or relatively quickly. For "slow" lane patients, the physician initiates work-ups and patients are transferred to the main ED. Split-flow models address the time-to-physician, patients who leave prior to clinical evaluation, and length of stay of patients.

   Dedicated fast-track units capitalize on the concept of segmentation, or grouping similar types of patients. A fast track is an area of the ED dedicated to low severity patients; they are widespread in the United States and have been show to improve ED flow.[14] More recently, this concept has been extended for uncomplicated moderate acuity patients with similar throughput results.[15] In the operations literature, segmenting these patients in dedicated units can improve flow by decreasing process variation as well as keeping these patients on the "fast" lane. Creating new space for fast-tracks also increases the capacity of the ED, improving the overall capacity.

3. **Immediate bedding and bedside registration**. Immediate bedding allows patients to bypass the activities of nursing triage and registration when beds in the ED are available. By moving registration to the bedside, immediately placing patients in a bed, this

intervention allows both the clinical team and the registration to occur simultaneously while bypassing the triage process. After all, triage, developed for soldiers on the battlefield in the 1700s, was meant to prioritize patients when demand for services outstripped their accompanying resources. Therefore, when beds are available, triage introduces additional activities that can delay patient care. The impact of this intervention in the peer-reviewed literature is varied given the heterogeneity of the intervention.[13]

4. **First-line orders (FLO)/triage-based care protocols.** FLO allow triage nurses to initiate work-ups based on their triage assessment and preestablished advance triage protocols without a new physician order. This intervention allows for a patient's work-up and treatment to begin while they wait for beds. By reducing the amount of time to initiate clinical work-ups, FLO have been shown in the literature to decrease the length of stay and improve ED flow.[13]

Output

Another method from operations research, computer simulation modeling, has demonstrated the impact of boarding on ED flow. While outflow is commonly cited as the major cause of ED crowding, interventions to address the flow of admitted patients from the ED are primarily focused on hospital-based interventions. The major causes for boarding admitted patients in the ED are inefficiencies rather than capacity constraints. Several hospital practices, such as reservation of empty beds for elective schedule, nonsmoothing of elective outpatient surgery schedules, and geographic pooling of beds, are examples of some common hospital procedures that contribute to the inefficiencies and lead to extended ED boarding.[16]

In the ED peer-reviewed literature, there are limited studies of interventions addressing the flow of patients from the ED. The majority of interventions that may address ED boarding and outflow are thus in hospital management journals and focus on optimization of inpatient bed utilization as a primary endpoint and are not directly applicable to the ED.

1. **Boarding in inpatient hallways.** Moving of admitted patients boarding in the ED to inpatient hallway beds reduces boarding hours in the ED and frees up ED beds.[16] While this intervention is frequently mentioned in the literature, the impact on ED crowding has not been published. However, the limited literature does support that this intervention can be safely done and that patients prefer boarding in inpatient hallways than in the ED.[17,18]

2. **Inpatient discharge timing and active bed management strategies.** Shifting the time of day that admitted inpatients get discharged from the hospital by a few hours has been shown to create inpatient capacity and reduce ED boarding.[19,20] The overall inpatient capacity saved is significant and a key focus off hospital administrators in creating capacity. In addition, inpatient bed management strategies have also been shown to decrease inpatient length of stay and ED boarding.

3. **Elective surgery management and procedure schedule smoothing.** Elective surgery and procedure scheduling contributes to the inefficiencies that lead to increased ED boarding. In most hospitals, the 5-day operating room schedule combined with surgeon preferences lead to high caseloads early in the week while remaining variable for the remainder of the week. Scheduling variability creates downstream spikes in demand for inpatient beds following elective procedures and reduces the availability of beds for

admitted ED patients. Some studies have described the role of smoothing elective surgery schedules and the impact on ED boarding.[18] Successful interventions actively manage elective surgeries by smoothing surgery schedules, expanding operating room schedules to 6 days, and canceling elective cases when hospitals have reached an established inpatient capacity. Similar results have been shown with elective procedures. For example, cardiac catheterization laboratories that perform angiography in one institution were found to increase ED crowding for chest pain patients requiring telemetry beds in the hospital. A computer simulation found that simply moving cardiac catheterization before noon had the same boarding-time effect as installing three additional hospital beds.

Discussion

Beyond identifying an intervention to improve ED patient flow is the entire process of implementation. Success in the implementation of an intervention to improve patient flow in the ED can be just as important as the selection of the intervention. Not only can the current intervention be compromised if poorly executed, but future implementations may be as well. Another vital issue affecting ED performance is how to evaluate the ED. Until now, the primary dimension of evaluation was through timeliness of care. However, the ED receives virtually no recognition for diagnosing a complicated, undifferentiated illness that may prevent future unnecessary healthcare visits. Instead, timeliness is the primary dimension used to evaluate the ED. Timeliness happens to be one of the dimensions that is easiest to measure but may have limited effect on the actual performance of the ED. Even with the sole focus on timeliness, improving performance in this area requires a much broader evaluation of the dimensions of emergency care delivery both internal and external to the ED. Moreover, as mentioned by the IOM report, there are six dimensions to deliver quality care. Moving beyond timeliness requires not only operational interventions but careful coordination with patients, their families, and caregivers. In addition, not only is the actual performance of the ED important, but forces that influence the arrival of patients at the ED and how patients move out of the ED also dramatically influence the ED's throughput. Given the multifactorial causes of crowding, addressing ED flow requires the ED management to engage hospital leadership to invest in changing ED as well as hospital processes.

References

1. Hoot NR, Aronsky D. Systematic review of emergency department crowding: causes, effects, and solutions. *Annals of Emergency Medicine.* 2008;52(2):136.

2. Bernstein SL, Aronsky D, Duseja R, et al. The effect of emergency department crowding on clinically oriented outcomes. *Academic Emergency Medicine.* 2009;16 (1):1–10.

3. Weiss SJ, Derlet R, Arndahl J, et al. Estimating the degree of emergency department overcrowding in academic medical centers: results of the national ED overcrowding study (NEDOCS). *Academic Emergency Medicine.* 2004;11(1):38–50.

4. Bernstein SL, Verghese V, Leung W, et al. Development and validation of a new index to measure emergency department crowding. *Academic Emergency Medicine.* 2003;10(9):938–942.

5. McCarthy ML, Aronsky D, Jones ID, et al. The emergency department occupancy rate: a simple measure of emergency department crowding? *Annals of Emergency Medicine.* 2008;51(1):24.

6. Hwang U, McCarthy ML, Aronsky D, et al. Measures of crowding in the emergency

department: a systematic review. *Academic Emergency Medicine.* 2011;18(5):527–538.

7. Wang H, Robinson RD, Bunch K, et al. The inaccuracy of determining overcrowding status by using the national ED overcrowding study tool. *The American Journal of Emergency Medicine.* 2014;32 (10):1230–1236.

8. Asplin BR, Magid DJ, Rhodes KV, et al. A conceptual model of emergency department crowding. *Annals of Emergency Medicine.* 2003;42(2):173–180.

9. Moskop JC, Sklar DP, Geiderman JM, et al. Emergency department crowding, part 1: concept, causes, and moral consequences. *Annals of Emergency Medicine.* 2009;53 (5):605–611.

10. Soremekun OA, Terwiesch C, Pines JM. Emergency medicine: an operations management view. *Academic Emergency Medicine.* 2011;18(12):1262–1268.

11. Derlet RW, Kinser D, Ray L, Hamilton B, et al. Prospective identification and triage of nonemergency patients out of an emergency department: a 5-year study. *Annals of Emergency Medicine.* 1995;25 (2):215–223.

12. Burke LG, Joyce N, Baker WE, et al. The effect of an ambulance diversion ban on emergency department length of stay and ambulance turnaround time. *Annals of Emergency Medicine.* 2013;61(3):311.

13. Wiler JL, Gentle C, Halfpenny JM, et al. Optimizing emergency department front-end operations. *Annals of Emergency Medicine.* 2010;55(2):160.

14. Soremekun OA, Shofer FS, Grasso D, et al. The effect of an emergency department dedicated midtrack area on patient flow. *Academic Emergency Medicine.* 2014;21 (4):434–439.

15. Soremekun OA, Shofer FS, Grasso D, Mills AM, Moore J, Datner EM. The effect of an emergency department dedicated midtrack area on patient flow. *Academic Emergency Medicine.* 2014;21(4):434–439.

16. Rabin E, Kocher K, McClelland M, et al. Solutions to emergency department "boarding" and crowding are underused and may need to be legislated. *Health Affairs.* 2012;31(8):1757–1766.

17. Viccellio P, Zito JA, Sayage V, et al. Patients overwhelmingly prefer inpatient boarding to emergency department boarding. *The Journal of Emergency Medicine.* 2013;45(6):942–946.

18. Viccellio A, Santora C, Singer AJ, et al. The association between transfer of emergency department boarders to inpatient hallways and mortality: a 4-year experience. *Annals of Emergency Medicine.* 2009;54 (4):487–491.

19. Howell E, Bessman E, Kravet S, et al. Active bed management by hospitalists and emergency department throughput. *Annals of Internal Medicine.* 2008;149 (11):804–811.

20. Howell E, Bessman E, Marshall, R. Hospitalist bed management effecting throughput from the emergency department to the intensive care unit. *Journal of Critical Care.* 2010;25 (2):184–189.

Bringing the Patient Voice into Emergency Care

Marc A. Probst and Erik P. Hess

Introduction

In recent years, there has been an increased emphasis placed on the importance of patient engagement in both chronic and acute care. Patient engagement can be broadly defined as active patient involvement in their healthcare to strengthen their influence on medical decisions and behaviors.[1] A key component of patient engagement is shared decision-making (SDM). SDM is defined as a process by which patients and providers consider outcome probabilities and patient preferences and reach a healthcare decision based on mutual agreement.[2] An SDM approach to clinical decisions in the emergency department (ED) is a reliable way to have the patient's voice heard with regard to their values, preferences, and unique circumstances. In this chapter, we describe concepts underlying SDM, review the existing literature on patient decision aids and SDM in the ED setting, and offer three clinical vignettes to illustrate the process of SDM in emergency care.

What Is Shared Decision-Making?

SDM is an approach in which clinicians actively bring the patient's voice into the medical encounter. Although the patient's role has classically been relegated to providing a history of the present illness and answering specific clinical questions, patients can have a more active role through asking questions, voicing concerns, and expressing values and preferences. Charles, Gafni, and Whelan described a conceptual model of SDM in the context of medical encounters for potentially life-threatening chronic conditions.[3] They proposed four key characteristics of SDM: (1) at least two participants must be involved – physician and patient (or surrogate); (2) both parties share information; (3) both parties build consensus regarding the patient's preferred treatment; and (4) a mutual agreement is reached on the treatment to pursue. They describe a spectrum from paternalistic, physician-directed decision-making to fully informed, patient-directed decision-making, with SDM lying in the middle. The purported benefits of such an approach include increased patient satisfaction, increased adherence to treatment, and improved functional status.

SDM is also appropriate for ED care. All ED encounters entail clinical decisions, be they diagnostic, therapeutic, or dispositional (i.e., whether the patient is admitted or discharged from the ED). For many of these clinical decisions, only one action is medically reasonable, for example, obtaining an electrocardiogram for a patient with symptoms suggestive of acute myocardial ischemia, administering intravenous antibiotics for a patient in septic shock, or hospital admission for severe acute decompensated heart failure. For these types of decisions, the physician should offer a professional recommendation as to the medically appropriate course of action and seek to obtain consent, provided palliative care or end-of-life decision-making is

Table 6.1 Informed Consent versus Shared Decision-Making

	Informed Consent	Shared Decision-Making
Medically reasonable options	One	Two or more
Explanation of risks and benefits	Necessary	Necessary, with consideration to selecting among management options
Use of decision aid	Optional (if available)	Optimal (when available)
Compassionate persuasion	Appropriate	Inappropriate
Process of deliberation	Typically unilateral (physician)	Collaborative by definition (patient and physician)

not a contextually appropriate consideration. If the patient is hesitant or refuses, the physician should employ compassionate persuasion, without coercion, to convince the patient based on the ethical principle of beneficence. Obtaining informed consent in a scenario with one best medical option does *not* constitute SDM (see Table 6.1). However, there are numerous clinical scenarios in which the best course of action is either uncertain or in equipoise with an alternative course of action. SDM is appropriate for clinical scenarios in which there is more than one medically reasonable course of action.[4] Take, for example, the patient with a mild form of an acute medical illness (e.g., pneumonia, pancreatitis, or pyelonephritis) who can be managed in the hospital or at home with expedited follow-up. The most appropriate disposition may depend on the patient's social support, personal values, access to medical care, and competing priorities, among others. All of these factors depend on the patient's unique personal circumstances that he or she is most suitable to assess. Thus, eliciting this information and involving the patient in the medical decision-making process through SDM is key to providing high-quality, patient-centered care.

More recently, Hess et al. have adapted this model to the emergency care context.[5] These authors highlight the unique practical and contextual challenges that the ED presents, including the acute time-sensitivity of certain decisions, occasional lack of decision-making capacity on the part of the patient, frequent absence of surrogate decision-makers, frequent interruptions, lack of an established rapport between patient and physician, and limitations of the scientific evidence base, among others. On the other hand, there are often scenarios where SDM is not appropriate. Situations requiring emergent medical intervention (e.g., cardiac or respiratory arrest in a patient known to be "full code") would generally not be appropriate for SDM given the acute time-sensitivity at hand. Similarly, any patient without decision-making capacity (e.g., due to dementia, delirium, intoxication, or psychosis) would not be appropriate to engage in SDM. These, and other limitations, are described in more detail below. Nonetheless, there are many scenarios in the ED in which SDM may be appropriate for diagnosis, treatment, or disposition.[6]

Patient Decision Aids

Patient decision aids are evidenced-based tools designed to help patients participate in healthcare decisions.[7] It is important to note that decision aids *supplement*, rather than replace, clinical counseling and explanation of healthcare options. In general, decisions aids should explicitly state the decision to be considered, provide objective information about the health condition, and describe the different clinical options and the potential outcomes associated with each. Further, decision aids should help patients clarify how their values and preferences impact the healthcare decision at hand.[8]

In the outpatient setting, in which care is delivered over a longer period of time, decision aids can be used before, during, or after a clinical encounter as a tool to facilitate SDM. As emergency care is largely unscheduled and episodic, it is generally not feasible to present patients with a decision aid prior to the ED encounter, although it may be feasible for patients with certain complaints to consult a decision aid while waiting to be evaluated by an emergency physician, either in the waiting room or in an ED bed.

A key concept underlying the design and use of decision aids is that of risk communication. Risk communication between physicians and patients is often difficult, with or without the use of decision aids.[9] Barriers to effective risk communication using decision aids include limited patient literacy and numeracy. The average American patient reads at an 8th-grade reading level,[10] yet many decision aids have found to be written at levels substantially higher than that.[11] Patients may also have difficulty comprehending numerical information such as odds or probabilities if not presented in a clear, easy-to-understand manner. Limited understanding of risk may undermine the SDM process. Various strategies have been proposed to enhance patients' numerical understanding when facing medical decisions, including (1) presenting statistical information as an absolute risk, as opposed to a relative risk or number needed to treat, (2) highlighting incremental risks distinct from baseline risks, and (3) using pictographs to communicate risk and benefit information (see Figure 6.1).[11]

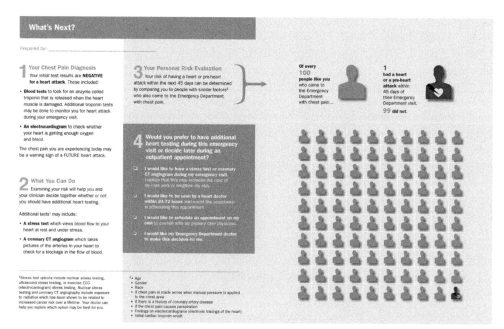

Figure 6.1 The Chest Pain Choice decision aid. Reproduced from Anderson et al.[26] Used with permission of Mayo Foundation for Medical Education and Research, all rights reserved.

Multiple studies have evaluated the impact of decision aids on various patient-centered outcomes. Patient-centered outcomes have been defined as "health outcomes meaningful and important to patients and caregivers," for example, pain scores or days of work missed.[12] These stand in contradistinction to physiological measures (e.g., hemoglobin A1c) and clinician-reported measures. A recent systematic review of published randomized controlled trials on this topic demonstrated that decision aids increased knowledge, improved the accuracy of risk perception, and increased the proportion of patients choosing an option congruent with their values.[8] Further, decision aids resulted in less decisional conflict, reduced patient passivity, and fewer patients who remained undecided postintervention. Use of certain decision aids was associated with decreased intensity of care and improved patient–physician communication, with a possible increase in the duration of the patient encounter.[8] It is reasonable to assume that most of these effects could be extrapolated to ED-based decision aids. However, substantially less research in this setting exists at the current time.

SDM in the Emergency Care Setting

At the time of writing, there were 11 published SDM studies conducted in the ED setting.[6,13–22] This list includes studies of decision aids, also known as decision support interventions (DSIs), previously reported in a systematic review,[23] as well as SDM studies that have been published since the review was completed. Three studies[14–16] were conducted in the pediatric population, with the remaining seven studies focused on adults.[6,13,17–22,24] Three studies[14,15,22] sought to increase patient engagement in care decisions through improving the informed consent process; five studies reported the development or effect of use of a DSI to facilitate SDM[13,16–19]; and two studies were surveys of practicing emergency physicians to assess their perceptions on the frequency with which they engage patients in SDM[6] and emergency conditions and decisions for which SDM might be appropriate.[24] Only two studies reported the effect of use of a decision aid during the clinical encounter on clinical outcomes and decisional quality.[17,18]

Two surveys of emergency physicians assessing the frequency of perceived use of SDM and the appropriateness of SDM for emergency decisions have been published.[6,21] The first study engaged two multispecialty focus groups to explore decision-making around resource utilization, diagnostic imaging utilization, and SDM to design a survey. Respondents included 435 emergency physicians from 29 states.[6] Emergency physicians reported that there was more than one reasonable management option in over 50 percent of their patients and taking an SDM approach in 58 percent of such patients. The second survey conducted a cross-sectional survey of 709 emergency physicians attending the 2014 American College of Emergency Physicians annual meeting to assess the perceived appropriateness of SDM for different categories of ED management (testing, treatment, and disposition).[24] SDM was perceived to be most frequently appropriate for invasive procedures, followed by computed tomography (CT) scanning and disposition. Use of intravenous tissue plasminogen (tPA) for acute ischemic stroke was felt to be most frequently appropriate for SDM, followed by lumbar puncture to evaluate for possible subarachnoid hemorrhage and cranial CT for pediatric minor head injury.

Most parents of febrile children at risk for occult bacteremia opted for no investigations and preferred to be involved in the decision-making process regarding their child.[14] In another study it was reported that most parents of children with small lacerations preferred infiltrated lidocaine over topical anesthesia, nonsedation over sedation, and to be involved in care decisions regarding their child.[15] A touch-screen tablet-based DSI was designed for use by adult patients and their clinicians during the ED visit to come to a shared decision on whether to undergo head CT or further observation after a minor head injury.[19] This DSI is currently undergoing feasibility and usability testing. A COMPuterized Decision Aid for Stroke ThrombolysiS (COMPASS) has been developed to provide decision support for clinicians caring for patients with acute ischemic stroke regarding whether t-PA is indicated, whether a contraindication for t-PA is present, and to communicate the risks and benefits of thrombolysis to patients and/or their surrogate decisionmakers.[13] Preliminary testing of this computerized decision aid demonstrated it to be both feasible and acceptable to patients and their relatives and clinicians. A quantitative pretest probability instrument estimates the 45-day risk of acute coronary syndrome (ACS) in ED chest pain patients.[17] These investigators reported greater patient satisfaction regarding the explanation of their problem and a safe reduction in resource utilization in patients who were provided with a printout of their ACS risk compared with those who did not receive a printout. Another investigator developed a decision aid that incorporated the 45-day risk of ACS generated from the quantitative pretest probability instrument, information regarding their testing and diagnostic evaluation, and the available management options (Figure 6.1).[25] These investigators tested the efficacy of the decision aid in a single-center randomized trial and found that, compared with patients who received usual care, patients randomized to the decision aid had greater knowledge regarding their 45-day risk of ACS and the available management options, were more engaged in the decision-making process, had less decisional conflict related to choosing among alternative management options, and a 19 percent lower rate of observation unit admission for cardiac stress testing.[18] There were no adverse events in either arm of the trial.

Two multicenter trials to test the effectiveness of a decision aid on clinical outcomes, decisional quality, and safety are ongoing. The Chest Pain Choice multicenter randomized trial was recently conducted in six EDs across the United States.[18,26] Recruitment for this trial is complete, and data analysis is ongoing. The Head CT Choice trial, a multicenter trial testing the effectiveness of a decision aid in parents of children with minor head injury, is also being conducted in seven EDs across the United States.[27] Results are anticipated to be available in 2017. In the following case vignettes, we will describe three conditions in which emergency clinicians might utilize an SDM approach with their patients.

Clinical Vignettes

Case 1: A 6-Year-Old Girl with Minor Head Trauma

A 6-year-old, otherwise healthy girl is brought to the ED by her parents 3 hours after sustaining blunt head trauma. She was playing on the jungle gym in a nearby park when she accidentally fell 4 feet, hitting her head first on the ground. There was a brief witnessed loss of consciousness that lasted less than 30 seconds. She cried on awakening and was able to walk home unassisted. One hour after the fall, she vomited once spontaneously but exhibited normal behavior otherwise. This prompted the father, a retired police officer, to bring her to the ED for evaluation.

On examination in the ED, the child is alert and oriented. She is seated on the gurney and appears tired, but is interactive. Her speech, balance, and gait are within normal limits. There is no visible evidence of trauma; no laceration, scalp hematoma, or signs of basilar skull fracture. She has no midline cervical tenderness to palpation. The rest of the physical exam is unremarkable. The father is worried that his daughter may have sustained a concussion or, worse, bleeding in her brain.

Case discussion. The primary clinical decision that needs to be made here is one of diagnostic testing: does this patient need an immediate head CT or careful observation in the ED and/or at home? One could argue, using high-quality evidence, that both of these options are medically reasonable given the clinical information at hand. The physician could simply make this decision unilaterally without taking into account the patient's or parent's wishes. Alternatively, the physician could allow the patient/parent's voice to be heard by employing SDM. The first step would be to verbally acknowledge that a clinical decision, with more than one reasonable option, needs to be made. The second step is to describe the options and their potential outcomes using available evidence. In this case, information about the probability of clinically significant traumatic brain injury (i.e., requiring intervention or having long-term neurological consequences), the logistics of a CT scan, the small but relevant risks of radiation in a young child, the potential for incidental findings, and the time and cost associated with each could all be discussed. The validated clinical decision instrument put forth by the Pediatric Emergency Care Applied Research Network (PECARN) for pediatric blunt head trauma would be useful to inform this discussion.[28] Step three is to elicit the values, preferences, and circumstances of the patient/surrogate. Finally, in step four, the patient and physician come to a mutually agreed-on decision and carry out the corresponding clinical action. Critical, throughout this process, is for the physician to create a relaxed environment that is conducive to open dialogue, question-asking, and deliberation on the part of the family. This requires particular interpersonal and communication skills in order to alleviate the potential power differential that can exist between lay parents and physicians and to educate the parent without using medical jargon. This SDM process can be done informally, via unstructured dialogue, or more formally, using a patient decision aid.[27]

Case resolution. You return to the bedside and engage the father in SDM, explaining that the patient has indeed sustained a concussion, based on the history and physical exam. The risk of a serious injury is roughly 1 percent based on her two PECARN risk factors: loss of consciousness and vomiting. The radiation from a CT does incrementally increase the risk of cancer in the long term, the exact magnitude of which is controversial and difficult for most people to grasp. Observation in your ED typically entails 2–4 hours, while a CT could be obtained in under 1 hour. In the event of a neurological deterioration in the ED, a CT could be obtained with a small delay in diagnosis but likely no change in ultimate clinical outcome. The father asks whether sedation would be needed to obtain the CT and whether concussions can have long-term consequences. You address both of these concerns adequately. Finally, the father expresses his concern over the radiation exposure and opts for a period of observation in the ED, and then at home. The patient slowly improves over the period of the next 4 hours and is discharged home with an uneventful recovery. The family leaves informed and empowered; they are confident they made a decision consistent with their values and preferences.

Case 2: 3-Year-Old Male with Fever and Otalgia

A 3-year-old, otherwise healthy boy is brought in to the pediatric ED by his mother for fever and ear pain for 3 days. His rectal temperature at home was 101.2°F today. He received oral acetaminophen and subsequently defervesced. He intermittently reports right ear pain to his mother, and has some mild nasal congestion. He has no nausea, vomiting, cough, sore throat, or other respiratory symptoms. The review of systems is otherwise unremarkable. On physical exam, the child appears well and is alert and interactive. The oropharynx and lungs are unremarkable. The left tympanic membrane (TM) exam is within normal limits, while the right TM exhibits erythema and mild bulging without perforation or discharge. There is no evidence of external ear infection. The mother is concerned since he has been waking up at night, difficult to console. Both mother and patient have been sleeping poorly as a result. The child has no known drug allergies and is on no medications.

Case discussion. Acute otitis media (AOM) is the most common condition for which antibiotics are prescribed to children.[29] However, AOM has a high rate of spontaneous resolution, with similar rates of complications with or without antibiotic therapy. This condition can have a viral or bacterial etiology; differentiating between the two is often challenging for the clinician. Resistance to antibiotics is a major, long-term public health risk and is associated with overuse of antibiotics. More conservative treatment for fever and otalgia using ibuprofen often effectively controls the symptoms without need for antibiotics. While antibiotics can accelerate the resolution of symptoms, they are associated with increased cost, side effects (e.g., vomiting, diarrhea, or rash), and allergic reactions. In this case, the patient appears to have nonsevere AOM. Medically reasonable courses of action include (1) supportive care with ibuprofen alone, (2) supportive care plus oral antibiotics, or (3) a hybrid of the two, using a wait-and-see prescription (WASP). The WASP approach involves writing a prescription for antibiotics and instructing the parent to fill it only if the child is not better, or is worse, in 48 hours. This approach has been shown to decrease antibiotic use without adversely affecting clinical outcomes.[30]

Case resolution. Once the evaluation of the child is complete, you begin by explaining to the mother how the constellation of signs and symptoms is consistent with AOM, also known as a middle ear infection. Further, you explain the possible causes (viral vs. bacterial), describe the natural history of the disease, and provide an opportunity for questions. You then acknowledge the clinical decision that needs to be made with regard to medical therapy. Since no ED-based patient decision aids are available, you use open dialogue to elicit values and preferences and use categorical descriptions of probabilities to communicate risk. The mother asks about the cost of the antibiotics and the duration of therapy. You explain that amoxicillin is generally low cost and would be given twice a day for 7 days. The mother prefers to have the option of initiating antibiotics if her child does not improve in 2 days but also wishes to avoid unnecessary antibiotics, if possible. You give her a prescription date for 2 days in the future as well as specific return precautions. The mother's wishes have been incorporated into the decision to use a WASP strategy through SDM, and, furthermore, she will be in a position decide whether or not to initiate antibiotics 48 hours from now. The family leaves informed and empowered; they are confident that they have made a decision consistent with their values and preferences.

Case 3: 58-Year-Old Female with Acute Chest Pain

A 58-year-old female with a history of sporadic smoking and hypertension presents to the ED with acute anterior chest pain for 1 day. The pain has been intermittent, lasting 20–30 minutes. The last episode occurred roughly 2 hours prior to arrival. It is associated with mild dyspnea, but no diaphoresis, nausea, vomiting, or dizziness. The pain is nonradiating and nonexertional. She has never had this pain before and has never had any provocative cardiac testing performed. She is divorced and lives with her mother, who suffers from Alzheimer's dementia. She works at a local university as a chemistry professor. She takes two oral antihypertensives daily. Recently, she has been under increased psychological stress while contemplating placing her mother in a nursing home. On physical exam, she is calm and cooperative, is pain free, and has normal vital signs. Her heart and lung exam are unremarkable with no chest wall tenderness. Her initial electrocardiogram demonstrates a normal sinus rhythm with T-wave flattening in the lateral precordial leads but no ST-segment deviations. Her chest x-ray and first set of cardiac biomarkers are negative. She is eager to get home to care for her elderly mother.

Case discussion. Acute chest pain is the second most frequent common reason to present to the ED in the United States.[31] Due partly to medicolegal concerns, clinicians often initiate formal diagnostic testing for acute coronary syndrome (ACS) at very low risk thresholds. These diagnostic pathways are associated with substantial costs, radiation exposure, and potential false-positive test results.[32] Unstructured risk communication surrounding chest pain and ACS probability is variable and often ineffective.[9] Thus, patients often undergo advanced diagnostic testing without a clear understanding of their personalized risk of ACS. Recent studies have sought to objectively calculate and communicate risk of ACS with patients and physicians in an effort to reduce resource utilization.[17] Building on this, a patient decision aid referenced earlier (see Figure 6.1) was developed in order to formally engage patient in SDM surrounding the decision to be admitted after a nondiagnostic ED visit for acute chest pain.[18] As discussed above, this decision aid was evaluated in a randomized control trial and was shown to increase patient knowledge and engagement in decision-making while decreasing admission rates to the observation unit with no change in clinical outcomes.

Case closure. You return to the bedside equipped with a paper-based, personalized version of the Chest Pain Choice tool to facilitate an SDM conversation. Based on her eight key clinical variables and the negative initial troponin, this patient's 45-day risk of ACS was estimated to be 3 percent. After guiding her through the text of the decision aid and looking at the graphical representation of risk (see Figure 6.1) together, she better understands the nature and magnitude of the risk and her options going forward. This stimulates further questions, which you are glad to answer for her, including what the risks of stress testing are, how quickly she will obtain the results, and how quickly she will be discharged the following day. She is lecturing at the university at 4 PM and does not want to have to cancel her class. She understands that the option to go home is appropriate only in the event that her subsequent cardiac biomarkers are normal as well. She requests to make a phone call while waiting for the next blood draw. The second troponin is also negative. In the interim, she has called her ex-husband to attend to her elderly mother and elects to stay in the observation unit overnight for a cardiac stress test in the morning. She prefers to expedite the test and gain certainty regarding the etiology of the chest pain. She also has nothing scheduled the following morning, making it a good time to undergo further testing.

Limitations of SDM

There are often scenarios in which SDM is *not* appropriate. First, if only one medically reasonable option exists, informed consent, with compassionate persuasion as needed, should be obtained without attempts at bona fide SDM. Second, if a patient lacks decision-making capacity (e.g., due to altered mental status, acute psychosis, or advanced dementia), SDM is no longer an option, unless an appropriate surrogate decision-maker is present. If no surrogate is available, the clinician should unilaterally make the best medical decisions for the patient based on what is known or presumed about the patients' wishes. Third, a patient may elect to not be involved in the decision-making process, due to personal, social, or cultural reasons, and may prefer that the clinician make the medical decision unilaterally. Although practicing SDM is generally benign, there are some potential risks, including increasing patient anxiety by providing excessive information or by requesting that they become involved in a decision in which they do not feel comfortable being involved. Having to make medical decisions can place a psychological burden on patients, especially in times of acute stress/illness. These harms can be mitigated by the clinician through sensitive communication and a gradual, step-wise progression into the SDM process. Last, SDM does require a certain amount of time for conversation and deliberation. Given the time pressures faced by the emergency clinician, SDM can be attempted only for a small subset of all the medical decisions made in the ED.

Conclusion

Contemporary medicine, along with improving health at the population level and reducing per capita costs, is placing increasing emphasis on the patient experience of care (quality and satisfaction). Shared decision-making is a key domain of healthcare quality and is an effective way of bringing the patient voice into the medical encounter. Decision aids, patient-centered decision tools used to facilitate SDM, have been shown to improve patient's knowledge, the accuracy of risk perception, patient engagement, and the quality of the decision-making process. Despite contextual challenges inherent in healthcare delivery in the ED setting, limited evidence suggests that SDM is feasible and safe and may improve patients' experience of care while curtailing unnecessary resource use.

References

1. Coulter A. *Engaging Patients in Healthcare*. New York: Open University Press, 2011.

2. Frosch DL, Kaplan RM. Shared decision making in clinical medicine: past research and future directions. *American Journal of Preventive Medicine*. 1999;17:285–294.

3. Charles C, Gafni A, Whelan T. Shared decision-making in the medical encounter: what does it mean? (or it takes at least two to tango). *Social Science & Medicine*. 1997;44:681–692.

4. Barry MJ, Edgman-Levitan S. Shared decision making: the pinnacle of patient-centered care. *The New England Journal of Medicine*. 2012;366:780–781.

5. Hess EP, Grudzen CR, Thomson R, et al. Shared decision-making in the emergency department: respecting patient autonomy when seconds count. *Academic Emergency Medicine*. 2015;22:856–864.

6. Kanzaria HK, Brook RH, Probst MA, et al. Emergency physician perceptions of shared decision-making. *Academic Emergency Medicine*. 2015;22:399–405.

7. Elwyn G, O'Connor A, Stacey D, et al. Developing a quality criteria framework for patient decision aids: online international Delphi consensus process. *BMJ*. 2006;333:417.

8. Stacey D, Legare F, Col NF, et al. Decision aids for people facing health treatment or screening decisions. *The Cochrane Database of Systematic Reviews*. 2014;1: CD001431.

9. Newman DH, Ackerman B, Kraushar ML, et al. Quantifying patient–physician communication and perceptions of risk during admissions for possible acute

coronary syndromes. *Annals of Emergency Medicine.* 2015;66:13–18.

10. Kirsch IS JA, Jenkins L, Kolstad A. *Adult Literacy in America: A First Look at the Results of the National Adult Literacy Survey.* National Center for Education Statistics, 1993.

11. Lin GA, Fagerlin A. Shared decision making: state of the science. *Circulation: Cardiovascular Quality and Outcomes.* 2014;7:328–334.

12. Frank L, Basch E, Selby JV. Patient-centered outcomes research I. The PCORI perspective on patient-centered outcomes research. *JAMA.* 2014;312:1513–1514.

13. Flynn D, Nesbitt DJ, Ford GA, et al. Development of a computerised decision aid for thrombolysis in acute stroke care. *BMC Medical Informatics and Decision Making.* 2015;15:6.

14. Yamamoto LG. Application of informed consent principles in the emergency department evaluation of febrile children at risk for occult bacteremia. *Hawaii Medical Journal.* 1997;56:313–317, 320–312.

15. Yamamoto LG, Young LL, Roberts JL. Informed consent and parental choice of anesthesia and sedation for the repair of small lacerations in children. *The American Journal of Emergency Medicine.* 1997;15:285–289.

16. Karpas A, Finkelstein M, Reid S. Parental preference for rehydration method for children in the emergency department. *Pediatric Emergency Care.* 2009;25:301–306.

17. Kline JA, Zeitouni RA, Hernandez-Nino J, et al. Randomized trial of computerized quantitative pretest probability in low-risk chest pain patients: effect on safety and resource use. *Annals of Emergency Medicine.* 2009;53:727–735.

18. Hess EP, Knoedler MA, Shah ND, et al. The chest pain choice decision aid: a randomized trial. *Circulation: Cardiovascular Quality and Outcomes.* 2012;5:251–259.

19. Melnick ER, Lopez K, Hess EP, et al. Back to the bedside: developing a bedside aid for concussion and brain injury decisions in the emergency department. *EGEMS.* 2015;3:1136.

20. Melnick ER, Shafer K, Rodulfo N, et al. Understanding overuse of computed tomography for minor head injury in the emergency department: a triangulated qualitative study. *Academic Emergency Medicine.* 2015;22(12):1474–1483.

21. Probst MA, Kanzaria HK, Frosch DL, et al. Perceived appropriateness of shared decision-making in the emergency department: a survey study. *Academic Emergency Medicine* 2016;23(4):375–381.

22. Merck LH, Ward LA, Applegate KE, et al. Written informed consent for computed tomography of the abdomen/pelvis is associated with decreased CT utilization in low-risk emergency department patients. *Western Journal of Emergency Medicine.* 2015;16(7):1014–1024.

23. Flynn D, Knoedler MA, Hess EP, et al. Engaging patients in health care decisions in the emergency department through shared decision-making: a systematic review. *Academic Emergency Medicine.* 2012;19:959–967.

24. Probst MA, Kanzaria HK, Frosch DL, et al. Appropriateness of shared decision making in the emergency department: a survey study. *Academic Emergency Medicine.* 2016;23(4):375–381.

25. Pierce MA, Hess EP, Kline JA, et al. The chest pain choice trial: a pilot randomized trial of a decision aid for patients with chest pain in the emergency department. *Trials.* 2010;11:57.

26. Anderson RT, Montori VM, Shah ND, et al. Effectiveness of the chest pain choice decision aid in emergency department patients with low-risk chest pain: study protocol for a multicenter randomized trial. *Trials.* 2014;15:166.

27. Hess EP, Wyatt KD, Kharbanda AB, et al. Effectiveness of the head CT choice decision aid in parents of children with minor head trauma: study protocol for a multicenter randomized trial. *Trials.* 2014;15:253.

28. Kuppermann N, Holmes JF, Dayan PS, et al. Identification of children at very low

risk of clinically-important brain injuries after head trauma: a prospective cohort study. *Lancet.* 2009;374:1160–1170.

29. Lieberthal AS, Carroll AE, Chonmaitree T, et al. The diagnosis and management of acute otitis media. *Pediatrics.* 2013;131: e964–999.

30. Spiro DM, Tay KY, Arnold DH, et al. Wait-and-see prescription for the treatment of acute otitis media: a randomized controlled trial. *JAMA.* 2006;296:1235–1241.

31. McCaig LF, Burt CW. National hospital ambulatory medical care survey: 2002 emergency department summary. *Advance Data.* 2004 Mar 18;(340):1–34.

32. Foy AJ, Liu G, Davidson WR Jr., et al. Comparative effectiveness of diagnostic testing strategies in emergency department patients with chest pain: an analysis of downstream testing, interventions, and outcomes. *JAMA Internal Medicine.* 2015;175:428–436.

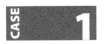

Expanding the Role of Observation Care

Christopher W. Baugh, Christopher G. Caspers, and Anthony M. Napoli

Introduction

The concept of observation in health care is not new. More than 2,300 years ago, Hippocrates said "leave nothing to chance, overlook nothing: combine contradictory observations and allow enough time – a great part, I believe, of the art of medicine is to be able to observe."[1] His wise words on the value of the "tincture of time" ring true today – patients often require extended time for additional diagnostics and treatments to arrive at a more accurate decision around the need for subsequent inpatient care or other interventions. When available and well operated, an observation unit provides a patient-centered setting and model of care to match patient needs with healthcare resources.

In 1972, the first mention of observation appeared in the modern medical literature with the description of a dedicated unit for the care of pediatric patients.[2] Since that time, hundreds of papers have been published illustrating the benefits of observation units, including reductions in inpatient hospitalization, lower costs, greater standardization of care, and improved patient satisfaction. The earliest and most compelling clinical case for observation care was the risk stratification of patients with chest pain or suspected anginal equivalents.[3,4,5] Since coronary disease is such a common and morbid condition in Western societies, accurate identification and exclusion of disease is imperative. Innovations in cardiac biomarker and stress testing technology have been able to improve our ability to assess these patients, yet chest pain remains the single most common condition among observation patients – representing nearly 20 percent of visits.[6]

In the United States (US), payer policy (more specifically, Medicare) has been a dominant force around defining observation care. Medicare describes observation as a "well-defined set of specific, clinically appropriate services, which include ongoing short term treatment, assessment, and reassessment before a decision can be made regarding whether patients will require further treatment as hospital inpatients or if they are able to be discharged from the hospital ... usually in less than 24 hours. In only rare and exceptional cases do reasonable and necessary outpatient observation services span more than 48 hours."[7] This was further clarified in 2013 when the "two midnight rule" was introduced, wherein Medicare expects patients requiring less than two midnights of hospital care (with very few exceptions) to be classified as observation patients.[8]

Aside from the above time frames, no payer has defined the exact setting or model of care required to deliver observation services in the hospital; observation care takes on a variety of appearances across time and hospital location. As a result of these complexities and frequent payer policy changes, the concept of observation has been a persistent source of confusion among patients and providers. In its most basic form, observation is simply an outpatient billing status. In the United States this is accomplished via an order to start the observation visit and the creation of an observation medical record. Patients can be physically located anywhere in the hospital, but as a generally accepted best practice, it is described as a dedicated observation unit in this chapter. Hospitals may use various names for an observation unit, such as a "clinical decision unit," "rapid diagnostic unit," or "short stay unit." A dedicated unit contains beds specifically allocated for observation patients, is usually a closed unit (i.e., run by one specialty), and employs specific protocols of care developed for common conditions encountered by observation patients (e.g., chest pain, dehydration, asthma).

Problem/Innovation

New York University Langone Medical Center (NYULMC) is an urban, tertiary care, academic medical center with an annual visit volume of about 65,000 located on the Lower East Side of Manhattan. It is a Comprehensive Stroke Care Center, ST-elevation myocardial infarction (STEMI) center, and National Cancer Institute Designated Cancer Center. The majority of patients presenting to the NYULMC emergency department (ED) are commercially insured. Like other hospitals across the US, in 2009 NYULMC was experiencing pressure to develop an alternative means to manage short-stay inpatient admissions. Recovery Audit Contractors (RACs), whose mission is to identify and recover improper Medicare payments through the detection and collection of overpayments on healthcare services, created pressures for hospitals to avoid short inpatient stays, a prime target for RAC audits. These pressures resulted in hospitals expanding their observation services as an alternate delivery model for short-stay hospital admission.[9]

In 2009, NYULMC implemented observation services using the same model as the majority of US hospitals at that time. This model consisted of no geographic cohorting of hospitalized patients placed in observation status. Patients placed on observation status were placed on traditional inpatient services scattered throughout various hospital wards. Patients were placed in observation status at the time of ED disposition if they were deemed to require short-term hospitalization. This review was performed during the ED evaluation when the decision to admit was made. The admitting hospital service then assumed the primary management role of the patient and the patient was transferred to a traditional inpatient medical/surgical hospital ward.

Observation services delivered in this model were characterized by several, now well-known, pitfalls that resulted in reduced hospital flow efficiency, poor patient outcomes related to prolonged hospitalization, and higher costs when compared with observation services delivered in a dedicated unit. In the former model, providers used traditional inpatient workflows to care for patients in observation status, such as once-daily rounding, infrequent reassessments, and variable care plans depending on the discretion of the inpatient team. Observation patients were physically intermixed among more acutely ill and medically complex inpatients, but the distinction of observation versus inpatient class was not readily apparent to providers. Thus, it was difficult to prioritize the less acute, less complex observation patients by the medical teams who were simultaneously managing both inpatients and observation patients in this distributed-bed model.

Then on October 29, 2012, Hurricane Sandy hit and a public health disaster in New York City ensued. The storm completely destroyed the NYULMC ED, forcing it to close and discontinue all clinical operations. In response, the ED at NYULMC implemented an urgent care center (UCC) with an associated ED-run observation unit (EDOU) in a new location within the medical center. Prior to this, the ED was frequently operating at maximum capacity and lacked the space for beds and clinical staff to care for patients requiring subsequent observation services, despite an interest in delivering these services from the ED as a known best practice model.

Planning for the EDOU required the ED to assume the responsibility of delivering a new model of healthcare. The Department of Emergency Medicine lacked expertise in observation medicine, and operational planning required a widespread educational effort. Local champions sought the counsel of nationally recognized content matter experts in observation medicine, who advised the leadership team and shared experiences with the providers. Clinical protocols were adapted for use from the American College of Emergency Physicians (ACEP) Observation Medicine section website and other observation units. A core multidisciplinary leadership team was assembled that included emergency physicians, nurses, physician assistants (PAs), administrators, cardiologists, neurologists, and other ancillary services. Relationships were established with ancillary and consulting services in order to optimize patient throughput and share the vision of observation medicine as a new model of healthcare delivery. An expanded emphasis in coordinating the care plan between the ED provider and primary care providers, care managers, and social workers was implemented in order to create effective discharge planning from the EDOU.

The investment in leadership and the degree of change management required to effect such a transformative change deserves particular attention. On both an institutional and departmental level at NYULMC, the ED was traditionally a place where care was episodic and brief relative to other points of care during a traditional hospitalization. As such, ED clinical staff were accustomed to caring for patients for several hours prior to dispositioning the patient home or transitioning the patient to an inpatient team for subsequent care. With the introduction of the EDOU, ED providers were suddenly confronted with being responsible for patient care and for managing acute disease processes for up to 24–48 hours, which many considered beyond their scope of training. Additionally, there was a lack of understanding and familiarity with observation medicine as a unique form of healthcare delivery, and many viewed it simply as a substitution of class status for reimbursement for equivalent "inpatient" care. This required distinguishing the difference between observation medicine as a type of healthcare delivery versus observation status, which is simply a billing class. Some providers were even apprehensive as to the motivation for exploring this care model given negative press highlighting observation status as a cost-shifting risk and a threat to the patient from a financial perspective when delivered inappropriately. This concern was partially valid, but emphasizing that such risks could be mitigated through the use of a cost-effective, best practice model of delivering observation services in a dedicated, protocol-driven space was paramount. At the same time, leadership assumed the responsibility of monitoring out-of-pocket costs during the early implementation phases to anticipate the possibility of significant out-of-pocket expenses, which did not occur. Concerns external to the ED existed as well. These included the perceived threat that private practice (non-hospital-employed) physicians had to the ED caring for patients who were traditionally admitted to the hospital and cared for by them. This required policy change and institutional support of the ED, as well as commitment by the ED providers to collaborate with private physicians when patients were placed in the EDOU to coordinate management plans and care transitions. Ultimately, a major culture change began during the planning phase that would carry throughout the implementation as we began providing a new type of longitudinal care for the first time. It was stressed that the EDOU was a strategic initiative for the medical center, and the ED was fortunate to be at the center of it.

On January 14, 2013, 77 days after Hurricane Sandy, the department operationalized 9 observation beds as part of the 35-bed UCC on a repurposed wing of the main hospital building following the destruction of the ED. The UCC was established in two geographically distinct locations, due to destruction of the physical plant of the ED by flooding from the storm. The UCC operated for the ensuing 14 months in the absence of the ED. The arrival area of the UCC was located on the ground level of the hospital near the main entrance. This area was staffed by emergency medicine nurses, physicians, and PAs. Patients who arrived at the ground level were triaged and a medical screening examination was performed. Low acuity patients remained in this location for the duration of their evaluation. Higher acuity patients were screened for stability and then transported to the second area of the UCC on a repurposed wing of the 16th floor of the hospital building. This second area was a 35-bed unit on a traditional inpatient ward, refitted for an UCC. Patients completed their UCC work-up and were dispositioned to inpatient, observation, or discharge status. All patients placed in the EDOU originated from the UCC. Patients dispositioned to the EDOS were placed in a physically separate 9-bed area for further evaluation and management at the discretion of the ED attending based on predefined inclusion and exclusion criteria.

Patients were placed into the EDOU following UCC management if they met criteria for placement into ED observation per guidelines (Table CS1.1). Once in the observation unit, patients were managed by emergency physicians and PAs. The unit was staffed with medical/surgical nurses at a ratio of three to four patients per nurse. All patients received care according to clinical protocols that outlined components of management such as antibiotics, pain medication, diagnostic studies, and consultations. Some protocols required collaboration with other services. For example, the chest pain protocol required partnering with cardiology to develop a stress test algorithm and expedite interventions based on these results, while the transient ischemic attack protocol required partnering with neurology to determine stroke risk factor modification and neuroimaging strategies.

The EDOU consistently demonstrated more favorable outcomes and served as a more cost-effective care model for observation services than observation services delivered by other departments at NYULMC. As a result, on May 5, 2014, the EDOU expanded from a 9-bed to 15-bed unit. The expansion was marked by a reduction in exclusion criteria in an

Table CS1.1 Inclusion and Exclusion Criteria for Emergency Department Observation Unit (as of January 2013)

Inclusion Criteria

Patients requiring the active management of their condition following the initial UCC visit to determine the need for inpatient admission or discharge

Exclusion Criteria

No clear working diagnosis

No clear management plan

Acute exacerbation of psychiatric condition

Acutely altered mental status

Hemodynamic instability

Sepsis

Requirement for nursing evaluation more frequently than every 4 hours

Agitated, combative, or acutely intoxicated patient (may be placed in observation unit after clinical sobriety achieved in UCC)

effort to add the psychosocially complex patient population to ED observation. Typically, such patients are excluded from ED observation services on a national level. Initially, there was an increase in length of stay and inpatient conversion rate due to the lack of adequate resources in the EDOU to arrange timely, complex care transitions out of the hospital. For example, inclusion of nonambulatory patients (e.g., nonoperative pelvic fracture) and patients with cognitive impairment (e.g., chronic dementia) required robust care coordination by social work and care management in order to ensure safe care transitions out of the hospital. To gain support for these resources, leadership from these disciplines was engaged and asked to pilot workflows that sent individuals to the unit during morning rounds. Eventually, a team consisting of social work, care management, physical therapy, home care agency liaisons, providers, and nurses learned to prioritize and effectively discharge these patients.

The EDOU continued to operate at full capacity for the months following the expansion to 15 beds while maintaining a length of stay that was less than 24 hours and an inpatient conversion rate of less than 20 percent. The number of clinical protocols was expanded to account for new conditions being placed in the EDOU, and postprocedural observation workflows were developed with modalities such as interventional cardiology, electrophysiology, and endoscopy.

At that point, the institution again considered expanding the size of the EDOU. A revenue analysis was performed that demonstrated a revenue risk when observation services were delivered outside the EDOU. This was attributed to the standardized workflows and protocolized care in the EDOU, which ensured optimal efficiency and reimbursement for the work performed and minimized the need for dropped charges. Patients receiving observation services outside the EDOU often lacked justification for ongoing observation services, resulting in a greater amount of dropped charges and higher costs relative to the EDOU. For these reasons, the decision was made to consolidate hospital observation services at NYULMC into the EDOU and expand the cohort from 15 to 35 beds. In the fall of 2014, the ED leadership was asked to initiate planning to expand the EDOU in order to manage the increased volume of observation visits to more than 30 beds. This necessitated the creation of many new protocols, workflows, and a reevaluation of all current processes to ensure compatibility on a larger scale. The EDOU nurse manager, administrative director, and PA leadership led several interdisciplinary work groups of front-line staff to focus on protocol development, new workflows such as more efficient rounding, a new patient placement process into the EDOU, and a multidisciplinary care coordination huddle to prioritize resolving discharge barriers. Regular meetings were initiated and included leaders from other departments, such as cardiology, neurology, radiology, and ancillary services. Other groups focused on unit structure and geographic provider/nurse team assignments, logistics, and revamping documentation to make interaction with the electronic health record more efficient. With this expansion, the vast majority of observation services would now be delivered from the EDOU.

The expansion of EDOU to 35 beds was completed on August 3, 2015. A distinct observation medicine division was formed in the ED with dedicated observation medicine attending physicians and leadership. These dedicated providers would work a progressively greater proportion of EDOU shifts than the larger core emergency medicine providers, who worked in the EDOU much less frequently and were inherently less familiar with the workflows of the EDOU. The dedicated attending physicians and PAs quickly became familiar with the day-to-day workflows and managing the conditions in the EDOU and more readily adhered to workflows and clinical protocols. This familiarity resulted in optimal performance throughout the expansion as well as flexibility as new workflows and protocols were piloted. Additionally, as the care became more complex, the dedicated attending physicians developed a strong foundation in observation medicine, and the changes were less disruptive to their workflows.

At the time of the expansion, more than 30 clinical protocols were in use to care for the approximately 750 patients per month who were placed in the unit. The observation-to-inpatient conversion rate for patients in ED observation versus non-ED observation was 17 percent versus 42 percent, respectively, with the 30-day admit to inpatient following EDOU discharge remaining less than 4 percent. Patient satisfaction scores remained in the 99th percentile.[10]

Discussion

The creation of a dedicated observation unit has tremendous potential to favorably impact all healthcare stakeholders – patients, providers, hospitals, and payers. Two key stakeholders required to start an observation unit are senior hospital leadership and providers from both the ED and inpatient services. Leaders in the realm of observation medicine have demonstrated great efficiencies in grouping observation patients such that observation medicine workflows are now being embraced by providers and administrators alike. Observation care is traditionally not directly viewed as a profit center and hospital beds are a scarce and valuable resource, so it can occasionally be difficult to gain administrator buy-in given competing programs (e.g., establishing a bariatric surgery service, adding an endoscopy suite). However, expanded ED observation units and their associated efficiencies improve inpatient hospital bed capacity and thereby free up beds for such initiatives via creation of a backfill opportunity. In a fixed payment model, the increased efficiency associated with these units also reduces costs and improves profitability (or reduces the loss) involved in such cases. Additionally, concerns about "claw backs," that is, insurance company demands for financial refunds for overcharging for "inappropriate" inpatient admissions or hospital readmissions in observation-status patients, have led US hospital administrators to invest in physician advisors and case managers to more accurately designate hospitalized patients as observation status according to US payer policy.[11] The dedicated unit provides the most appropriate setting to care for the increasing population of hospitalized patients newly designated as being of "observation" status.

The rise of observation care over the past several decades has nurtured a best practice for delivering care to the observation patient that promises to be a true innovation: the dedicated ED observation unit that uses condition-specific protocols of care. Typically located within or immediately adjacent to an ED, these units can have as few as 5 and as many as 30 or more beds staffed for the explicit purpose of observation care. In most cases, ED staff continue to care for patients in these units, working with relevant specialty services to develop and maintain protocols to ensure evidence-based diagnostics and treatment for common conditions such as chest pain, syncope, dehydration, asthma, cellulitis, transient ischemic attack, abdominal pain, and many others. More mature and complex units maintain over 20 different protocols. The typical rate of subsequent inpatient admission is about 20 percent and the average length of stay is about 15 hours, with an average 30 percent reduction in overall length of stay as compared with equivalent patients managed by inpatient providers.[9,12] Attending physicians direct a team of advanced practice providers (APPs) and nurses via structured rounds and ongoing collaborative decision-making. When the dedicated unit is run by the ED, registered nurses from the ED typically staff the unit. Typical nurse-to-patient ratios range between 1:4 and 1:6, which are more efficient than inpatient ratios.

Every study comparing observation care provided in a dedicated, protocolized observation unit has shown a clinical and/or financial benefit when compared with hospitalization and care by inpatient providers. Observation care in a distributed model (patients hospitalized in observation status anywhere throughout the hospital, and not cohorted) without any protocol is simply labeled as such but is functionally no different from inpatient care.[13] The inpatient model was not created for short-stay patients, and is thus understandably ill-suited to provide this care with optimal efficiency. Herein lies the opportunity – a dedicated observation unit in a hospital with sufficient annual ED visit volume to sustain a dedicated unit (typically 5–10 percent of visits in an ED with at least 30,000 visits) can be transformative.[14] The dedicated observation unit provides a home for patients previously falling into one of three categories: (1) patients previously admitted to an inpatient service, managed inefficiently, typically with a hospital length of stay well over 30 hours, (2) patients discharged home from the ED too soon, and (3) patients with extended ED stays. Therefore, the dedicated observation unit could (1) create new capacity in the inpatient wards and the ED, (2) improve patient safety and satisfaction, and (3) reduce hospital costs through efficient resource utilization. All of these outcomes are of critical importance to healthcare leaders today and in the future, and all of these outcomes have been demonstrated in previous studies.

In addition to finding space for an observation unit, administrators must also finance the staff working in the new unit. At NYULMC, the expansion of the observation medicine program required an increase in dedicated staffing in order to preserve performance when the ED assumed responsibility of delivering observation services. In addition to obvious staffing costs such as nurses, medical assistants, and unit clerks, other staffing costs typically include case managers and even APPs. APPs provide front-line care for observation patients and allow the attending physician to remain involved at key times in the patient stay (i.e., morning or afternoon rounds) without necessitating a continuous physician presence on the unit. Of note, many of these costs are already borne by the institution if the observation patients would have been hospitalized elsewhere. However, grouping these patients in a protocol-driven unit often results in simply shifting staffing resources from inpatient to outpatient, but the reduced length of stay results in efficiency gains. At NYULMC, not only were the efficiency gains realized when the ED assumed responsibility for delivering observation services, but the inpatient resources that were formerly delivering observation services were redistributed to inpatient care, which was a better match for their associated costs and productivity on the inpatient wards.

Political support from senior administrators and providers is another critical component of a successful observation unit, especially in the formative period. Change creates fear among providers who believe an observation unit will negatively impact them. Specialists may fear that the observation unit will take away patients from their service or place a strain on their consultants. Nurses and doctors with an emergency medicine background staffing the new unit fear that they will be taking care of patients with unfamiliar problems that are out of scope of their prior training and clinical experience. A cohesive leadership team of stakeholders who believe in the benefits of an observation unit need to assuage these fears and support their staff to help them understand the positive impact all their work will create. Creating multidisciplinary protocols, engaging specialists and support staff (i.e., case management, physical therapy, pharmacy, interpreter services, housekeeping, security, transport, etc.), and both defining and sharing key metrics are all necessary activities to support front-line staff. Typically, this work takes a minimum of 6–9 months prior to opening a new unit and must continue indefinitely afterward as new protocols are added and continued quality assurance and review is a necessity.

As the baby boom generation reaches retirement age, expected demographic shifts will increase the age of patients seeking care. Older patients with more complex presentations will increase the demand for bed hours in the ED; this demand is forecasted to be much higher in the inpatient setting.[15] Even if visit volumes remain relatively flat, we should anticipate hospital capacity challenges. Since adding inpatient beds is extraordinarily costly and often takes years to complete, the dedicated ED observation unit offers an alternative strategy to accommodate the future demands for inpatient bed hours. Reducing the length of stay for hospitalized patients is perhaps the most efficient solution to capacity constraints; in addition, bundled payments in the US and elsewhere create an incentive for early discharge or transfer. However, providers have been working on improving inpatient efficiency for years and the increased age and complexity of inpatients in the future leave little room to expect remarkable gains. In addition, these same inpatient providers are often in charge of providing care to lower acuity observation patients. Grouping observation patients in accelerated diagnostic and treatment units, such as the ED observation unit, offers the ability to efficiently manage these patients while not sacrificing the attention necessary for the more complicated inpatients. As a result, avoidance of inpatient admission altogether is a valuable strategy, as long as the observation unit does not come at the expense of congesting the capacity to provide acute care in the ED. In addition to other outpatient pathways that enable care in the home setting (e.g., visiting nurses, intravenous therapies at home), the observation unit is another increasingly attractive resource to ensure that patients who may not need inpatient care are kept away from that setting.

Hospital leaders typically repurpose underutilized space already available within the hospital to create the space needed for an observation unit. However, it is important to consider common pitfalls that can make a dedicated unit less effective. First, since observation units typically have a low census in the mid-afternoon (after morning discharges and prior to evening arrivals), some hospitals fill their empty observation unit beds with inpatients boarding in the ED. Many hospitals have significant boarding times, and thus this strategy will have a significant downstream impact. In the evening, as the demand for observation beds starts to increase, those beds will now be occupied, resulting in inpatient admission of patients otherwise eligible for observation unit care. This practice effectively sabotages the functional capacity of the observation unit and will negatively impact metrics of operational efficiency; as a result, it is a practice best to avoid. In addition, patients with an acute psychiatric illness are often seen as an attractive target for observation units. However, they frequently have prolonged lengths of stay, and the requirements of their care require additional resources (e.g., security, social workers) not traditionally present in a typical ED observation unit.

Last, the provision of efficient, protocol-driven observation care is optimally driven by a single overseeing physician. Closed units, led by emergency physicians in consultation with other services, have been shown to yield the greatest efficiency. An open unit, wherein multiple attending physicians from throughout the hospital can directly manage patients in the observation unit, creates unwarranted variations in care, competing priorities, and their attendant inefficiencies. The experience at NYULMC supports this concept, wherein the initial delivery model of observation services was provided in an open "unit" or scatter bed model, until it was transitioned to a closed model within the ED and a best-practice model was adopted. Additionally, providers working in the observation unit need to be supported with patient exclusion criteria and clear plans of care to ensure they are working within their scope of practice. These exclusion criteria also allow leadership to match the scope of the observation services with the available resources. For example, at NYULMC, exclusion criteria were initially required to avoid placing patients with significant psychosocial barriers to discharge into the EDOU, until a more robust care management and social work presence became available in the EDOU to assist with patient care. As the EDOU grew, the exclusion criteria were systematically reduced and the scope of services expanded. This change was achieved by continuous development and revision of condition-specific protocols and education, working with consulting services and addressing care concerns. Finally, patient out-of-pocket costs have been a frequent concern of patients and their advocates in relation to observation care. A 2013 report from the Office of the Inspector General found that the average patient expense among Medicare beneficiaries for an observation visit was $528, versus $725 for short inpatient admissions.[16] The observation cost even included the cost of home medications – a frequent source of concern impacting patient expense. Overall, 94 percent of observation patients had a lower expense than the inpatient deductible amount, and only 0.6 percent of visits included an observation stay during at least 3 days in the hospital followed by skilled nursing facility care without a Medicare benefit.[16] This analysis reveals that while there are cases where patients can be exposed to high out-of-pocket costs associated with observation care, they are quite rare and should not influence the decision to use an observation visit for its intended purpose: to efficiently manage a short hospital stay, avoid an inpatient admission, and facilitate a safe discharge home. Such a risk of high out-of-pocket costs is further minimized when observation services are delivered in a protocol-driven, dedicated observation unit, where length of stay and variability in care is minimized. One testament to this is the high patient satisfaction scores in the EDOU at NYULMC. One would argue that if patients were being exposed to high out-of-pocket costs, they would be less satisfied with their care. The patient satisfaction scores for the EDOU at NYULMC are consistently in the 99th percentile, and grievances for patient bills are essentially nonexistent across more than 15,000 patient visits.[9]

As we look ahead to the future of observation care, one would expect government and payment reforms to continue to push the setting of care toward less resource-intensive settings for many diagnoses (or low-risk subsets of a particular diagnosis): from inpatient to observation, and from observation to home. For example, emergency physicians now routinely manage as outpatients certain conditions (e.g., asthma, migraines, pyelonephritis) previously admitted for inpatient care. In addition, for the first time, in 2016, Medicare introduced bundled payments for facility observation charges in their 2016 outpatient prospective payment system final rule. This significant shift from fee-for-service to bundled payments incentivizes hospitals to perform only essential diagnostics and treatments for observation patients, pushing more care to outpatient clinic follow-up.[17]

One good example of this push toward outpatient management and accelerated observation care is the most common observation unit diagnosis: chest pain. As new, highly sensitive troponin assays become more widely available, we will see increased use of accelerated diagnostic protocols relying on a delta troponin (calculated change in troponin value trended over time) in as little as 1–2 hours with very high sensitivity.[18] Furthermore, recent risk stratification tools, such as the HEART (history, ECG, age, risk factors, troponin level) score a risk stratification algorithm, in combination with short-interval serial bio-markers, are also allowing clinicians to identify low-risk patients who may be eligible for discharge from the ED.[19,20] As new evidence and specialty society guidelines around these accelerated diagnostic protocols in low-risk patients evolves, one could easily imagine the lowest risk patients no longer needing an observation stay to exclude acute myocardial ischemia as the cause of their symptoms.[21] Will higher risk chest pain patients take their place? Perhaps novel observation protocols, like those helping clinicians identify patients at low risk for pulmonary embolism for observation care, will be added. Novel conditions related to growing patient populations of geriatrics and oncology are also likely areas of future growth for observation services. Both of these populations (which also overlap considerably) are particularly vulnerable to the risks of inpatient hospitalization but are also high utilizers of healthcare. This makes them an ideal cohort for care in the observation unit – promising safe but expedited care.

As our current healthcare system evolves, stakeholders will increasingly demand improved outcomes at a lower cost. The dedicated observation unit meets this challenge by shifting the site of care to a less resource-intensive setting while also using evidence-based protocols to ensure proper patient selection and evidence-based management. Financial and operational pressures on the healthcare system will persist, creating more demand for observation services to become integrated into EDs as a standard setting and model of care in the future.

References

1. Lyons AS. Hippocrates. Available at www.healthguidance.org/entry/6338/1/Hippocrates.html; 2013. Accessed February 25, 2013.

2. Gururaj VJ, Allen JE, Russo RM. Short stay in an outpatient department: an alternative to hospitalization. *American Journal of Diseases of Children.* 1972;123(2):128–132.

3. Graff LG, Dallara J, Ross MA, et al. Impact on the care of the emergency department chest pain patient from the chest pain evaluation registry (CHEPER) study. *American Journal of Cardiology.* 1997;80 (5):563–568.

4. Gaspoz JM, Lee TH, Weinstein MC, et al. Cost-effectiveness of a new short-stay unit to "rule out" acute myocardial infarction in low risk. *Journal of American College of Cardiology.* 1994;24(5): 1249–1259.

5. Farkouh ME, Smars PA, Reeder GS, et al. A clinical trial of a chest-pain observation unit for patients with unstable angina. Chest Pain Evaluation in the Emergency Room (CHEER) Investigators. *New England Journal of Medicine.* 1998;339 (26):1882–1888.

6. Venkatesh AK, Geisler BP, Gibson Chambers JJ, et al. Use of observation care in US emergency departments, 2001 to 2008. *PLoS ONE.* 2011;6(9):e24326.

7. Medicare Payment Advisory Committee. A data book: healthcare spending and the Medicare program. 2011:112.

8. Center for Medicare and Medicaid Services. Frequently asked questions: 2 midnight inpatient admission guidance and patient status reviews for admissions. 2013; 2014. Available at www.cms.gov/Research-Statistics-Data-and-Systems/Monitoring-Programs/Medical-Review/Downloads/QAsforWebsitePosting_110413-v2-CLEAN.pdf. Accessed September 9, 2015.

9. Baugh CW, Venkatesh AK, Bohan JS. Emergency department observation units: a clinical and financial benefit for hospitals. *Health Care Management Review.* 2011;36 (1):28–37.

10. Chandra A, Sieck S, Hocker M, et al. An observation unit may help improve an

institution's Press Ganey satisfaction score. *Clinical Geriatric Medicine.* 2011;10 (2):104–106.

11. American Hospital Association. Exploring the impact of the RAC program on hospitals nationwide. Available at www.aha.org/content/13/ 12Q4ractracresults.pdf. Accessed December 29, 2015.

12. Mace SE, Graff L, Mikhail M, et al. A national survey of observation units in the United States. *American Journal of Emergency Medicine.* 2003;21(7):529–533.

13. Ross MA, Hockenberry JM, Mutter R, et al. Protocol-driven emergency department observation units offer savings, shorter stays, and reduced admissions. *Health Affairs.* 2013;32(12):2149–2156.

14. Graff LG. Observation medicine: the healthcare system's tincture of time. Available at www.acep.org/Physician-Resources/Practice-Resources/ Administration/Observation-Medicine/. Accessed December 29, 2015.

15. Pallin DJ, Allen MB, Espinola JA, et al. Population aging and emergency departments: visits will not increase, lengths-of-stay and hospitalizations will. *Health Affairs.* 2013;32(7):1306–1312.

16. Office of the Inspector General. Hospitals' use of observation stays and short inpatient stays for Medicare beneficiaries, 2013. OEI-02-12-00040.

17. Centers for Medicare and Medicaid Services (CMS). 2016 Medicare OPPS final rule. Available at www.cms.gov/Medicare/ Medicare-Fee-for-Service-Payment/ HospitalOutpatientPPS/Hospital-Outpatient-Regulations-and-Notices-Items/CMS-1633-FC.html?DLPage=1& DLEntries=10&DLSort=2&DLSortDir= descending. Accessed December 29, 2015.

18. Reichlin T, Schindler C, Drexler B, et al. One-hour rule-out and rule-in of acute myocardial infarction using high-sensitivity cardiac troponin T. *Archives of Internal Medicine.* 2012;172(16):1211–1218.

19. Backus BE, Six AJ, Kelder JC, et al. Chest pain in the emergency room: a multicenter validation of the HEART Score. *Critical Pathways in Cardiology.* 2010;9(3):164–169.

20. Mahler S, Riley R, Hiestand B, et al. The HEART pathway randomized trial: identifying emergency department patients with acute chest pain for early discharge. *Circulation: Cardiovascular Quality and Outcomes.* 2015;8(2):195–203.

21. Prasad V, Cheung M, Cifu A. Chest pain in the emergency department: the case against our current practice of routine noninvasive testing. *Archives of Internal Medicine.* 2012;172(19):1506–1509.

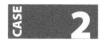

CASE 2

An Innovative Strategy to Streamline Care for Behavioral Health in the Emergency Department

Michael Turturro, Leslie Zun, and Jack Rozel

Introduction

Behavioral health patients frequently use the emergency department (ED) when they are in crisis. Up to 10 percent of all ED patients have one or more behavioral health complaints.[1] The fragmentation of the care for these patients is significant, where frequently patients receive care from multiple facilities and providers.

When it comes to ED care, many EDs do only a medical clearance and do not have the resources to conduct a formal psychiatric evaluation to determine the need for admission. Many departments rely more on in-house psychiatry consultants or in some cases an outside service, such as telepsychiatry, to provide an assessment for admission. Some hospitals have inpatient psychiatric units and outpatient services; however, many do not. For those requiring inpatient admission, locating an appropriate inpatient service is often difficult because of the limited number of dedicated psychiatric beds within the community. For those being discharged, many EDs may not have up-to-date information for available community-based behavioral health services. Care fragmentation has been made worse because of the long history of a contraction of inpatient and outpatient psychiatric resources in the United States. Between 1970 and 1998 inpatient psychiatric beds in the United States dropped by about 50 percent. The number of people coming for care in ambulatory mental health settings increased more than 300 percent, from 1,202,098 in 1969 to 3,967,019 in 1998. A testament to the lack of resources was a study of ED directors in California: in 2006, 23 percent of EDs reportedly routinely sent patients with behavioral health complaints home without being seen by a mental health professional.[2]

Outside the ED, the care system for mental illness is similarly underresourced, fragmented, and overcrowded. Faced with declining resources out of the hospital to manage mental health conditions as well as difficulty in navigating complex healthcare systems, patients in need of mental health treatment frequently resort to or are referred to EDs due to lack of alternative sites to receive care. The end results are long waits for care and boarding of these patients – sometimes on the order of days – in EDs while appropriate sites for care are identified. According to a 2015 survey conducted by the American College of Emergency Physicians, 80 percent of emergency physicians felt that systems currently in place in their communities and surrounding regions are not providing optimal care for patients with mental health needs; in a 2008 survey 79 percent of emergency physicians reported boarding of psychiatric patients in their EDs,[1] a situation that has worsened over time.[3]

Innovation

Below we describe a hospital and community that engaged in an intervention that successfully linked patients with mental health needs to community resources and help standardize care with the ED.

Background

The 2008 closure of a local state-run long-term mental health facility (Mayview State Hospital in Allegheny County, Pennsylvania) and reductions of regional inpatient mental health beds had an immediate effect on mental health patients turning to the ED for care at the University of Pittsburgh Medical Center (UPMC) – Mercy. Over the 4-year period following these closures, patients arriving at the ED requesting behavioral health and substance abuse treatment increased by 325 percent, while ED volume grew by only 22 percent. Admissions for mental health conditions increased by 95 percent, while inpatient capacity remained the same, resulting in an increase in patients boarding as well as longer boarding times in the ED, often exceeding 48 hours. Average wait times for behavioral health patients until first evaluation by a clinician tripled. The entire ED had been under duress as a result of this situation, with a behavioral health intake unit within the ED operating over capacity and behavioral health patients being boarded in the general ED space. This adversely affected the care for all ED patients and caused dissatisfaction among patients, families, and ED staff. Hospital costs for security and trained patient observers for behavioral health patients had increased. Patients admitted to inpatient units with concomitant chemical dependency were also not being managed optimally, resulting in patient deterioration (e.g., poorly controlled ethanol withdrawal) and potentially avoidable critical care transfers.

Interventions

Based on recurrent observations of behavioral health patients boarding in the ED and increased expenditures to protect the safety of these patients in the ED (e.g., need for patient observers to ensure that patients do not harm themselves or elope), and adverse impacts on patients, hospital leadership agreed that is was necessary to intervene. A multidisciplinary team was assembled to pinpoint the underlying factors involved in the high volumes of patients with behavioral health complaints, identify opportunities to more efficiently manage patients, and optimize existing resources for these patients outside the hospital. Major areas of focus were the following:

1. Partnering with a community-based crisis center to provide urgent patient evaluation by crisis clinicians in the ED. The major focus of these evaluations was to determine behavioral health and social service needs as well as to seek safe alternatives to hospitalization, with a goal of managing patients in the community whenever feasible. To fund this initiative, ED social work positions were converted to crisis clinician positions, allowing three staff from the crisis center to provide 12–16 hours per day of coverage. These staff supported the ED by expediting discharges of patients presenting with behavioral health needs best suited to community intervention, including linkage to outpatient, crisis, respite, and related services.

2. Regionalization of inpatient bed capacity including facilitated communication between sites with inpatient units to identify available beds in real time. More recently, the health system has begun to develop a single point of contact for behavioral health bed management, including processing and expediting referrals from community and hospital providers. Capacity includes capturing clinical and medical necessity information, processing prior authorization, reviewing medical stability, and handling legal status as well as transportation to appropriate psychiatric units.

3. Direct referrals from the ED to existing outpatient programs such as partial hospitalization programs, respite programs, and post-ED follow up appointments.
4. Reducing inpatient length of stay by utilization review training of ED and inpatient staff with postdischarge planning commencing immediately following inpatient admission. This is reevaluated daily between hospital behavioral health, case management, and social services leadership and local outpatient resources.
5. Training of dedicated staff to perform structured substance abuse assessments with recommended disposition (Table CS2.1) while optimizing referrals to ambulatory detoxification programs. The focus of this intervention was to select the patients who would most benefit from detoxification in the hospital and refer patients who could safely detoxify from substances in an outpatient setting. In addition, inpatient nursing staff was trained in detoxification assessments and protocolized treatment (Box 2.1 and Box 2.2) to reduce the risk of patient deterioration.
6. Training of hospitalist and house staff on recognition and management of withdrawal syndromes, including the use of symptom-based protocols (Box 2.1 and Box 2.2)

Table CS2.1 Pennsylvania Client Placement Criteria Admission Overview

Dimensions	Level 1A: Outpatient	Level 1B: Intensive Outpatient	Level 2A: Partial Hospitalization	Level 2B: Halfway House	Level 3A: Medically Monitored Inpatient Detox
Acute Intoxication or withdrawal	Minimal to no risk of withdrawal	Minimal to no risk of withdrawal	Minimal risk of severe withdrawal	Minimal to no risk of withdrawal	High risk of severe withdrawal, daily use of substance with physical dependence but without psychiatric or medical disorder
Biomedical conditions and complications	Stable enough to permit participation	Not severe enough to warrant inpatient admittance but may distract from recovery efforts.	Not severe enough to warrant 24-hour observation; relapse could severely exacerbate conditions	Conditions do not interfere with treatment and do not require monitoring outside this level; OR relapse would severely aggravate existing condition	Medical condition severely endangered by continued use; requires close medical monitoring but not intensive care

Table CS2.1 *(cont.)*

Dimensions	Level 1A: Outpatient	Level 1B: Intensive Outpatient	Level 2A: Partial Hospitalization	Level 2B: Halfway House	Level 3A: Medically Monitored Inpatient Detox
Emotional/ behavioral conditions and complications	Nonserious, transient emotional disturbances; mental status allows full participation	Able to maintain behavioral stability between contacts; symptoms do not obstruct participation	Inability to maintain behavioral stability over 72-hour period; OR mild risk of dangerous behavior; OR history of dangerous behavior	Conditions do not interfere with treatment and disorders may be treated concurrently; at least one serious emotional/ behavioral problem is present	Psychiatric symptoms interfere with recovery; moderate risk of dangerous behaviors; impairment requires 24-hour setting; self-destructive behavior related to intoxication
Treatment acceptance/ resistance	Willing and cooperative; requires only monitoring and motivation rather than structure	Willing and cooperative; requires only monitoring and motivation rather than structure	Structured milieu required due to denial or resistance but not so severe as to require residential setting	Cooperative and accepts need for 24-hour structured setting	N/A
Relapse potential	Able to maintain abstinence with support and counseling	Needs support and counseling; difficulty postponing immediate gratification	Likely to continue use without monitoring and intensive support; OR difficulty maintaining abstinence despite engagement in treatment	Unaware of relapse triggers; impulsivity; would likely relapse without structured setting	N/A
Recovery environment	Supportive living environment or environment in which stressors can	Not optimal but has supportive living environment or motivation to establish one;	Exposure to usual daily activities makes recovery unlikely; OR inadequate support for	Lack of supportive persons in living environment; significant stressors; OR logistic barriers	Living environment makes abstinence unlikely

Table CS2.1 (cont.)

Dimensions	Level 1A: Outpatient	Level 1B: Intensive Outpatient	Level 2A: Partial Hospitalization	Level 2B: Halfway House	Level 3A: Medically Monitored Inpatient Detox
	be managed so that abstinence can be maintained	available supports willing to help facilitate recovery	recovery from significant others; OR estrangement from potential support in living environment	to treatment at less intensive level of care	

Dimensions	Level 3B: Medically Monitored Short-Term Residential	Level 3C: Medically Monitored Long-Term Residential	Level 4A: Medically Managed Inpatient Detoxification	Level 4B: Medically Managed Inpatient Residential
Acute intoxication or withdrawal	Minimal to no risk of severe withdrawal	Minimal to no risk of withdrawal with ongoing postacute withdrawal symptoms	Risk of severe withdrawal, with cooccurring psychiatric or medical disorder requiring medical management; OR overdose requiring medical management; OR only available setting that meets client's management needs	Minimal to no risk of withdrawal
Biomedical conditions and complications	Continued alcohol and other drug use places client in possible danger of serious damage to physical health	Continued alcohol and other drug use places client in danger of serious damage to physical health	Complications of addiction require daily medical management; OR medical problem requires diagnosis and treatment; OR recurrent seizures	Imminent danger of serious physical health problems requiring intensive medical management
Emotional/ behavioral conditions and complications	Psychiatric symptoms interfere with recovery; moderate risk of dangerous behaviors; impairment	Two of: disordered living skills, disordered social adaptation, disordered self-adaptiveness, disordered	Emotional/ behavioral complications of addiction require daily medical management; OR risk of dangerous behavior; OR	Two of: psychiatric complications of addiction, concurrent psychiatric illness, dangerous

Table CS2.1 (*cont.*)

Dimensions	Level 3B: Medically Monitored Short-Term Residential	Level 3C: Medically Monitored Long-Term Residential	Level 4A: Medically Managed Inpatient Detoxification	Level 4B: Medically Managed Inpatient Residential
	requires 24-hour setting; self-destructive behaviors related to intoxication	psychological status	substance use would have severe mental health consequences	behaviors, mental confusion or other impairment of thought process
Treatment acceptance/ resistance	24-hour intensive program needed to help client understand consequences and severity of addiction	24-hour intensive program needed to help client understand consequences and severity of addiction	N/A	N/A
Relapse potential	Inability to establish recovery despite previous treatment in less intensive settings; unable to control use in face of available substances in environment	Inability to establish recovery despite previous treatment in less intensive settings; unable to control use in face of available substances in environment	N/A	N/A
Recovery environment	Social elements unsupportive or highly stressful; coping skills inadequate to conditions	Social elements unsupportive or highly stressful; coping skills inadequate to conditions; OR antisocial lifestyle	N/A	N/A

Results

In the first year following these interventions, the following improvements were noted:

1. An estimated 28 percent of what would have been mental health admissions were avoided, and patients were safely directed to other levels of care.
2. Transfers of admitted patients to other sites with available space increased by 81 percent.
3. Referrals to outpatient programs increased by 160 percent.
4. Outpatient referrals for substance abuse treatment increased 10-fold.
5. Mean ED length of stay for patients admitted for mental health services decreased by 71 percent; for patients referred to outpatient mental health treatment, ED length of stay

Box 2.1 Clinical Opiate Withdrawal Scale (COWS)

Resting pulse rate (beats per minute) measured after patient is sitting or lying for 1 minute

0 Pulse rate 80 or below
1 Pulse rate 81–100
2 Pulse rate 101–120
4 Pulse rate >120

Sweating (over past 1/2 hour not accounted for by room temperature or patient activity)

0 No report of chills or flushing
1 Subjective report of chills or flushing
2 Flushed or observable moistness on face
3 Beads of sweat on brow or face
4 Sweat streaming off face

Restlessness (observation during assessment)

0 Able to sit still
1 Reports difficulty sitting still but is able to do so
3 Frequent shifting or extraneous movement of legs or arms
5 Unable to sit still for more than a few seconds

Pupil size

0 Pupils pinned or normal size for room light
2 Pupils moderately dilated
5 Pupils so dilated that only the rim of the iris is visible

Bone or joint aches (if patient was having pain previously, only the additional component attributed to opiate withdrawal is scored)

0 Not present
1 Mild diffuse discomfort
2 Patient reports severe diffuse aching of joints or muscles
4 Patient is rubbing joints or muscles and is unable to sit still because of discomfort

Runny nose or tearing (not accounted for by cold symptoms or allergies)

0 Not present
1 Nasal stuffiness or unusually moist eyes
2 Nose running or eyes tearing
4 Nose constantly running or tears streaming down cheeks

Gastrointestinal upset (over last 1/2 hour)

0 No gastrointestinal symptoms
1 Stomach cramps
2 Nausea or loose stool
3 Vomiting or diarrhea
5 Multiple episodes of diarrhea or vomiting

Tremor (observation of outstretched hands)

0 No tremor
1 Tremor can be felt but not observed
2 Slight tremor observable
4 Gross tremor or muscle twitching

Yawning (observation during assessment)

Box 2.1 (*cont.*)

0 No yawning
1 Yawning once or twice during assessment
2 Yawning three or more times during assessmnet
4 Yawning several times per minute

Anxiety or irritability

0 None
1 Patient reports increasing irritability or anxiousness
2 Patient obviously irritable or anxious
4 Patient so irritable or anxious that participation in the assessment is difficult

Gooseflesh skin

0 Skin is smooth
3 Piloerection of skin can be felt or hairs standing up on arms
5 Prominent piloerection

Score

5–12 Mild
13–24 Moderate
25–36 Moderately severe
More than 36 severe withdrawal

Box 2.2 Withdrawal Assessment Scale (WAS) for Ethanol and Benzodiazepine Dependence

Temperature (per axilla)

$0 = {<}37.0°C$
$1 = 37.0–37.5°C$
$2 = 37.6–38.0°C$
$3 = {>}38.0°C$

Pulse (beats per minute)

$0 = {<}90$
$1 = 90–95$
$2 = 96–100$
$3 = 101–105$
$4 = 106–110$
$5 = 111–120$
$6 = {>}120$

Respiratory rate (breaths per minute)

$0 = {<}20$
$1 = 20–24$
$2 = {>}24$

Blood pressure (diastolic mmHg)

$0 = {<}95$
$1 = 95–100$

Box 2.2 (cont.)

2 = 101–103
3 = 104–106
4 = 107–109
5 = 110–112
6 = >112

Nausea and vomiting

0 = None
2 = Nausea/no vomiting
4 = Intermittent nausea/dry heaves
6 = Nausea/dry heaves/vomiting

Tremor (arms extended, fingers spread)

0 = No tremor
2 = Not visible – can be felt fingertip to fingertip
3 = Moderate with arms extended
4 = Severe even with arms not extended

Sweating (observation)

0 = No sweat visible
2 = Barely perceptible, palms moist
4 = Beads of sweat visible
6 = Drenching sweats

Tactile disturbances

0 = None
2 = Mild itching or pins and needles or numbness
4 = Intermittent tactile hallucinations (e.g., bugs crawling)
6 = Continuous tactile hallucinations (feels things constantly)

Headaches ("Does it feel like a band around your head?")

0 = Not present
2 = Mild
4 = Moderately severe
6 = Severe

Auditory disturbances (loud noises, hearing voices)

0 = Not present
2 = Mild harshness or ability to frighten (increased sensitivity)
4 = Intermittent auditory hallucinations
6 = Continuous auditory hallucinations

Visual disturbances (photophobia, seeing things)

0 = Not present
2 = Mild sensitivity (bothered by light)
4 = Intermittent visual hallucinations
6 = Continuous visual hallucinations

Hallucinations

0 = None
1 = Minimal visual, auditory, or tactile

Box 2.2 (*cont.*)

2 = Nonfused auditory and visual
3 = Fused, auditory and visual

Clouding of sensorium
0 = Oriented

2 = Disoriented to date by no more than 2 days
3 = Disoriented to date
4 = Disoriented to place (reorient if necessary)

Quality of contact

0 = In contact with examiner
2 = Seems in contact but is oblivious to environment
4 = Periodically becomes detached
6 = Makes no contact with examiner

Anxiety ("Do you feel nervous?" – observation)

0 = No anxiety, at ease
2 = Appears anxious
4 = Moderately anxious
6 = Overt anxiety (equal to panic)

Agitation (observation)

0 = Normal activity
2 = Somewhat more than normal activity
4 = Moderately fidgety and restless
6 = Pacing or thrashing about constantly

Thought disturbances (flight of ideas)

0 = No disturbance
2 = Plagued by unpleasant thoughts constantly
4 = Does not have much control over nature of thoughts
6 = Thoughts come quickly and in a disconnected fashion

Convulsions (seizures of any kind)

0 = No
6 = Yes

Flushing of face

0 = None
2 = Mild
4 = Severe

Score

<10 No further action needed
10–14 Administer prn dose of benzodiazepine
>14 Administer prn dose of benzodiazepine and call house staff to reassess

If there are any concerns or changes in patient status, call house staff to reassess.

decreased by 50 percent; wait time for all patients requesting mental health treatment decreased by 78 percent.

6. Mean ED length of stay for patients admitted for substance abuse treatment decreased by 70 percent; for patients referred to outpatient substance abuse treatment, ED length of stay decreased by 50 percent; wait time for all patients requesting substance abuse treatment decreased by 78 percent.

In the 3 years since these interventions began, boarding of behavioral health patients has remained low, and ED lengths of stay for mental health patients have decreased by an additional 18 percent, despite a 7 percent increase of patients presenting to the ED for mental health evaluations. Crisis clinician evaluations have increased by 25 percent over this same time period. Hospital leadership, the medical director of the county crisis network, and the chair of the department of psychiatry have remained unflappable champions in continuously improving the quality and efficiency of care provided to patients with mental health or addiction needs who present to the ED.

Program Challenges

Funding for the county crisis network is under constant threat of state and county budget cuts. Since the crisis network is specific to Allegheny County, referral to residential services is not available for patients who present to the ED from neighboring counties. The opioid abuse crisis has not abated, and there has been an increase in patients requesting opioid detoxification. Most of these patients are able to successfully be referred to outpatient programs with medications to control withdrawal symptoms in the interim (Box 2.3) with naloxone distributed in the case of relapse.

Box 2.3 Opioid Detox Starter Pack

Clonidine 0.1 mg (2 tabs): take one q 12 hr prn
Hydroxyzine 25 mg PO (4 tabs): take one q 6 hr prn
Ondansetron 4 mg (4 tabs): take one q 6 hr prn
Lomotil (8 caps): take two q 6 hr prn
Trazodone 50 mg (#3)

Discussion

EDs have been burdened with ever-increasing numbers of behavioral health patients. A recent study from the Centers for Disease Control demonstrated that approximately 10 percent of ED patients present with a psychiatric complaint.[1] Many of these patients may need an inpatient bed or outpatient resources, both of which have been contracting in the last two decades. This contraction has led to the problem of boarding psychiatric patients in the ED.[5] The problem of psychiatric boarding has been compounded by not only the lack of ED capability to see additional patients but also the concern about the lack of dedicated ED resources, experienced personnel, and protocols for dealing with the specific needs of this patient population.

The lack of resources for psychiatric patients in many communities has led not only to boarding of psychiatric patients in EDs for hours all over the country, but also, in some cases, to potentially inappropriate disposition decisions. A study of medical directors of EDs in California described frequently sending patients home without psychiatric consultation because one was not available in a timely fashion in their community.[2] Adult and pediatric patients are frequently admitted to medical floors instead of psychiatric ones because of the lack of availability of psychiatric beds.[5] In one unfortunate case, a psychiatric patient waited 38 days in an ED for an inpatient bed.[6]

The solutions to this problem are not simple. It is not in the purview of this chapter to discuss the societal and governmental solutions for these patients. Rather, it is best to focus on what emergency medicine can do to resolve the demands placed on our specialty. EDs can work on several elements of care: before the patient arrives at the ED, while the patient is in the ED, and after the decision is made to admit.

Before the Patient Arrives at the ED

Dramatic results can happen when providers in an area get together to improve care of the psychiatric patient in their community, as illustrated in this case. The results are impressive and demonstrate that the community can come together to improve the care of behavioral health patients if resources are dedicated to improving processes. However, few comprehensive solutions like this exist on the community level, as described in this case. Barriers can be difficult to overcome to motivate healthcare and community mental health providers, those in substance use treatment facilities, law enforcement and emergency medical services personnel, and those in the legal system to provide multiple levels of care for psychiatric patients who commonly present to EDs. San Antonio is a city that serves as another example where multiple these parties came together to provide healthcare, mental health, emergency, homeless, and substance use treatment services.[7] San Antonio developed a three-pronged approach that includes care for substance use disorders, short-term psychiatric care, and resources for the homeless patients.

It should also be considered whether EDs are the best place for patients with primary behavioral health emergencies. In many cases, these patients may be better served by services focused on caring for patients in crisis. These include crisis call centers, crisis management teams, respite centers, living rooms, and other drop-in services. These provide focused services to meet the patients' needs at home or in the community. Although these services may be valuable for some patients with mental illness, it is not appropriate for those who have had significant decompensation in their psychiatric illness or medical complaints. Some communities have crisis call centers, teams that go to the patients, and community mental health resources that are better equipped to determine the need for an ED visit.

While in the ED

Another issue that tends to delay the patients in the ED is the emergency physicians who have the tendency to depend heavily on mental health workers or psychiatric services to determine the patient's need for admission. In many cases, it may not be unreasonable for the emergency physician to perform a mental health assessment of the patient to determine the need for admission. This process is not dissimilar to that for other patients. A clinical focused history together with the use of collateral information and an appropriate mental status evaluation provides the basis for admission determination. As payment models change, there may be further pressure on emergency physicians to keep patients out of the hospital.

In addition, there are other means to care for patients who have mental health illness after care in the ED. Some patients may go home after evaluation in the ED. However, many times in the ED, emergency physicians are asked to intercede when there is a dispute at the nursing home, jail, group home, or residency. Emergency physicians are often compelled to admit these patients to the hospital because the ED may lack the resources and time to adjudicate these decisions. Criteria for psychiatric admission from the ED are not well defined and need further development. Most emergency physicians use danger to self, danger to others, and inability to care for oneself as the criteria for admission. It is easy to determine to admit a patient who has a serious suicide attempt but not so easy if the patient only has suicidal ideation. The same thought process can be made for patients with homicidal ideation. It is not so easy to determine if patients can care for themselves, especially for patients who have schizophrenia or other behavioral health problems that impact activities of daily living. However, information to make the most appropriate decision is often limited by a lack of comprehensive knowledge about a patient's prior care, uneven ability to consult with the psychiatric caregivers, and often an inability to obtain psychiatric medical records. Many patients may benefit from being discharged home with care instructions or referral to community mental health resources, living rooms, or crisis centers. For others, crisis stabilization units may be the means to provide diagnostic certainty, needed observation, and short-term treatment.[8] Not unlike other types of observation, these patients may to stay in these units for 23 hours or less with intense medical and psychiatric care. Regionalization of crisis stabilization units has reduced wait time for psychiatric patients in the ED waiting for psychiatric dispositions. For example, Zeller and others found that the ED boarding time was reduced to 1 hour 48 minutes and that only 24.8 percent needed admission after this service was implemented.[9]

There are some tools available to determine a patient's need for admission. However, although the Suicide Prevention Resource Center has developed a tool to assist in suicide assessment, currently no tool has been validated that provides for a safe disposition decision for patients with suicidal ideation.[10,11,12]

After the Decision to Admit to the Hospital

Once a decision is made to admit a patient to an inpatient psychiatric unit, there is often little intervention that occurs in the ED. The patient waits for a bed until one is available. Few of these patients receive treatment while they are waiting for a bed. Although no studies have examined the benefit of initiating treatment in the ED, it is reasonable to assume that it would not be much different from that which occurs in psychiatric observation or a crisis stabilization unit. If treatment is initiated in the ED, it is possible that the inpatient stay might be shortened. Not only is it possible to start pharmacologic treatment in these patients without or without a psychiatric consultation, especially if they stopped taking their medicines, but also there are other therapeutic interventions performed by psychiatry or social work. This might include some crisis interventions, peer mentoring, or talk therapy.

After the decision to admit, the ED facility and staff are not well equipped to deal with patients with behavioral health problems. EDs are loud, bright, and chaotic places that do not place the patient in a low-stimulation, comfortable environment. In addition, negative staff attitudes toward patients with behavioral health problems may adversely affect patient care. Studies have documented that there is concern about little training in behavioral emergencies in emergency medicine residencies or psychiatric residencies, gaps in detecting patients with substance use disorder, lack of education in care of psychiatric patients, mental health patients managed inadequately, shortage of services to treat these patients, societal attitudes and personal biases, crowding, caregiver lack of confidence in skills and experience, and a lack of guidelines.[12] Focused efforts to mitigate these concerns have not been widespread.

Much work remains to be done across the country when it comes to the ED care of psychiatric patients. What is clear is that additional work is needed to partner with community service providers, provide a friendly environment of care, and refine admission criteria.

References

1. Emergency department visits by patients with mental health disorders – North Carolina, 2008–2010. *MMWR*. 2013 Jun 14;62(23):469–472. American College of Emergency Physicians Psychiatric and Substance Abuse Survey 2008. Available at www.acep.org/uploadedFiles/ACEP/ newsroom/NewsMediaResources/ StatisticsData/Psychiatric%20Boarding% 20Summary.pdf. Accessed December 13, 2015.

2. Baraff LJ, Janowicz N, Asarnow JR. Survey of California emergency departments about practices for management of suicidal patients and resources available for their care. *Academic Emergency Medicine*. 2006 Oct;48(4):452–458.

3. Schumacher Group: 2010 Survey Hospital Emergency Department Administrators. Available at http://schumachergroup.com/ _uploads/news/pdfs/ED%20Challenges% 20and%20Trends%2012.14.10.pdf. Accessed March 13, 2016.

4. Commonwealth of Pennsylvania Department of Drug and Alcohol Programs. Pennsylvania's Client Placement Criteria for Adults. Available at www.ddap.pa.gov/ Manuals/PA%20Client%20Placement%20 Criteria%20(PCPC)%20Edition%203% 20Manual.pdf. Accessed December 13, 2015.

5. Mansbach, JM, Wharff E, Austin SB, Ginnis K, Woods ER. Which psychiatric patients board on the medical service? *Pediatrics*. 2003;111(6 Pt. 1):e693–698.

6. Armour S. South Carolina psychiatric patient stuck 38 days in ER. www.bloomberg.com/news/articles/2013- 07-18/south-carolina-psychiatric-patient- stuck-38-days-in-er. Accessed April 3, 2016.

7. Hnatow D. Providing care for the acute mentally ill: a community response. *Urgent Matters Patient Flow Enewsletter*. 2005;2(6). Available at http://urgentmatters.org/e- newsletter/318774/318775/318777.

8. Breslow, RE, Klinger, BI, Erickson, BJ. Crisis hospitalization on a psychiatric emergency service. *General Hospital Psychiatry*. 1983;15:307–315.

9. Zeller, S, Calma, N, Stone, A. Effects of regional psychiatric emergency service on boarding of psychiatric patients in area emergency departments. *The Western Journal of Emergency Medicine*. 2014;15:1–6.

10. Suicide Prevention Resource Center. Caring for adult patients with suicide risk: a consensus guide for emergency departments. Available at www.sprc.org/ ed-guide. Accessed April 3, 2016.

11. Bengelsdorf H, et al. A crisis triage rating scale: brief dispositional assessment of patients at risk for hospitalization. *The Journal of Nervous and Mental Disease*. 1984;172:424–430.

12. American Association of Community Psychiatry. Locus: level of care utilization system for psychiatric and addiction services. Available at www.ct.gov/dmhas/ lib/dmhas/publications/CSPLOCUS.pdf. Accessed April 3, 2016.

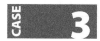

The Geriatric Emergency Department

Ula Hwang and Christopher R. Carpenter

Introduction: Our Aging Population and the Disconnect with Emergency Care

An aging society presents unique emergency management challenges for providing prompt, thorough clinical care worldwide. Optimal outcomes for medical illness and surgical trauma depend on accurate diagnoses and timely consultation, but older adults often display atypical symptoms clouded by the complexities of comorbid disease, including age-related physiologic changes and undiagnosed organ dysfunction. The contemporary emergency department (ED) was designed to manage acute medical issues in populations of all ages, but the time-intensiveness and complexity of geriatric evaluations has traditionally been relegated to inpatient settings.[1] Concerns about healthcare costs and efficacy have produced a policy environment in which inpatient access is increasingly being constrained by payers because of escalating costs, so the onus is on emergency medicine to transform itself and develop protocols that provide more intensive, yet efficient, geriatric evaluations in the future.[2]

It is projected that older adults (age 65+) will utilize the ED more than any other age group.[3] Once in the ED, they are more likely to have testing, longer lengths of stay in the ED, higher ED charges, and to be admitted (specifically to the intensive care unit).[4,5,6,7,8] Despite this high volume of care, older adults often receive a lower quality of care than younger patients.[9,10,11] They are at greater risk for iatrogenic injuries, including adverse drug events and catheter-associated urinary tract infections, and have poorer post-ED discharge outcomes, including ED revisits, hospitalizations, and death.[12,13,14,15]

Emergency medicine seeks to promote health, accelerate recovery from disease and injury, and ease the end-of-life process. However, the complexity of older adult emergencies, combined with an amalgamated healthcare web leading to challenging gaps in care transitions, leave modern EDs to contribute at times to unsatisfactory outcomes for the aged.[16] It is not uncommon for dementia and delirium to be unrecognized; fall victims to not receive guideline-appropriate management; acute pain to be undertreated; and palliative care resources to be underutilized.[17,18] These deficiencies occur across healthcare systems internationally, providing an extraordinary opportunity to advance the science and humanism of emergency medicine for older adults around the world.

Societal expectations for more geriatric-friendly emergency care manifest in several forms. First, the concept of an ED solely designed to target care for aging adults was first described in 2007; the number of hospitals claiming to provide geriatric-friendly resources has increased annually since 2009.[19,20] Second, geriatric-specific core competencies for emergency medicine trainees have evolved.[21] Core competencies represent the minimal skill set that learners must attain and demonstrate to be deemed clinically competent for a domain of expertise. The geriatric emergency medicine core competencies include six domains (atypical presentation of disease, trauma including falls, cognitive and behavior disorders, emergency intervention modifications, medication management, and transitions of care) with 26 specific recommendations. For example, one competency for cognitive and behavioral disorders is to "Assess and document current mental status and any change from baseline in every elder, with special attention to determining if delirium exists or has been superimposed on dementia."[21] Third, Geriatric ED (GED) Guidelines have been developed and widely endorsed. The 2014 GED Guidelines are the product of an interorganizational, interprofessional, and interdisciplinary effort. A team of clinicians representing emergency physicians, geriatricians, and emergency nurses from the American College of Emergency Physicians (ACEP), American Geriatrics Society (AGS), Emergency Nurses Association, and Society for Academic Emergency Medicine (SAEM) convened as the Geriatric Steering Committee and reviewed the literature and provided best evidence recommendations for essential geriatric emergency care. Protocols for clinical care, trained staff, and physical modifications for geriatric patients in the inpatient and outpatient settings have been shown to be successful in the reduction of delirium, iatrogenic complications, cost, hospital length of stay, and transfer to long-term care facilities, while improving patient-centered outcomes. The goal is to introduce these models and protocols to patients in the ED. The recommendations fall in the six general categories of staffing, transitions of care, education, quality improvement, equipment/supplies, and policies/procedures/protocols and were proposed, subsequently reviewed and approved by the memberships and boards of directors of the participating national organizations.[22] Professional medical organizations have endorsed the GED Guidelines to provide recommendations and sample clinical protocols, staff training, infrastructure components, and quality improvement metrics that ensure older adult emergency care based on geriatric principles. The GED Guidelines are not intended to promote older-adult-only EDs, which would be logistically and financially unsustainable for many healthcare systems; instead, they illustrate approximately 40 pragmatic examples that any ED can adapt in part or in whole based on personnel and space resources to "geriatricize" care for potentially vulnerable patients based on implementation science principles.

Case Study: GEDI WISE

Early programs that have implemented the GED Guidelines include three hospitals that participated in GEDI WISE (Geriatric ED Innovations in Care through Workforce, Informatics and Structural Enhancements). GEDI WISE was a Round One US Centers for Medicare and Medicaid Services (CMS) Health Care Innovation Award program.[23] This is a clinical demonstration program that occurred at Mount Sinai Medical Center in New York, NY; Northwestern Memorial Hospital in Chicago, IL; and St. Josephs Regional Medical Center in Paterson, NJ from 2012 to 2016.[24] GEDI WISE clinical implementation goals are aligned with those of CMS, which are to facilitate better health care, better health, and lower healthcare costs for older patients (age 65+) seen in the ED.

The hospitals improved the quality of geriatric emergency care by focusing resources and attention on enhanced staffing (with expansion of clinical roles by existing or additional staff), implementing protocols targeted at identifying and assessing older adults at greater risk for increased hospital utilization or geriatric syndromes, and creating policies and staffing models that supported better care transitions from the ED back to the community with the goal of safely reducing avoidable hospital admission.

Staffing/Administration

Optimal geriatric care relies on interdisciplinary efforts to provide clinical care that is not only effective, but also addresses the overall functional and psychosocial needs of the older adult. These are goals not typically taught, addressed, nor operationalized in traditional ED models of care. In shifting the care protocols with a geriatric approach, usually focused on care transitions, there would be geriatric education training of the emergency physicians, specialized nurses, social workers, case managers, pharmacists, designated professionals to coordinate geriatric services, physical therapists, and, if available, geriatric consultants. With dedicated geriatric EDs, the following positions should exist: a geriatric emergency department medical director and a GED nurse manager, both of whom would qualify by completing geriatric-appropriate training and oversight responsibilities that ensure geriatric performance improvement programs as described in the guidelines.[25] Additionally, staff physicians and nurses working in the geriatric ED should complete a minimum of 4 hours of annual continuing medical education focused on geriatric-specific education. Other staff that should be considered include social workers, case managers, pharmacists with geriatric certification, and physical or occupational therapists for patients while in the ED. The resources and feasibility of establishing such staffing and administration, however, may not be readily or easily found in most EDs. Thus it is important to increase geriatric-focused education and training to ensure that high-quality care is delivered by all staff in an ED that may care for older patients.[25]

With the GEDI WISE model, all three hospitals implemented geriatric emergency care programs with the expansion of responsibilities by already existing interdisciplinary staff. For example, at Mount Sinai, which had originally had three preexisting ED-based social workers and two ED-based pharmacists, the positions were augmented with funding for an additional social work and a pharmacist position. However, clinical care education and training of geriatric-specific assessments focused on functional status, home safety assessments, and accessibility to primary care were provided to all the social workers so they could better target and manage transitions of care.[26] Similarly, even with the addition of a geriatric ED pharmacist to the staff, all ED pharmacists received Geriatric Pharmacy certification and became skilled at providing targeted medication reconciliation in identifying potentially inappropriate medications for older adults seen in the ED. With this model, even with a subsequent reduction in numbers of dedicated clinical staff positions, the existing ED staff had their clinical skills augmented by enhanced geriatric emergency care capabilities.

Follow-Up and Transitions of Care

A common goal of most geriatric EDs is to reduce likelihood of admissions, and it was one of the goals for GEDI WISE hospitals. Hospitalizations are costly and significantly associated with poorer outcomes for older adults with evidence of increased rates of delirium, nosocomial infections, iatrogenic complications, and subsequent functional decline.[27,28] Attempts to screen older patients who might be at risk for adverse events may help direct targeted interventions and more efficient resource utilization earlier on while a patient is still in the ED, initiate earlier care coordination, and potentially and safely avert a hospital admission. Recommendations from the guidelines to facilitate transitions of care, especially from the ED to the community, include having specific geriatric discharge protocols that allow for clear communication, understanding, and transfer of patient information not only to the patient, but also to family and caregivers; establishment of appropriate and timely patient follow-up; and coordination of these care transitions by the interdisciplinary team staffed above to the patients primary caregiver.[25]

All three GEDI WISE hospitals created new clinical nursing positions in the EDs focused on transitions of care. The goal of transitional care nurses (TCNs) is improve care coordination for older ED patients such that they may be safety discharged from the ED back to the community.[29] The TCNs target patients based on recent hospitalization discharges, ED clinician request, or identification of seniors at risk (ISAR) scores, which are completed at triage to identify patients at risk for subsequent hospitalizations. By working with the support of interdisciplinary staff (i.e., social workers, case managers, pharmacists, physical therapists, visiting nurse services), the TCN facilitates discharge care coordination for older patients that may avoid a hospital admission and establishes possible home care and follow-up or even direct admissions from the ED to skilled nursing or subacute rehabilitation facilities.[30]

Policies, Procedures, and Protocols

Many of the above recommendations with regard to goals of improved care coordination and transitions of care, however, are not unique to the older adult. Patients of all ages would benefit if such programs were available in all EDs. Nonetheless, because of their multi-morbidity and risk for functional and cognitive impairment, older adults are more likely to have greater benefit from such programs. Many suggested protocols and procedures are provided in the GED Guidelines, along with early evidence-based tools and algorithms that could easily be incorporated into the ED evaluation. Although the prognostic ability of many risk-screening tools is mixed and more reliable tools are urgently needed, these tools nonetheless provide information about elder patient capabilities for self-care and risks of subsequent hospital and ED utilization. Examples of screening tools, protocols for reducing risk of iatrogenic complications and incorporating palliative care, and common presentations and challenges that should be addressed when caring for older patients are provided in the guidelines.[25,30]

Older patients can also have geriatric syndromes that would greatly benefit from ED-based interdisciplinary approaches for screening, assessment, evaluation, and follow-up. These include evaluation for falls risk, delirium, and polypharmacy medication management.

Falls

One-third of adults over age 65 fall each year, and falls represent the leading cause of traumatic mortality in older adults. Noninjurious falls represent an opportunity to reduce future falls that can cause life-threatening injury since one-third of fallers will fall again within 6 months. Noninjurious falls also reduce activity, quality of life, mobility, and functional independence for some. Despite the prevalence and potential implications of standing level falls, fall victims rarely receive guideline-directed care that includes identification of intrinsic and extrinsic risk factors with appropriate documentation, referrals, and patient education when issues are identified. For example, less than 15 percent of fall victims receive referrals to prevent future falls.[18] Since current practice patterns do not incorporate guidelines into fall management, educational strategies, institutional protocols, and quality improvement metrics that promote recognition of future fall risk and preventive interventions into clinical care are important. Efficient implementation into practice requires institutional assessment of cultural capacity to change, feasibility and adaptability of fall screening and interventions based on institutional resources, and sustainability.

Delirium

Approximately 10 percent of geriatric patients in ED settings suffer delirium during an episode of care, yet 75 percent are unrecognized by providers.[17] Failure to diagnose or treat acute delirium diminishes the accuracy of the ED history and physical exam, while increasing hospital length of stay and ED returns. Adapting delirium screening for different EDs necessitates linking nurse and physician education with triage and reassessment protocols and access to inpatient resources for appropriate monitoring of hypoactive and hyperactive delirium patients. The GED Guidelines provide valid, accurate, and feasible delirium screening instruments for ED settings.[25]

Polypharmacy

Over 80 percent of all older adults take a medication; almost a third of older adults take at least five prescriptions concurrently.[32] Polypharmacy is the principal risk factor in adverse drug events.[33] The Beers Criteria is a list of potentially inappropriate medications (PIM) for older adults in general and those with certain diseases, with updated iterations of this listing since it was first proposed in 2003. The most recent update was in 2015.[34] These drugs are associated with poorer health outcomes and in general should be avoided in older patients. Emergency clinician education and awareness of these PIMs; establishing policies and protocols to review high-risk medications, such as blood thinners or antiglycemic agents that have been show to increase risk of hospitalization in older adults; and facilitating staffing review of accurate patient medication lists and management by physicians, nurses, and pharmacists in the ED are all recommended pathways to reduce poor outcomes that commonly result from polypharmacy and high-risk medications.[25,35]

With the GEDI WISE model, policies and protocols were implemented to facilitate screenings and assessment for increased risks of falls, delirium, and adverse drug events at all three hospitals. Protocols were developed with assessments tasked to certain staff for completion. ED nurses and technicians were trained to screen for falls risk with the Timed Up and Go test.[36] Nurses were trained to evaluate for presence of delirium with the Confusion Assessment Method by testing cognitive function and querying for changes from baseline cognitive status. Pharmacists completed careful review of current baseline medications for risk of adverse drug events.[37] To facilitate the screenings, documentation templates were created and incorporated into the electronic health records and integrated with geriatric-specific track boards of screening results. This would provide the interdisciplinary teams with the ability to quickly identify patients needing additional evaluation and care coordination. For example, patients noted to be on anticoagulants or diabetic medications had an in-depth review of their medications by the geriatric ED pharmacist.[35] Those with a high risk of falls were seen by a physical therapist for early processing of potential physical therapy referral. With these policies and protocols targeted at geriatric syndromes, the goal was to transform the standard approach of adult emergency care to one that was geriatric focused.

With GEDI WISE, the program has continued at all three sites post-CMS funding because of the value seen by the hospitals of the care provided to older patients. Additionally, early planning to embed training and implementation into the roles of both preexisting and newly added staff allowed for these care models to continue even if staffing was reduced. Therefore, training all the staff to have geriatric certification or knowledge of geriatric emergency policies and protocols (e.g., all the pharmacists, or social workers, or

TCNs), rather than having dedicated positions completing these tasks, allows for the sustaining of targeted geriatric care programs even when staffing is reduced or limited.

Discussion

Innovation Process: Promoting Spread

To transform our current model of ED care to one that addresses the geriatric needs, we will need more than just nationally endorsed guidelines and recommendations delineating best practices. This "innovative" care will require dissemination and implementation into clinical care. One such approach that has been developed to promote the GED Guidelines was the "Geriatric ED Boot Camp."[38] In a joint organizational effort by ACEP, AGS, and SAEM that was funded by the John A. Hartford Foundation, a pilot boot camp program was implemented between 2013 and 2014 to geriatricize EDs. With the boot camp, geriatric emergency medicine faculty are able to bring education content from the guidelines to hospitals dedicated to improving the quality of geriatric emergency care. At a 1-day onsite conference, the faculty delivers geriatric-specific education and an array of tools and resources to help the hospital promote a preidentified quality improvement initiative, such as better transitions of care or detection and management of delirium. By hosting the conference at the hospital, this promotes attendance, networking, and collaborations between essential interdisciplinary staff (physicians, nurses, social workers, case managers, pharmacists, physical therapists, etc.) at the institution with the shared goal of devising a team-based quality improvement project. It is hoped that such innovated models of dissemination and implementation will deliver and spread the GED model of care to hospitals throughout the country. The goal is to promote practice change of our current model of emergency care to one that also addresses the unique but growing needs of older adults.

Two availability challenges must be overcome to ensure widespread access to emergency care that adheres to geriatric principles. First, most geriatric research is not conducted in ED settings. In addition, many studies purposely exclude frail older adults to simplify patient recruitment and avoid confounding comorbidities. Consequently, the GED Guidelines lack high-quality evidentiary support, so additional research is essential to understand the effectiveness of alternative management approaches for subsets of older adults.[39] Second, the proportion of geriatricians is dwindling and is entirely insufficient to meet the needs of an aging society. This means that nongeriatrician medical specialties will often lack access to geriatricians for educational content and timely consultations. Emergency medicine providers will therefore need to rely on experts in and core competencies derived from within their specialty to attain and maintain proficiency with older adult emergency care.[21,25] The AGS recognized this reality in the 1990s, which led to the concept of "geriatrics by stealth," whereby medical and surgical specialties develop experts in older adult healthcare within their specialty, funded by numerous research and educational grants.

Another challenge to widespread implementation of the GED Guidelines to promote innovative healthcare delivery to aging adults in ED settings is the skepticism from within emergency medicine. Some providers oppose any division of emergency medicine because their vision of an effective ED is to provide timely care to any patient, anywhere, anytime. These opponents view efforts to improve care for subpopulations of pediatric, geriatric, cardiac, trauma, or stroke patients as divisive, expensive, and likely nonsustainable for emergency medicine. Nonetheless, some (but not all) studies suggest that credentialed trauma and cardiac centers provide more evidence-based care with better outcomes. There is currently no published evidence suggesting that EDs improve older adults' outcomes, reduce costs, or alleviate suffering by adhering to the GED Guidelines, but since the guidelines were just published in 2014 this is hardly surprising. The absence of evidence is not evidence of absence, but studies are needed to understand which recommendations work for which patients at what cost.

Others oppose the GED Guidelines due to concerns that they reach beyond the scope of emergency medicine. Most emergency providers did not choose emergency medicine to become de facto geriatricians, yet the GED Guidelines encourage these providers to effectively manage geriatric syndromes such as falls, delirium, and polypharmacy. Incorporating geriatric-friendly protocols into the typical ED will require additional training and resources, but observational studies suggest that failure to do so increases ED returns, admissions, and functional decline while diminishing patient satisfaction.[40,41]

Disclosure

The GEDI WISE project described in this chapter is supported by Grant 1C1CMS331055-01-00 of the Department of Health and Human Services (DHS), Centers for Medicare and Medicaid Services (CMS). Its contents are solely the responsibility of the authors and have not been approved by the DHS, CMS.

References

1. Carpenter CR, Platts-Mills TF. Evolving prehospital, emergency department, and "inpatient" management models for geriatric emergencies. *Clinical Geriatric Medicine*. 2013;29(1):31–47.

2. Hwang U, Shah MN, Han JH, Carpenter CR, Siu AL, Adams JG. Transforming emergency care for older adults. *Health Affairs*. 2013;32(12):2116–2121.

3. Tang N, Stein J, Hsia RY, Maselli JH, Gonzales R. Trends and characteristics of US emergency department visits, 1997–2007. *JAMA*. 2010;304:664–670.

4. Strange G, Chen E. Use of emergency departments by elder pateints: a five-year follow-up study. *Academic Emergency Medicine*. 1998;5:1157–1162.

5. Wofford JL, Schwartz E, Timerding BL, Folmar S, Ellis SD, Messick CH. Emergency department utilization by the elderly: analysis of the national hospital ambulatory medical care survey. *Academic Journal of Emergency Medcicine*. 1996;3(7):694–699.

6. Hamdy RC, Forrest LJ, Moore SW, Cancellaro L. Use of emergency departments by the elderly in rural areas. *South Medical Journal*. 1997;90(6):616–620.

7. Singal B, Hedges J, Rousseau E, et al. Geriatric patient emergency visits part 1: comparison of visits by geriatric and younger patients. *Annals of Emergency Medicine*. 1992;21:802–807.

8. Baum SA, Rubenstein LZ. Old people in the emergency room: age-related differences in emergency department use and care. *Journal of American Geriatric Society*. 1987;35(5):398–404.

9. Magid DJ, Masoudi FA, Vinson DR, et al. Older emergency department patients with acute myocardial infarction receive lower quality of care than younger patients. *Annals of Emergency Medicine*. 2005;46 (1):14–21.

10. Hwang U, Belland LK, Handel DA, et al. Is all pain treated equally? A multicenter evaluation of acute pain care by age. *The Journal of Pain*. 2014 Dec;155(12):2568–74.

11. Hwang U, Platts-Mills TF. Acute pain management in older adults in the emergency department. *Clinical Geriatric Medicine*. 2013;29(1):151–164.

12. Hastings SN, Smith VA, Weinberger M, Oddone EZ, Olsen MK, Schmader KE. Health services use of older veterans treated and released from Veterans Affairs medical center emergency departments. *Journal of the American Geriatric Society*. 2013;61 (9):1515–1521.

13. Hastings SN, Oddone EZ, Fillenbaum G, Sloane RJ, Schmader KE. Frequency and predictors of adverse health outcomes in older Medicare beneficiaries discharged from the emergency department. *Journal of Medical Care*. 2008;46(8):771–777.

14. McCusker J, Cardin S, Bellevance F, Belzile E. Return to the emergency department among elders: patterns and predictors. *Academic Emergency Medicine*. 2000;7 (3):249–259.

15. Grunier A, Silver MJ, Rochon PA. Emergency department use by older adults: a literature review on trends, appropriateness, and consequences of unmet health care needs. *Medical Care Research and Review*. 2011;68(2):131–155.

16. Schnitker L, Martin-Khan M, Beattie E, Gray L. Negative health outcomes and adverse events in older people attending emergency departments: a systematic review. *Australasian Emergency Nursing Journal*. 2011;14:141–162.

17. Han JH, Zimmerman EE, Cutler N, et al. Delirium in older emergency department patients: recognition, risk factors, and psychomotor subtypes. *Academic Emergency Medicine*. 2009;16 (3):193–200.

18. Tirrell G, Sri-On J, Lipsitz LA, Camargo CA, Kabrhel C, Liu SW. Evaluation of older adult patients with falls in the emergency department: discordance with national guidelines. *Academic Emergency Medicine*. 2015;22(4):461–467.

19. Hwang U, Morrison RS. The geriatric emergency department. *Journal of the American Geriatrics Society*. 2007;55 (11):1873–1876.

20. Hogan TM, Olade TO, Carpenter CR. A profile of acute care in an aging America: snowball sample identification and characterization of United States geriatric emergency departments in 2013. *Academic Emergency Medicine*. 2014 21(3):337–346.

21. Hogan TM, Losman ED, Carpenter CR, et al. Development of geriatric competencies for emergency medicine residents using an expert consensus process. *Academic Emergency Medicine* 2010;17(3):316–324.

22. Carpenter CR, Hwang U, Rosenberg M. New guidelines enhance care standards for elderly patients in the ED. *ACEP Now*. 2014;33:14–16, 28.

23. Centers for Medicare and Medicaid Innovation. Health Care Innovation Award project profiles. 2012. Available at http://innovation.cms.gov/Files/x/HCIA-Project-Profiles.pdf, http://innovation.cms.gov/initiatives/Health-Care-Innovation-Awards/New-York.html. Accessed August 18, 2014.

24. Hwang U, Rosenberg MS, Dresden SM. Geriatrics emergency department: The GEDI WISE Program. In Malone M, Capezuti E, Palmer RM, eds., *Geriatrics Models of Care: Bringing "Best Practice" to an Aging America*. 2015:201–209.

25. Rosenberg M, Carpenter CR, Bromley M, et al. Geriatric emergency department guidelines. *Annals of Emergency Medicine*. 2014;63(5):e7–e25.

26. Hamilton C, Ronda L, Hwang U, et al. The evolving role of geriatric emergency department social work in the era of health care reform. *Social Work Health Care*. 2015;54(9):849–868.

27. Chin MH, Jin L, Karrison TG, et al. Older patients' health-related quality of life around an episode of emergency illness. *Annals of Emergency Medicine*. 1999;34 (5):595–603.

28. Creditor MD. Hazards of hospitalization of the elderly. *Annals of Internal Medicine*. 1993;118:219–223.

29. Aldeen AZ, Courtney MC, Lindquist LA, Dresden SM, Gravenor SJ. Geriatric emergency department innovations:

preliminary data for the geriatric nurse liaison model. *Journal of the American Geriatrics Society*. 2014;62(9):1781–1785.

30. McCusker J, Bellavance F, Cardin S, Belzile E, Verdon J. Prediction of hospital utilization among elderly patients during the 6 months after an emergency department visit. *Annals of Emergency Medicine*. 2000;36(5):438–445.

31. Carpenter CR, Shelton E, Fowler S, et al. Risk factors and screening instruments to predict adverse outcomes for undifferentiated older emergency department patients: a systematic review and meta-analysis. *Academic Emergency Medicine*. 2015;22(1):1–21.

32. Qato DM, Alexander GC, Conti RM, Johnson M, Schumm P, Lindau ST. Use of prescription and over-the-counter medications and dietary supplements among older adults in the United States. *JAMA*. 2008;300(24):2867–2878.

33. Cooper JA, Cadogan CA, Patterson SM, et al. Interventions to improve the appropriate use of polypharmacy in older people: a Cochrane systematic review. *BMJ Open*. 2015;5(12):e009235.

34. American Geriatrics Society 2015 Beers Criteria Update Expert Panel. American Geriatrics Society 2015 updated Beers Criteria for potentially inappropriate medication use in older adults. *Journal of the American Geriatrics Society*. 2015;63 (11):2227–2246.

35. Budnitz DS, Lovegrove MC, Shehab N, Richards CL. Emergency hospitalizations for adverse drug events in older Americans. *New England Journal of Medicine*. 2011;365 (21):2002–2012.

36. Centers for Diease Control and Prevention (CDC). The timed up and go (TUG) test. Stopping Elderly Accidents Deaths and Injuries. Available at www.cdc.gov/steadi/pdf/tug_test-a.pdf. Accessed March 7, 2016.

37. Inouye SK, Van Dyke C, Alessi C, Balkin S, Siegal A, Horowitz R. Clarifying confusion: the confusion assessment method. A new method for detection of delirium. *Annals of Internal Medicine*.1991;15:941–948.

38. Carpenter CR, Biese K, Hogan TM, Hwang U, Malone M, Melady D. Geriatric ED boot camp offers collaborative onsite educational outreach pilot. *ACEP Now*. 2014; 14–16, 28.

39. Carpenter CR, Gerson L. Geriatric emergency medicine. In: LoCicero J, Rosenthal RA, Katic M, Pompei P, eds., *A Supplement to New Frontiers in Geriatrics Research: An Agenda for Surgical and Related Medical Specialties*. The American Geriatrics Society, 2008:45–71.

40. Mion LC, Palmer RM, Meldon SW, et al. Case finding and referral model for emergency department elders: a randomized clinical trial. *Annals of Emergency Medicine*. 2003;41(1):57–68.

41. McCusker J, Verdon J, Tousignant P, de Courval LP, Dendukuri N, Belzile E. Rapid emergency department intervention for older people reduces risk of functional declinde: results of a multicenter randomized trial. *Journal of the American Geriatrics Society*. 2001;49(10):1272–1281.

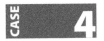

4 How the United Kingdom Responded to the 4-Hour Rule

Suzanne Mason and Michael J. Schull

Introduction

Demand for emergency care is rising in many jurisdictions, and the causes are not clearly understood. Many explanatory factors have been proposed, alone or in combination, that include poor access to alternatives such as primary care; behavioral change where patients more commonly expect immediate, one-stop, medical assessment and care; and an aging population with more complex health needs. In addition, increased social mobility and a lack of robust social care structures make patients more likely to access emergency care rather than rely on their social networks. One result has been increasingly long waiting times and crowding of emergency departments (EDs) in many countries, a problem that frequently attracts substantial attention from the press and public.

Many jurisdictions have adopted policies aimed at reducing crowding in EDs. The evidence for many interventions is often weak, and local implementation and adaptations combined with limited evaluations challenge efforts to understand their effect and generalizability. Interventions have typically focused on (1) modification of help-seeking behavior of patients, (2) increasing availability of alternative pathways of care for patients, (3) improving the processes of care once patients are in the ED, (4) making departure from the ED easier by increasing access to inpatient beds (e.g., access block), or (5) finding alternatives to inpatient care (e.g., rapid-access follow-up clinics post-ED discharge).

Many jurisdictions have dealt with high levels of demand for ED services and crowding through a performance management approach focused on total ED length-of-stay (often referred to as "ED waiting time"). In 2004, the UK government was the first to introduce an ED waiting time target for hospitals, mandating that 98 percent of patients should be seen, treated, and discharged from the ED within a maximum of 4 hours.[1] The 98 percent 4-hour cutoff was not based on any good research evidence, and this target had not previously been demanded anywhere else in the world. As a result of its introduction, overall performance with respect to meeting this target improved. Though the United Kingdom was the first to set a throughput target for ED visits, New Zealand, Australia, and Canada have since implemented similar targets for their ED patients.[2,3,4] The 4-hour target was designed to improve crowding and patient outcomes by reducing the time patients spend in EDs. No one denied that many patients spent longer than needed in our EDs. This was more often because of a lack of an inpatient bed, not because they were receiving essential treatment. It was not clear whether putting a cap on time would improve patient outcomes.

Monitoring of the 4-Hour Target

The UK Department of Health took a keen interest in monitoring and reporting the performance against the target of each English NHS Acute Trust, or service that delivers healthcare. Figures were submitted weekly by individual Trusts, and these were reported nationally each week. This showed a gradual increase in the ability of Trusts to deliver the target performance. Between 2004 and 2005, financial incentives were provided by the Department of Health for organizations that showed consistent improvement on the target until the target was deemed to be fully implemented at 98 percent. In order to support

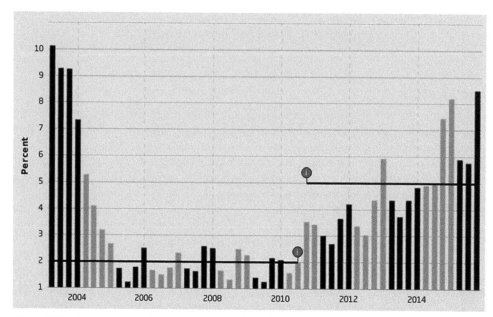

Figure CS4.1 Percentage of patients spending more than 4 hours in the emergency department from arrival to admission, transfer, or discharge. The two disks represent the point when the target changed from 98 percent to 95 percent. Reproduced with permission from the King's Fund.

hospitals in improving their processes of care, the Emergency Services Collaborative, established prior to implementation of the target, allowed representatives of hospitals to discuss best practices for improving flow within both the ED and the rest of the hospital. Acute Trusts that were found to be performing poorly against the target were identified and inspected by organizations such as the Care Quality Commission and Monitor, with a view to making suggestions on why performance was lower than expected, and what measures could be taken by Trusts to improve. National performance has changed over time and progress on the target was made from 2004 to a gradual deterioration in performance in 2010 once the goal was relaxed to 95 percent in 2010 (see Figure CS4.1).

Changes Made to Meet the 4-Hour Target

In order to achieve the 4-hour target, EDs undertook a number of process improvement efforts that were not cost neutral. These were partly documented through a survey of English EDs in 2006 where 111 out of 198 EDs responded (56 percent).[5] The commonest efforts taken were mainly related to an increase in staffing. The survey found that many EDs introduced additional senior doctor hours (39 percent of ED respondents) and the creation of a "4 hour monitor" role (37 percent of ED respondents) that consisted of an individual responsible for watching the clock and identifying patients who would breach the target. Other improvements included the ability to gain access to existing emergency beds (36 percent of EDs respondents), additional nonclinical staff hours (such as portering and reception staff; 33 percent of ED respondents), additional nursing hours (29 percent of ED respondents), and triage undertaken by senior staff (28 percent of ED respondents). However, in 32 percent of EDs responding, no changes were made to usual practice. The survey authors found that the biggest influence on improved performance was the number of interventions rather than the specific nature of these interventions taken by a department.

Impact of the 4-Hour Target on Patients in England

In order to explore the impact that the 4-hour target was having on patients, routine data were analyzed in a subsequent study to examine the distribution of total time patients spent in the ED. Data were available from 83 English EDs for the month of April in 2004 ($n =$ 428,953 patient episodes). Figure CS4.2 shows the distribution of time in the ED by disposition category (i.e., admitted and discharged patients). The median total time in the ED for discharged patients was 96 minutes (98th centile = 341 minutes); 91.0 percent ($n =$ 283,894) of these patients spent <220 minutes in the department, with a further 3.6 percent ($n = 11,161$) spending 220–239 minutes. However, patients admitted from the ED had a median total time of 183 minutes (98th centile = 625 minutes). The distribution of total time in the department for admitted patients shows the most striking anomaly, with 64.0 percent ($n = 60,315$) of patients spending <220 minutes in the department and a further 12.3 percent ($n = 11,563$) spending 220–239 minutes. Patients spending 220–239 minutes in the department were also significantly older than those spending <220 minutes there.[6] This distribution demonstrates a trend toward the admitted patients (who are sicker and older) benefiting the least from the introduction of the target. It also demonstrates that EDs played to the target with a large proportion of patients being recorded as moving out of the ED in the last 20 minutes before the target time passes.

The 4-hour standard has reduced the time that patients spend in the ED, but it has not promoted other aspects of quality defined by the World Health Organization in 2006.[7] It lacks equity across patient groups, with important groups, such as those in critical care, the elderly, and mental health patients seeming to be the most disadvantaged. There are concerns that the standard may result in "effort substitution" (where the activity measured takes precedence over equally valuable care.) If the 4-hour target were a medicine or medical device, then a much more rigorous evidence base would have been required to justify the effort and expense. There is only weak and inconsistent evidence that the 4-hour

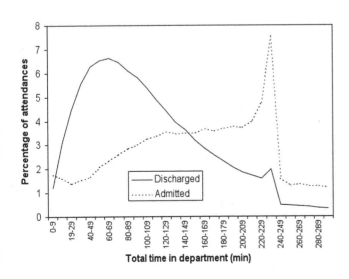

Figure CS4.2 Distribution of total time in department for episodes resulting in admission or discharge.

standard was associated with reduced inpatient mortality among emergency admissions in the United Kingdom, and the stronger study designs, such as that of Mason and colleagues, showed no impact on 7-day mortality.[8] The Australian picture is more positive. The evaluation of the introduction of the National Emergency Access Target found it was associated with a decrease in mortality, from 1.12 percent to 0.98 percent.[9] Though this change is small, in a high-volume system it reflects a significant and substantial health benefit. For example, in the US system with 140 million ED visits annually, a 0.14 percent change in 7-day mortality equates to 196,000 lives saved each year. Mason also showed that the intradepartmental mortality rate was unchanged,[8] though this represents only a small number of the deaths among emergency admissions. Royce demonstrated that there is no convincing association between hospital standardized mortality ratio performance and 4-hour standard performance.[10]

Impact of the 4-Hour Target on the Organization

Further in-depth work with 15 EDs identified that the 4-hour target did encourage change, and a number of new processes were introduced that were felt to be beneficial to patient care. These included introducing measures such as streaming of patients according to their acuity level on arrival, early ordering of laboratory tests, increased senior doctor front door triage of patients, and the introduction of clinical decision units where patients could continue their investigations without being admitted to a hospital bed and while also "stopping the clock." Key lessons from the implementation of the target were learned, and these included the following:[11]

- Emphasizing the responsibility of the whole organization
- Maintaining the focus on improving patient care
- Embracing opportunity
- Involving all stakeholders

The "targets and terror" regimes that have emerged over the past 20 years in the UK health service drive top-down healthcare targets by applying stringent time deadlines and financial penalties and by ultimately in threatening job losses at the senior management level. Now there is a focus on immediate, easily measurable, process interventions to provide quantifiable evidence of performance. This has forced organizations to divert their professional, largely value-driven staff away from "doing the right thing" to achieving externally imposed goals instead. In 2010 the Department of Health announced a relaxation of the 98 percent 4-hour standard to 95 percent along with the introduction of a dashboard of clinical quality indicators.[12] This was undertaken following a decision by the Secretary of State for Health at the time, who recognized that the target did little to improve quality of care. It was decided to take a more balanced approach by measuring and reporting a dashboard of quality indicators that would produce a broader picture of the ED. The indicators included a new 4-hour target of 95 percent, as well as time to treatment, time to initial assessment, proportion of patients leaving the ED without being seen, reattendance rates, and total time in ED. These measures were felt to be a broader representation of patient experience, ED performance, and quality. However, they were not developed using robust methods nor evaluated for their ability to reflect important processes or outcomes such as safety and quality of care.

Having reliable data that are widely available, can be interrogated and manipulated from our EDs and the wider urgent and emergency care system, and that have universal meaning to each of these settings is probably the single biggest challenge. Whatever we choose as our outcome or process measures, we need to be able to record and benchmark our activity in order to measure current activity and inform future improvements. The UK's experience with the 4-hour target has led to a better understanding of the challenges that measuring performance can present.

Measuring Performance in Emergency Medicine

Measuring performance and outcomes remains a tremendous challenge for emergency medicine. Outcomes for patients are based on the whole journey, from calling for help to leaving the healthcare system. The journey may involve a number of services and healthcare staff. To focus attention on one part of that journey – the ED – does not necessarily mean overall patient care and outcomes are improved. Furthermore, the evidence regarding individual performance measures can change over time and result in the need to alter or withdraw a measure. One example is the provision of antibiotics in the ED to pneumonia patients. In 2004, the Joint Commission issued a standard that required giving pneumonia patients an antibiotic within 4 hours of ED presentation.[13] This measure was proposed based on two large retrospective studies[14,15] in US Medicare patients. However, concerns regarding its implementation and subsequent evidence called into question the rationale for the measure and identified potential adverse consequences.[16,17] The measure was eventually withdrawn.[16,17] Such evolution in performance measures is expected and should be welcomed, and continued focus on new evidence is laudable. But it does create challenges for health systems that must adapt to changing performance frameworks, and can unintentionally fuel doubts among providers about using performance measures to drive quality improvement efforts.

Experience in Ontario, Canada

The early success in England after the introduction of the 4-hour target was one factor that helped motivate the province of Ontario to implement its own ED wait time targets in 2008.[18] Subsequent population-based evidence from Ontario demonstrated an association between crowding and the likelihood of death or admission to hospital within 7 days of ED discharge.[19]

However, as in the UK, the ED length-of-stay targets in Ontario (90 percent of low acuity patients spending less than 4 hours total time in the ED, and less than 8 hours for high acuity or admitted patients) were chosen based on expert opinion.[18] Yet in a follow-up study of discharged ED patients in Ontario, a higher proportion of ED patients meeting time targets was associated with reduced risk of death or admission following discharge. These data provide empiric support for the Ontario targets (see Figure CS4.3).[20]

Time spent in the ED is an important quality indicator, but it is not the only one. Efforts to improve ED waiting times might lead to improvement on other quality-of-care measures as a consequence of improved flow and efficiency in the department. However, they might have a negative effect by virtue of a singular emphasis on flow to the detriment of other aspects of quality of care. Finally, they might simply be independent, and improvement in waiting times might have no discernible effect on other measures of quality of care. This question was examined over a 3-year period in 11 Ontario EDs in a study that compared changes in quality of care for acute myocardial infarction, asthma, and pain management in minor fractures. Overall wait time performance had improved after the introduction of

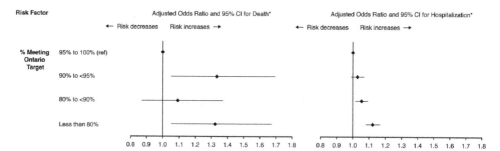

Figure CS4.3 Adjusted odds ratios (95% confidence intervals) for death and hospitalization within 7 days of an emergency department visit among all nonadmitted (seen-and-discharged and left-without-being-seen) high acuity patients (Canadian Triage and Acuity Scale levels 1 to 3).

waiting time targets compared with 13 EDs where it had not improved. Despite improvements in median ED waiting time of up to 63 minutes (26 percent) in the 11 wait-time improved sites, there was no difference when compared with the other quality-of-care measures in the 13 wait-time unimproved sites.[21] These findings suggest that successful strategies to address ED crowding will not necessarily be associated with improvements or worsening in other dimensions of quality of care. It is likely that other complex and hard-to-measure factors are also impacting the issue of quality, such as the confidence and competence of the treating physician, the skills and empathy of nursing staff, and the ability to communicate complicated health-related matters effectively to patients and their next of kin.

Discussion

The introduction of a time target in the United Kingdom led to a marked improvement in performance, with reduced ED wait times for the majority of patients. A more modest but significant improvement followed for Ontario. There is evidence that time targets can be associated with improved outcomes while simultaneously causing unintended consequences.[6,8,9,10] There is evidence that patients with minor conditions benefited the most from the time target, and those who were older, sicker, and required a hospital bed were more likely to be moved within the last few minutes of the target or to have breached it altogether. It is highly likely that older patients require more ED time in order to manage the often complex presentations and communications with patients and family and to ensure safe and robust discharge plans are put in place. In the United Kingdom, much of this management takes place in a clinical decisions unit, where the "clock" stops and patients requiring a more lengthy assessment can stay without taking up an acute hospital bed. In the United States, the increased popularity of the geriatric ED is facilitating the more prolonged management of patients in order to ensure safe discharge and reduce unplanned readmissions. However, further research is needed into the most appropriate ED skill and management strategies required to manage this growing and important patient group in a clinically and cost-effective way.

Simply mandating faster throughput of ED patients alone does not lead to better patient outcomes; the local response is also a critical factor for performance. Many clinicians in the United Kingdom, as in Ontario, saw the benefit of having the spotlight on the ED, with more resources and support being provided. In some cases, a whole hospital approach succeeded in redesigning patient flow and emergency care. In Ontario, hospitals reported the implementation of a whole series of measures to achieve wait time targets and improve care, including culture change, targeted staffing increases, and ED process improvement.[22] This suggests that wait time targets may be a necessary but not sufficient policy tool to motivate the implementation of a range of measures designed to reduce ED crowding. Whether the same could have been achieved in these jurisdictions without any wait time targets is unclear, but the practical experience in the United Kingdom and Ontario shows that targets were needed to motivate change. It remains the case that time is easy to measure, but other outcomes and process measures, such as clinical skills, are less easy to measure and quantify against a hard patient outcome and are therefore often ignored. However, somehow we need to harness the ability to measure all aspects of the patient experience to ensure our intervention can deliver successful improvements.

Since 2010 the United Kingdom has seen a gradual deterioration of performance as EDs once again struggle to cope with demand, crowding, and exit block. The latest figures show that, nationally, performance reached an all-time low of 93.4 percent of patients being seen within 4 hours, with the 95 percent target being met only during one month in 2015[23] (NHS England statistics). In addition, long waits for patients in the ED are rising, with increasing numbers breaching not only the 4-hour target, but 12 hours. Performance in Ontario has remained stable or improved slowly in recent years, with 87 percent of ED patients meeting targets, despite a seemingly inexorable rise in ED visit volumes.[24] The longest waits of all, not surprisingly, are experienced by admitted patients waiting for inpatient beds.[24] The problem of access block and long waits for inpatient beds for admitted ED patients remains a challenge in both England and Ontario.

It seems clear that wait time targets alone are not a solution to the ongoing rise in demand and complexity of patients presenting to the ED and that more work across the health system continuum is needed to provide integrated, easily accessible care for patients when they need it. NHS England is trying to redesign services to encourage signposting of patients to lower levels of care when appropriate and to encourage integration of care between the community and primary and secondary care networks. However, these proposals are in their infancy and have not been fully introduced or evaluated. Similar efforts are under way in Ontario.[25]

These developments are encouraging, as they suggest that policymakers are taking a broader view of the ED as an essential component of the healthcare system, and one where the best patient outcomes are likely to occur when high quality and timely care in the ED is preceded and followed by smooth integration with care in the community.

References

1. Department of Health. The NHS plan: a plan for investment, a plan for reform. 2000. Available at http://webarchive nationalarchives gov uk/. 010481829. Accessed March 18, 2016.

2. Ontario Ministry of Health and Long-Term Care. Ontario wait times: emergency room wait times – emergency room targets. Ontario Ministry of Health and Long-Term Care. 2015. Available at www.health.gov.on.ca/en/pro/programs/waittimes/edrs/targets.aspx. Accessed September 24, 2010.

3. National Health and Hospitals Network (NHHN), Australia. A national health and hospitals network for Australia's future. 2010. Available at www0.health.nsw.gov.au/resources/

Initiatives/healthreform/pdf/NHHN_
report3_RedBook.pdf. Accessed September
24, 2010.

4. New Zealand Ministry of Health.
    *Recommendations to Improve Quality and
    the Measurement of Quality in New
    Zealand Emergency Departments.*
    Wellington: Ministry of Health. 2009.
    Available at www.health.govt.nz/system/
    files/documents/publications/quality-ed-
    jan09.pdf. Accessed September 24, 2010.

5. Munro J, Mason S, Nicholl J. Effectiveness
    of measures to reduce emergency
    department waiting times: a natural
    experiment. *Emergency Medicine Journal.*
    2006;23(1):35–39.

6. Locker TE, Mason SM. Analysis of the
    distribution of time that patients spend in
    emergency departments. *BMJ.* 2005;330
    (7501):1188–1189.

7. The World Health Organization. Quality of
    care: a process for making strategic choices
    in health systems. 2006. Available at
    www.who.int/management/quality/
    assurance/QualityCare_B.Def.pdf.
    Accessed September 24, 2010.

8. Mason S, Weber EJ, Coster J, et al. Time
    patients spend in the emergency
    department: England's 4-hour rule – a case
    of hitting the target but missing the point?
    Annals of Emergency Medicine. 2012;59
    (5):341–349.

9. Geelhoed GC, de Klerk NH. Emergency
    department overcrowding, mortality and
    the 4-hour rule in western Australia.
    Medical Journal of Australia.
    2012;196:122–126.

10. Royce R. Four hours in A&E: what the
    target tells us about trusts. *Health Services
    Journal.* 2014. Available at www.hsj.co.uk/
    four-hours-in-ae-what-the-target-tells-us-
    about-trusts/5071094.fullarticle. Accessed
    June 4, 2014.

11. Weber EJ, Mason S, Carter A, et al.
    Emptying the corridors of shame:
    organizational lessons from England's
    4-hour emergency throughput target. *Annals
    of Emergency Medicine.* 2011;57(2):79–88.

12. NHS DoHUK. *Reforming Urgent and
    Emergency Care Performance Management.*

The National Archives, UK. 2011. Available
at http://webarchive.nationalarchives.gov
.uk/+/www.dh.gov.uk/en/Healthcare/
Urgentandemergencycare/DH_121239.
Accessed March 29, 2016.

13. Bromley M, Franklin A. Joint Commission
    to extend time to antibiotic administration.
    2014. Available at www.acep.org/Clinical–
    Practice-Management/Joint-Commission-
    to-Extend-Time-to-Antibiotic-
    Administration/. Accessed September 24,
    2010.

14. Meehan TP, Fine MJ, Krumholz HM, et al.
    Quality of care, process, and outcomes in
    elderly patients with pneumonia. *JAMA.*
    1997;278(23):2080–2084.

15. Houck PM, Bratzler DW, Nsa W, et al.
    Timing of antibiotic administration and
    outcomes for Medicare patients
    hospitalized with community-acquired
    pneumonia. *Archives of Internal Medicine.*
    2004;164(6):637–644.

16. Welker JA, Huston M, McCue JD.
    Antibiotic timing and errors in diagnosing
    pneumonia. *Archives of Internal Medicine.*
    2008;168(4):351–356.

17. Pines JM, Isserman JA, Hinfey PB. The
    measurement of time to first antibiotic
    dose for pneumonia in the emergency
    department: a White Paper and Position
    Statement prepared for the American
    Academy of Emergency Medicine. *Journal
    of Emergency Medicine.* 2009;37
    (3):335–340.

18. Ontario Hospital Association, Ontario
    Medical Association, Ontario Ministry of
    Health and Long-Term Care. Improving
    access to emergency care: addressing
    system issues. 2006. Available at
    www.health.gov.on.ca/en/common/
    ministry/publications/reports/improving_
    access/improving_access.pdf. Accessed
    March 18, 2016.

19. Guttmann A, Schull MJ, Vermeulen MJ,
    et al. Association between waiting times
    and short term mortality and hospital
    admission after departure from emergency
    department: population based cohort study
    from Ontario, Canada. *BMJ.* 2011;342:
    d2983.

20. Schull M, Vermeulen M, Guttmann A, et al. Better performance on length-of-stay benchmarks associated with reduced risk following emergency department discharge: an observational cohort study. *Canadian Journal of Emergency Medicine.* 2015;17(3):253–262.

21. Vermeulen MJ, Guttmann A, Stukel TA et al. Are reductions in emergency department length of stay associated with improvements in quality of care? A difference-in-differences analysis. *BMJ Journal of Quality & Safety.* 2016 Jul;25 (7):489–498.

22. Ovens H. ED overcrowding: the Ontario approach. *Academic Emergency Medicine.* 2011;18(12):1242–1245.

23. A&E crisis: NHS slips on four-hour waiting target in England. *The Telegraph.* 2016.

Available at www.telegraph.co.uk/news/ nhs/11990662/AandE-crisis-NHS-slips-on-four-hour-waiting-target-in-England.html. Accessed March 20, 2016.

24. Ontario Ministry of Health and Long-Term Care. Ontario wait times provincial summary. 2015. Available at www.ontariowaittimes.com/er/En/ ProvincialSummary.aspx?view=0. Accessed January 15, 2016.

25. Ontario Ministry of Health and Long-Term Care. Transforming Ontario's health care system: community health links provide coordinated, efficient and effective care to patients with complex needs. 2015. Available at www.health.gov.on.ca/en/pro/ programs/transformation/ community.aspx. Accessed January 15, 2016.

High-Cost Users

Using Information Technology to Streamline Care Plans

Dawn Williamson and Jody A. Vogel

Introduction

Information technology and systems are integral components of the healthcare system. In 2001, the Institute of Medicine (IOM) advocated the effective use of information technology in healthcare systems with the goal of improving healthcare quality, improving patient safety, and decreasing medical errors.[1,2] Subsequent significant legislation in the area of information technology included the Health Information Technology for Economic and Clinical Health Act of 2009. This legislation stated that the goal of healthcare information systems was not just the adoption of electronic medical records, but rather "meaningful use" of health information technology to improve the overall quality of healthcare.[3]

Use of information technology in the emergency department (ED) has the potential to significantly impact the delivery and quality of patient care while reducing unnecessary healthcare costs.[1,5] In 2009, the American College of Emergency Physicians released a White Paper indicating that health information technology offered ongoing opportunities to improve the quality of emergency care, promote patient safety, reduce medical errors, and enhance the efficiency of EDs.[1,4] The role of information technology and systems is especially important in the fast-paced ED where decisions regarding care may be associated with significant consequences and important information may not be readily available to the emergency healthcare provider.[1,5]

Given the cost and quality issues associated with frequent ED use, information technology is an important strategy in diverting patients to more appropriate levels of care. With the complex array of factors driving ED use, it is generally accepted that interventions to decrease ED use must be broad and multifaceted. One such approach are acute care plans (ACP), electronic documents that are targeted to provide guidance for ED clinicians. ACPs assist in addressing complex care issues and provide a continuity of care that links the patient back to outpatient caregivers.

ACPs are special treatment plans in a patient's record that have been integrated with information from the patient's primary care provider, case manager, or other clinician to help guide treatment decisions should the patient present to the ED. ACPs are flagged in the ED information system when a patient arrives at the ED, so that all providers are automatically notified of the plan. With an ACP, patients may avoid unnecessary testing or admission, as there is longitudinal documentation of the patient's risk factors, history, and care plan often developed by a multidisciplinary team.

Innovation

At the ED of the Massachusetts General Hospital (MGH), a large, urban, academic level-one trauma center with more than 102,000 patient visits annually, a process for developing electronic health record (EHR)-embedded ACPs was developed. High-utilizer patients represent 4 percent of the total patient population who receive treatment at this ED. Because a subset of high-utilizer patients comprises 17 percent of all ED visits and occupies 19 percent of ED

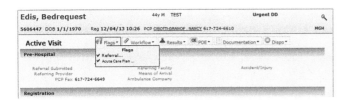

Figure CS5.1 Acute care plan flag.

bed hours, finding appropriate care for the complex needs of this population, which range from acute care to long-term case management, was deemed imperative by the leadership team. ACPs were created to address the lack of coordination among outpatient providers and ED providers when caring for patients who present frequently to the ED. A group of ED clinicians initially took on this issue as a quality improvement initiative. The first step was to identify patients who frequented the ED greater than ten times a year, then to gather patient information, which aided in identifying care needs for each patient.

The ACPs were then developed by multidisciplinary teams to communicate treatment plans for high-utilizer patients with input from outpatient care providers. The plans provide continuity of care and addressed issues such as who to call when the patient arrives at the ED, steps to facilitate evaluation, medication recommendations or restrictions, specific protocols to be followed, interventions to use to prevent admission, or issues that impact the transition back to home. The treatment plan specifically includes contact information for family or other support system members and gives guidance about patient disposition. The note has a template with standard fields to give guidance that is immediately helpful for the ED provider to implement on behalf of the patient.

These plans reside in the EHR system and are automatically flagged when a patient arrives at the ED by utilizing a software tool developed at MGH (Figure CS5.1). The patient's medical record is searched by an algorithm for notes titled "Acute Care Plan." The ED EHR receives information from the search and flags the patient's EHR. The ACP is then automatically viewable by the ED clinician. Education for ED staff about use of ACP is done on an ongoing basis by in-services and e-mail. Feedback from the clinicians regarding use of the ACP is elicited to help support the ongoing development and use of the plan. A report that lists patients who return frequently to the MGH ED is generated monthly and reviewed in the ED quality improvement (QI) meeting for active ACP development. Based on the report, instructional e-mails are sent to primary care providers that include the purpose of the ACP, with a template to follow to work to initiate development of a plan and enter it into the EHR (see Figure CS5.1).

Implementation of Acute Care Plans

A team was assembled to develop and communicate treatment plans to high-utilizer patients. At first the group consisted of a psychiatric clinical nurse specialist, ED social workers, and two ED case managers. This first group quickly expanded their meetings to include representation from a variety of disciplines, including nurse practitioners, physicians, staff nurses, outreach workers, and administrators. Each type of healthcare team member was able to add their expertise and leverage their expertise to identify all the resources available to the patient. This helped to shift the focus of treatment from episodic emergency care to long-term supportive treatment for the patients. At bimonthly meetings, treatment plans were developed for patients with the highest recent visits to the ED.

Other departments within the hospital saw value in the process, and soon began joining these treatment-planning meetings. During the meeting select participants would be designated to contact outpatient providers in order to collect collateral information and reengage outpatient teams.

With guidance from the ED QI team, a note template was developed within the electronic medical health system for documentation of the ACP (see Box 5.1). In developing the template, considerable thought was given to how to efficiently synthesize information to be immediately actionable to the ED provider team, often a distillation of a multitude of notes contained in the medical record. Outpatient providers were encouraged to write ACPs that clearly addressed who should be called when the patient arrives at the ED, steps to facilitate evaluation, medication suggestions, restrictions, specific protocols that should be followed, interventions that could be used to prevent admission, or issues that might impact a successful transition to home. Using the template, authors determined which information was relevant for each patient. Some ACPs were as simple as a phone number, while others provided complex treatment recommendations.

Box 5.1 Acute Care Plan

Note: Clinical management is ultimately determined at the discretion of the clinician caring for the patient
Ambulatory Care Team
(Primary care provider [PCP], registered nurse, social worker, visiting nurse service, hospice worker; contact information. If resident PCP, include preceptor as well.)
After Hours Clinical Contact
Key Specialists
(Specialist name and problem[s] managed – include only those with frequent involvement)
Key Caregivers/Contact Information
(Family members, in-home caretakers, day program contacts)

If patient presents for acute care, please consider:
Guide (remove instructions before you print for longitudinal medical record [LMR])
This section should highlight the four to five key points that will be useful to ED/inpatient clinicians at time of patient presentation, for example:

- *Particular member of ambulatory care team who should be called early in the course of evaluation (include title/role, contact information)*
- *Specific intervention that might prevent an admission or return to ED*
- *Any concrete steps/action plan that may facilitate evaluation and/or return home*
- *Contact specific outpatient provider for input (okay to page after-hours?)*
- *Admit to specific service/floor*
- *Pain medication recommendations/restrictions (be specific)*
- *Continue regular medications*
- *Consult pain service; other services*
- *Specific follow-up instructions if patient discharged home*
- *Notify specific clinician if patient discharged home*
- *Literacy issues that might impact safe/successful transition home*
- *Transportation issues that might impact timeliness of follow-up.*

(Patient should be aware of plan of care; should be reviewed and reinforced often with patient.)

Box 5.1 (*cont.*)

Current Clinical Management Plan
Immediate Active Problems (see LMR for detailed problem list)
  Guide (remove instructions before you print for LMR)
- *What problems has patient been presenting with recently?*
- *Which issues that are being actively managed could lead to an ED or inpatient visit?*
- *Which issues have required recent major medication changes?*

  Pain Management
  Pain/prescriptions managed by (provide name and contact information)
  Pain Management Care Plan
  Guide (remove instructions before you print for LMR)
  (Details, providers involved)
- *Specific pain management recommendations if pain is presenting symptom*
- *Details of any existing pain contract*
- *Follow-up plan and/or patient instructions if patient discharged home*
- *Clinician(s) to be contacted regarding patient follow-up if discharged home*
- *Pain management recommendations if patient admitted*
- *Any insurance or prescription issues*
- *Narcotics; person who is the prescriber for narcotics:*
  Name_____
  Contact information_____
  (must be able to be reached)

_____

Behavioral Health
Active Issues
  Behavioral Health Contract
  (Details, providers involved)
  Preferred Inpatient Unit

_____

Substance Abuse
Substance abuse history (include history of overdose, withdrawal, DTs)
- *Agree to detoxification: Yes or No*
- *Facility that usually agrees to accept patient (provide name)*
- *Banned from facilities (provide name[s])*

Treatment History
  Consider toxicology screen on presentation to ED/inpatient.

_____

Important Psychological and Psychosocial Elements
(Free form text)
  Is there a treatment contract in place?

_____

Prescription Issues
Guide (remove instructions before you print for LMR)
- *Special circumstances regarding medication delivery, specific pharmacy, hours of operation*
- *History of difficulty obtaining/affording prescriptions*

Box 5.1 (cont.)

Specific prescription problems that may interfere with care plan (health literacy issues, prior approval problems, etc.)

- *True allergies (allergic to everything but. . .)*

_____

Advance Care Planning
Healthcare professional
    (Name and contact information)
    Code status

_____

If patient is discharged home from ED:
Guide (remove instructions before you print for LMR)
    (Be as specific as possible, e.g., "E-mail PCP so s/he can arrange follow-up within XX days," or "Page PCP during business hours," etc.)

- *Patient to follow up with PCP/pain specialist within XX timeframe, how best to arrange*
- *Pain medication to be written for _____ days to maintain coverage until follow-up appt, OR patient should not receive pain medication from ED for chronic pain issues*
- *Care coordination practice based case manager*

If patient admitted to MGH (see above re: discharge from ED):
Referrals needed or made:
    Care plan endorsed by
    (PCP, also preceptor if resident PCP)
    Copy and paste the Continuity of Care plan into an LMR note; make sure
the label is "Acute Care Plan" so it can be recognized.

The ACP document remains in the EHR but needs to be copied, edited, and reentered in order to be flagged when the patient arrives at the ED. Any provider with access to patient documentation in the hospital EHR can update the ACP. Reminders are sent by e-mail to update the ACP as needed; in addition, primary care providers who work with the system receive automatic e-mails every time their patients are seen in the ED. Plans are considered "active" for 6 months; if not updated within this time frame they would no longer be automatically flagged in the EHR system. This was done to guard against outdated clinical information and acknowledge the likelihood of evolving treatment plans.

During a recent analysis, 119 MGH patients had an ACP. Among these, 41 (34%) were considered active and 78 (66%) had become inactive. For those high utilizers with an ACP, there was a 39 percent decrease in ED visit rates, resulting in a net decrease in 565 ED visits. Approximately 70 percent of all patients who had an ACP had a decrease in ED visit volume in the year following initiation of their ACP. In addition, 60 percent of patients with an active ACP had a decreased ED length of stay. The number of hospital admissions decreased by 48 percent for patients with an ACP, for a net decrease of 143 admissions. The effects appear to be sustained over time (years).

The cost of implementing the ACP was minimal but did require information system resources and care team members' time to create and update an ACP. The ACP does present a significant opportunity for cost savings to the healthcare system.

The effectiveness of the ACP is evident for Mr. S., a patient who is a paraplegic with bilateral below-the-knee amputations for osteomyletis and severe decubitus ulcers. He had a suprapubic tube and was homeless and wheelchair bound. The ACP was created by the patient's providers including his PCP, homeless outreach case manager, director of medical respite program, ED nurse, ED social worker, and ED physician during a conference in which the patient was present. The ACP encouraged use of a specialized shelter that could provide services for him with 24-hour-per-day access. Included in the plan was the name of and contact information for his outreach case manager. The case manager was available to meet the patient in the ED during the day or to provide assistance over the phone during the off hours. The plan specified that no new narcotic prescription was to be given from ED and that the PCP would be contacted to manage all opioid medications. If Mr. S did not meet the inpatient level of care for a hospital admission but required more skilled treatment than the shelter could manage, he could be admitted to a medical respite facility. Mr. S. had priority status for admission to the respite facility based on the ACP meeting. Gradually, after a few ED presentations, in which the ACP was followed, Mr. S. started to go to the shelter on his own instead of presenting to the ED. He worked with his case manager to obtain handicapped housing and eventually no longer returned to the ED. Three years later, he lives in his own apartment with visiting nurse services and is followed by his PCP and his case manager.

There are a number of lessons learned through the development of this program. The ACP requires buy-in from multiple partners in order to be successful. It relies on PCPs, other outpatient providers, ED case managers, ED nurses, and ED social workers in order to create the tool. Also, care team members need to continue to update the plans with relevant information. Although many of the ED providers within our system have used the tool, a number of the high-utilizer patients have PCPs outside our system, and it is often difficult to engage them in treatment planning. For these patients it often falls to ED nurses and social workers to formulate a plan, and then enter the ACP into the system. Last, while there has been consensus that the information in the ACPs is extremely useful to ED providers, there are times where the information is not actionable. For instance, during the overnight hours, our pain clinic is not open to see the patient. We have attempted to include providers and services that can be contacted 24 hours per day whenever feasible. In order to encourage the use of developed ACPs, PCPs within the system have a reported quality incentive measure in order to encourage PCPs of high utilizers to create and update ACPs. For ED physicians, a similar quality incentive measure was established to encourage providers to review ACPs.

Discussion

This ACP intervention for frequent ED visitors demonstrates the central and critical role that information technology can play in the coordination of care in the ED as a means to improve patient outcomes. The ACP intervention provided timely interdisciplinary treatment plans and important information regarding complex patients in an efficient and effective manner to the ED care team. This intervention led to improvements in the coordination of patient care for these complex, high-needs patients and was associated with an overall reduction in ED and inpatient utilization and healthcare costs.

A key factor in the ACP program's success was the accessibility of relevant and important information for frequent ED visitors from multiple care providers across the healthcare spectrum. Comprehensive information regarding complex patients is especially useful in the ED because generally emergency healthcare providers must make complex decisions regarding patient care with incomplete healthcare information.[6,7,8,9,10] While data suggest that ED physicians believe that longitudinal healthcare information would be beneficial, these physicians rate obtaining healthcare information from external sources as difficult or extremely difficult, and successful less than 50 percent of the time.[7,11,12] Due to the significant difficulties with accessing healthcare records, more than half of ED physicians report attempting to secure external healthcare records less than 10 percent of the time.[7,8,9,10,11,12] The facilitation of ready access to important healthcare information by the ACP is particularly relevant to the ED setting where longitudinal information from multiple care providers is often inaccessible due to a variety of patient and healthcare system factors.[8]

The importance and value of readily accessible interdisciplinary information and its potential to improve care is especially relevant for frequent ED visitors who are an at-risk, vulnerable population. Frequent visitors tend to be ill with complex medical conditions, have higher mortality than nonfrequent visitors, and often have psychosocial and financial concerns that impact their ability to successfully navigate the healthcare system.[13,14,15,16] The episodic treatment provided to frequent ED visitors contributes to fragmented, unco-ordinated care, as there is limited communication between the ED and facilities such as primary care offices, mental health practices, and specialty care practices. However, the ACP provided data to the ED care provider that included specialized treatment plans from the patient's PCP, case manager, or other clinician to help successfully guide ED treatment decisions and plans of care. These important data were accessed through the information technology system and readily available 24 hours per day, 7 days per week. The ACP provided integrated information from the healthcare providers who knew the patient best, thereby optimizing the patient's comprehensive medical care both in the ED and through-out the healthcare system.

The ACP program also offered the advantage of facilitating successful transitions of care between primary care and the ED. Transitions of care between the ED and other sectors of healthcare system are often associated with missing information, miscommunications, and limited or absent coordination of care. Data demonstrate that ED providers estimate that information gaps occur in up to a third of ED patient visits, with the missing information rated as very important or essential in half of the cases. These information gaps may lead to worse outcomes, including prolonged stays, increased costs, and the potential to comprom-ise the quality of patient care.[11] The ACP program specifically aided with increasing the efficiency of care by improving care transitions and potentially decreasing redundancy of efforts and healthcare costs while increasing patient satisfaction. This comprehensive approach to providing successful transitions of care will be essential to effectively facilitat-ing care coordination as healthcare reimbursement shifts from fee-for-service to account-able care organization initiatives and the US Department of Health and Human Services meaningful use requirements.[17]

Importantly, the ACP afforded a patient-specific approach to the management of frequent ED visitors. The care plan for each patient was completed by an interdisciplinary team and individualized to patient-specific care needs. The ACP also provided important information regarding patient-specific barriers to successful engagement with the health-care system and recommendations regarding how best to assist the patient with naviga-tion of the healthcare system. Future opportunities for ACP include eliciting patient participation in the determination of their plan in a patient-centered approach. This would enhance understanding of the goals of care for both patients and providers, potentially improving the satisfaction associated with both the provision and receipt of healthcare services.

The data on implementation of ACPs in other healthcare settings has demonstrated that ACPs are associated with a reduction in overall healthcare resource utilization. In a pre-postretrospective observational cohort study of 36 patients in the Community Resources for ED Overuse Program at the Henry Ford Health System, care plans created by the interdisciplinary team and accessible to all healthcare providers through the EHR were associated with a statistically significant reduction in ED visits, charges, laboratory testing, and total ED contact time (quantified as the product of the number of visits and length of stay at each visit).[18] In a single-center, prospective pragmatic study with retrospective data for comparison, care plans for 32 high-utilizing patients at St. Thomas' Hospital in London were associated with a significant decrease in median laboratory and radiology tests performed, number of ED visits, and hospital admissions.[19] In a single-center retrospective before-after study at the University of Chicago, multidisciplinary patient care plans for 50 selected high-utilizing ED patients showed a trend toward decreased ED visits.[20] In a single-center retrospective before-after study of 24 high-utilizing complex adult patients at Duke University Medical Center, multidisciplinary care plans implemented into the EHR were associated with a statistically significant decrease in hospital admissions, 30-day readmissions, and hospital costs. In this study, there was no significant change in ED visits and costs and no change in the inpatient length of stay.[21] The limitations of these studies include the single-center design with a small sample size and a pre-post analysis that may not account for potential healthcare utilization by high-utilizing patients at nearby healthcare facilities and may not incorporate changes in utilization among high-utilizing patients that may have occurred without any intervention.

If an institution is considering implementation of an electronic ACP to improve patient outcomes, important initial steps include an evidence-based, thoughtful program design with a robust methodologic strategy to evaluate the impact of the program on important patient outcomes. A critical step in the evaluation process is the identification of independent researchers at the onset of the program to help guide the development of rigorous methodology to successfully evaluate program outcomes. This is especially important in the high-utilizing population because existing data on these patients demonstrate that their high-utilizing status may be temporary with "regression to the mean" without any intervention.[22,23] For this reason, evaluation of any program for high-utilizing patients necessitates a valid comparison group, not just a before-and-after or pre-post design. Ideally, studies of high-utilizing patients would incorporate a randomized control trial design, but if this is not feasible, a valid control group with rigorous evaluation of the acute care program is necessary to successfully determine the true impact of the intervention on high-utilizing patients. This ACP program represents a key strength of the use of information technology to assist with the management of complex frequent ED visitors. The providers took a novel approach to providing integrated healthcare within the healthcare system, thereby improving patient care while simultaneously decreasing healthcare costs. As demonstrated by the innovative intervention outlined in this chapter, information technology can effectively aid healthcare providers in the management of complex patients, resulting in the timely provision of efficient, high-quality healthcare services.

References

1. Handel DA, Wears RL, Nathanson LA, Pines JM. Using information technology to improve the quality and safety of emergency care. *Academic Emergency Medicine.* 2011;18:e45–e51.

2. Institute of Medicine. *Crossing the Quality Chiasm: A New Health System for the 21st Century.* Washington, DC: National Academies Press, 2001.

3. Farley HL, Baumlin KM, Hamedani AG, Cheung DS, Edwards MR, Fuller DC, Genes N, Griffey RT, Kelly JJ, McClay JC, Nielson J, Phelan MP, Shapiro, JS, Stone-Griffith S, Pines JM. Quality and safety implications of emergency department information systems. *Annals of Emergency Medicine.* 2013;62:399–407.

4. American College of Emergency Physicians. Emergency department information systems: primer for emergency physicians, nurses, and IT professionals. 2009. Available at www.acep.org/WorkArea/DownloadAsset.aspx?id=45756. Accessed November 18, 2015.

5. Agency for Healthcare Research and Quality. Available at http://meps.ahrq.gov/mepsweb/data_stats/tables_compendia_hh_interactive. Accessed November 18, 2015.

6. Ben-Assuli O, Shabtai I, Leshno M. The impact of EHR and HIE on reducing avoidable admissions: controlling main differential diagnoses. *BMC Medical Informatics and Decision Making.* 2013;13:49.

7. Ben-Assuli O, Shabtal I, Leshno M. EHR in emergency rooms: exploring the effect of key information components on main complaints. *Journal of Medical Systems.* 2014;38:36.

8. Vest JR, Kern LM, Campion TR, Silver MD, Kaushal R. Association between use of a health information exchange system and hospital admission. *Applied Clinical Informatics.* 2014;5:219–231.

9. Stiell A, Forster AJ, Stiell IG, van Walraven C. Prevalence of information gaps in the emergency department and the effect on patient outcomes. *Canadian Medical Association Journal.* 2003;169:1023–1028.

10. Remen VM, Grimsmo A. Closing information gaps with shared electronic patient summaries: how much will it matter? *International Journal of Medical Informatics.* 2011;80:775–781.

11. Speedie SM, Park YT, Du J, Theera-Ampornpunt N, Bershow BA, Gensinger RA, Routhe DT, Connelly DP. The impact of electronic health records on people with diabetes in three different emergency departments. *Journal of the American Medical Informatics Association.* 2014;21:e71–e77.

12. Shapiro JS, Kanny J, Kushniruk AW, Kuperman G, and the New York Clinical Information Exchange Clinical Advisory Subcommittee. Emergency physicians' perceptions of health information exchange. *Journal of the American Medical Informatics Association.* 2007;14:700–705.

13. Ruger JP, Richter CJ, Spitznagel EL, Lewis LM. Analysis of costs, length of stay, and utilization of emergency department services by frequent users: implications for health policy. *Academic Emergency Medicine.* 2004;11:1311–1317.

14. Pines JM, Asplin BR, Kaji AH, Lowe RA, Magid DJ, Raven M, Weber EJ, Yealy DM. Frequent users of emergency department services: gaps in knowledge and a proposed research agenda. *Academic Emergency Medicine.* 2011;18:e64–e69.

15. Hunt KA, Weber EJ, Showstack JA, Colby DC, Callaham ML. Characteristics of frequent users of emergency departments. *Annals of Emergency Medicine.* 2006;48:1–8.

16. LaCalle E, Rabin E. Frequent users of emergency departments: the myths, the data, and the policy implications. *Annals of Emergency Medicine.* 2010;56:42–48.

17. Frisse ME, Johnson KB, Nian H, Davison CL, Gadd CS, Unertl KM, Turri PA, Chen Q. The financial impact of health information exchange of emergency department care. *Journal of the American*

Medical Informatics Association. 2012;19:328–333.

18. Stokes-Buzzelli S, Peltzer-Jones JM, Martin GB, Ford MM, Weise A. Use of health information technology to manage frequently presenting emergency department patients. *Western Journal of Emergency Medicine.* 2010;11:348–353.

19. Newton A, Sarker SJ, Parfitt A, Henderson K, Jaye P, Drake N. Individual care plans can reduce hospital admission rate for patients who frequently attend the emergency department. *Emergency Medicine Journal.* 2011;28:654–657.

20. Pillow MT, Doctor S, Brown S, Carter K, Mulliken R. An emergency department-initiated web-based multidisciplinary approach to decreasing emergency department visits by the top frequent visitors using patient care plans. *Journal of Emergency Medicine.* 2013;44:853–860.

21. Mercer T, Bae J, Kipnes J, Velazquez M, Thomas S, Setji N. The highest utilizers of care: individualized care plans to coordinate care, improve healthcare service utilization, and reduce costs at an academic tertiary care canter. *Journal of Hospital Medicine.* 2015;10:419–424.

22. Althaus F, Paroz S, Hugli O, Ghali WA, Daeppen J, Peytremann-Bridevaux I, Bodenmann P. Effectiveness of interventions targeting frequent users of emergency departments: a systematic review. *Annals of Emergency Medicine.* 2011;58:41–52.

23. Johnson TL, Rinehart DJ, Durfee J, Brewer D, Batal H, Blum J, Oronce CI, Melinkovich P, Gabow P. For many patients who use large amounts of health care services, the need is intense yet temporary. *Health Affairs.* 2015;34:1312–1319.

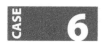

6   Emergency Care in an Integrated Healthcare Delivery System

The Kaiser Experience

Dana R. Sax, Jeffrey S. Selevan, and Wm. Wesley Fields

Introduction

Access to emergency department (ED) care without respect to the patient's ability to pay, including hospitalization for unstable conditions, was the first healthcare service to be protected under federal law in 1986 in the United States.[1] Prudent layperson laws extended these protections to persons with private health coverage soon thereafter in 1994, where the definition of an emergency medical condition was described as what would be considered an emergency by a "prudent layperson." Over the past 30 years as a result of universal access to EDs, hospital-based EDs have fulfilled several essential community services, from regionalized staging of life-threatening conditions to providing safety net care for vulnerable populations. ED visits have grown faster than population growth over the past two decades, and the intensity of ED resource utilization increased dramatically, along with the cost of ED care. The relative percentage of unscheduled hospital admissions originating from the ED has also steadily increased.[2-6] In addition, some research has linked expansion of health insurance coverage to greater ED utilization.[7] Greater life expectancy for Medicare beneficiaries, many with multiple chronic conditions, has also been shown to drive ED utilization and unscheduled hospital admissions.[8]

This chapter will discuss a health system that, despite several forces driving increased ED utilization, has developed strategies to help manage the demand for acute, unscheduled care services, including ED care, and has set national benchmarks for quality and limited population costs. As the US healthcare market shifts slowly to payment models that reward value over volume, it may be possible to learn from groups that have approached some of the broader issues in acute care through integrative approaches.

Case Study

Kaiser Permanente (KP) California is an example of acute care delivery that focuses on patient- and population-level health while being population cost efficient. In 2011, KP California, with almost seven million members, incurred significantly lower ED utilization than the State of California as a whole, and much lower than the United States. Furthermore, these findings were associated with fewer hospital admissions, lower length of stay, and fewer readmissions, while maintaining the highest quality standards.[11] After taking into account population morbidity as well as personal financial contributions to accessing ED services, KP may offer a model for how acute care might be better integrated in other domains through shared risk, financial alignment, and codesign of services between health plans, medical groups, and hospital systems.

This chapter uses the principal care delivery strategies of Kaiser Permanente California's acute care system as a business case study of how an organization can effectively support individual and population health while controlling costs. Central to KP California's ability to provide high-value care to its almost eight million members (as of 2015) is the alignment of financial incentives and care strategies between health plan, providers, hospitals, and members.

KP is the largest managed care operation in the United States and operates in eight states and the District of Columbia. In 2011, about 6,821,000 Californians, or 18 percent, were enrolled in the Kaiser Foundation Health Plan (approximately evenly split between northern and southern California regions of KP). Prior studies comparing KP members with other insured Californians found no difference with regard to age, race, or employment status, though KP members had lower mean income levels.[12]

KP's model of care focuses on improving individual patient health, promoting overall population health, and reducing per capita costs of care. A core strategy has been the alignment of financial incentives between the entities: multispecialty medical groups (Southern California Permanente Medical Group [SCPMG] and the Permanente Medical Group, Incorporated [TPMG] in northern California), Kaiser Foundation Hospitals (KFH), and the Kaiser Foundation Health Plan (KFHP). KP receives fixed prepaid premiums for the vast majority of its members; the shared strategy of these entities is to deliver affordable high-value care to keep patients enrolled and healthy. There are no financial incentives for providing ED care or hospitalizations when similar services can be delivered in a lower intensity and more convenient setting. In addition, cost sharing by KP California members for acute care services is low: in 2011, 86 percent of members had no deductible and 95 percent had a $100 or less copay for ED care.[13]

One key KP strategy of acute care is effective "demand management," that is, matching patient demand for acute care services to the most appropriate clinical setting. All KP members have access to advice nurses 24 hours per day and, through carefully vetted protocols and algorithms, are provided real-time clinical advice or directed to the most appropriate clinical setting. In some cases, especially those where the nurse thinks the patient may need ED services, calls are directed to an ED physician on call to help triage the patient to the best suited clinical site. This allows many complaints to be safely managed at home, in urgent but lower intensity (non-ED) settings or through next-day appointments. KP OnCall is Southern California's clinical advice center and is owned by KFH; SCPMG purchases this service from KFH to help manage acute care demand and coordinate care. Of the 850,000 calls fielded by KP OnCall in 2011, about 10 percent led to advice for home management, and another third are directed to same-day or next-day office follow-up appointments (Table CS6.1).

Another critical strategy has been the development of a comprehensive electronic health record (EHR), HealthConnect, to allow patients, providers, and hospitals to share information across clinical settings. HealthConnect is the largest private deployment of EHRs in the world,[14] has been implemented in every KP medical facility (more than 550 medical offices and 37 hospitals), and is available via smartphone. In 2011, members exchanged more than 12 million secure e-mails with caregivers and securely viewed more than 29 million lab test results online.[14] Outpatient use of HealthConnect has been associated with reductions in ED visits and hospitalizations for patients with diabetes,[15] and patient–clinician secure messaging was associated with significant improvements in Healthcare Effectiveness Data and Information Set (HEDIS) measures, including glycemic, cholesterol, and blood pressure control.[16] The EHR is also used to proactively identify and more closely follow high-risk members who may need more intense case management. While ED providers are not usually involved in patient follow-up and continuity of care in less integrated systems, KP ED providers use HealthConnect to reassess patients after discharge,

Table CS6.1 Southern California Kaiser Member Disposition Following KP OnCall Advice Nurse Assessment and Referral, 2011

Call type	Percentage of calls	Total number of calls
Other	21.3*	181,193
911	1.2	9,882
Pediatric urgent care	2.7	23,240
Home treatment	10.3	87,500
Urgent care	12.5	106,222
Emergency department	17.6	149,289
Office	34.4	291,727
Total	100	849,053

* About one-third of "other" calls are directed to a poison control center, one-third are nonclinical, and one-third involve calling a doctor. This information is based on personal correspondence between the authors of this chapter and Brad Schwartz, Medical Director of KP OnCall.

Source: Kaiser OnCall internal data provided by Brad Schwartz, Medical Director of KP OnCall.

answer patients' postdischarge clinical questions, place outpatient referrals to specialists (and many times direct book appointments), order further outpatient diagnostic studies, and message primary care providers to assure appropriate follow-up.

Health information through HealthConnect is also accessible to nonplan EDs when patients visit outside hospitals. Approximately 15 percent of KP member ED visits occur at non-KFH EDs. KP California's Emergency Prospective Review Program (EPRP) allows for smooth transitions of care for these offsite ED visits. The EPRP center is staffed 24 hours per day, 7 days per week, and 365 days per year by emergency physicians and ED/critical care nurses, and through the center, non-KP providers treating KP members at non-KP EDs have real-time telephonic access to Permanente emergency physicians and all existing medical records. This form of an interoperable health information exchange predates current EHRs and was available in the early 1990s for all KP Southern California members. When indicated, EPRP providers also help provide interfacility transfers (including critical care transport with a physician) to "repatriate" KP members to KP-owned facilities. The program has resulted in the transfer of high-risk patients without adverse impact on clinical outcomes or resource use.[17]

KP has also worked to develop smooth transitions of care across time and clinical settings within KP, with the ED recognized as pivotal along this continuum. From a care delivery system perspective, it is more efficient to obviate the need for the ED visit in the first place, and for the patient this is more convenient. Members who frequently need ED or hospital care for chronic disease management are identified and provided with more intensive inpatient and outpatient programs. Care managers – specialty trained nurses, social workers, or clinical pharmacists – support ED, inpatient, and primary care providers to manage patients with advanced disease or complex comorbidities. Care managers often work closely with ED providers to improve transitions of care and follow-up. In addition, development of the specialized care management teams has improved resource utilization and clinical outcomes. For example, a heart failure disease management program, which combines inpatient care management, ED, and inpatient follow-up via primary care and home health care visits, led to a 90-day heart failure readmission rate drop of 30 percent, significant decreases in ED visits, and lower mortality rates.[18] The program demonstrates how a hospital system (by supporting programs to avoid readmissions for insured patients), an insurance company (by investing in systems to support providers clinically), and physician groups (by adopting models to improve care) have worked together to improve population health management.

Along the same line, KP California has adopted a philosophy of higher intensity of ED care across the board, particularly when inpatient hospitalization is a consideration. This approach recognizes the relative facility cost differential between an ED visit and an inpatient admission, which are many-fold higher.[5,19] The strategy is to support greater disease management in the ED or observation units via increased diagnostic and treatment capabilities and specialist consultation. While rapid throughput is a priority for patients with low-acuity conditions and patients who immediately require admission to the hospital, throughput is less of a priority for patients with undifferentiated conditions requiring extensive diagnostic work-ups. This allows for a more extensive diagnostic work-up or satisfactory treatment/resolution of a presenting complaint in the ED, often negating the need for hospitalization.

More intensive ED care, often with patients who have been directed to the ED through the advice nurse system, often lead to longer ED lengths of stay and, on average, fewer patients seen per hour for KP emergency physicians than in other community EDs. This likely partly explains the lower admission rates at KFH hospitals than at non-KFH hospitals in California and across the country for Medicare and private patients (Table CS6.2).[10,20,21] Lower ED admission rates may be associated with a clinical culture within the medical group that encourages ED providers and their consultants to provide more intensive services before making a decision to admit, and a compensation system that does not discourage these clinical practices. This includes the extensive use of advanced diagnostic testing, consultations by specialists, ED disease management or observation periods, arrangement of follow-up appointments, and next-day electronic or telephone communication with patients. Physician compensation is largely based on clinical time and not units of service provided (visits or relative value units). There are modest physician compensation incentives for meeting clinical goals, group norms, and ensuring patients have a good experience. While investing in intense ED work-ups may be expensive, this strategy is promoted and supported by the health plan, providers, and hospital system because of the shared belief that it helps control overall population health costs, while not negatively impacting outcomes. As opposed to rewarding higher patient volume per provider and faster ED throughput, this strategy emphasizes provision of care in a more resource-efficient manner by supporting EDs to intensely evaluate and manage patients who in other settings might have been admitted to the hospital. While the Kaiser population may not be exactly comparable to a broad population of non-Kaiser patients, Table CS6.2 demonstrates lower utilization of ED services and admission rates among KP California members as compared with California and national averages.[9,19,20]

Finally, the core tenet and KP's overarching philosophy is the alignment of financial incentives between providers, hospitals, and the health plan. KFH, medical groups, and KFHP share accountability for the allocation of resources and services, facilities, and special programs to meet goals that are mutually beneficial to patients. Innovation, cross subsidization between entities, and shared decision-making promote collaboration between entities

Table CS6.2 Emergency Department Utilization and Hospital Admission Rates for the United States, California, and Kaiser Permanente (KP) California Members, 2010 and 2011

	Population[9]	Utilization rates per 1,000 people	Admission rates after ED evaluation
US population (2010)[19]	308,745,538	418	15.3%
Total	268,477,546	398	10.2%
<65	40,267,984	548	40.3%
≥65			
Non-KP California (2011)[20]	30,826,342	334	15.7%
Total	27,616,821	314	10.9%
<65	3,509,490	456	41.7%
≥65			
KP California (2011)[9]	6,821,382	244	13.2%
Total	5,926,085	206	8.2%
<65	895,297	496	27.1%
≥65			

Notes: Statistics on national and California-specific ED utilization and admission rates come from publicly available datasets. For national data, we used the Healthcare Cost and Utilization Project's National Emergency Department Sample (NEDS), the largest all-payer ED database in the United States.[20] The most recent year in which data were available from the NEDS was 2010. For California data, we used the 2011 State of California's Office of Statewide Health Planning and Development Emergency Department and Ambulatory Surgery Data (treat and release patient visits) and Patient Discharge Data (admitted patient visits).[21] Data on KP's utilization and admission rates is from the Management Information and Analysis department at KP California.[9]

that in other settings may have competing priorities. For example, the telephone advice system in southern California (KP OnCall) was purchased and owned by KFH, but provides the medical groups and members a service to manage demand for acute care safely, timely, and cost effectively, often avoiding unnecessary admissions in an "insured" population. Another example is KHFP's multibillion-dollar investment in HealthConnect for the benefit of KFH, the medical groups, and its members. Yet another is the medical groups' decision to provide (at their expense) 24-hour in-hospital coverage of all major primary specialties (e.g., pediatrics, internal medicine, obstetrics and gynecology, general surgery) and access to other specialty consultation in the ED. ED providers are encouraged to thoroughly evaluate and manage patients who in other settings might be admitted from the start. This greater intensity of ED care helps KFH limit potentially avoidable admissions and provides members with timely access to specialist care and disease management services in the ED and ambulatory care setting. The financial benefit of these efforts would accrue to the health plan, at the expense of the providers, in most other healthcare systems in the United States. Ultimately the patient benefits from cross subsidization.

This collaboration also allows for financial and risk-sharing agreements between KFHP and the KP medical groups to promote appropriate utilization without financially rewarding the denial of covered medically necessary care, nor incentivizing the provision of potentially avoidable care. Medical groups retain full accountability for all clinical care decisions. The contractual relationship between the medical groups and KFHP places significant limits on the amount that can be retained by the medical group when its revenue exceeds budgeted expenses. KP recognizes that clinical outcomes may be negatively affected by withholding covered clinically indicated care, leading ultimately to greater expenses, and

KFHP and the KP medical groups share in these downside financial risks, just as they recognize that misaligned financial incentives for utilization can lead to avoidable (and possibly harmful) care.

Discussion

Taken together, the elements of KP represent an industrial design for acute care integration that may be modeled by other accountable care organizations. Many individual elements deserve replication to validate their effectiveness in other systems. Yet some might argue that there are significant barriers to their wider adoption in the US healthcare system, which remains fragmented and often poorly aligned. While considering how KP's strategies may be applied in other systems, the first step is to "disintegrate" three major healthcare industries to understand potential challenges and opportunities.

First, it is worth a brief mention of how payment models and risk pooling work in most systems to cover healthcare costs. Most members of private plans contribute far more in premiums than they receive in health care services for any actuarial period. Cross subsidy within risk pools allow insurers to maintain sufficient resources to cover the costs of care for the relatively small number of members who generate the most financially significant medical events – plus administrative overhead, reinsurance, and capital reserves. Government-sponsored programs cross subsidize even more dramatically, with taxpayers providing sufficient revenue to cover the costs of care to US residents covered by programs such as Medicare and Medicaid. Historically, hospital systems cross subsidized the cost of services to the uninsured and underinsured by collecting more generous payments from commercial plans for services to their patients. Hospital-based physicians participating in ED staffing or backup engaged in similar billing and contracting practices, increasingly with cross subsidization of their professional services from the hospital directly. Indeed, one of the stated rationales of the Affordable Care Act was to disrupt this vicious cycle of cost shifting.

Therefore, a question regarding wider adoption of the KP acute care model may be: what are the conditions under which stakeholders are more willing to share risk and capital by cross subsidies across industries, rather than within entities and silos?

Health plans. Insurance providers are most likely to provide capital and share risk when they recognize an opportunity to reduce medical costs and improve patient outcomes or experience. Based on the KP data, this would appear to be most likely for ED-based programs aimed at reducing avoidable admissions, the largest single cost center for most healthcare programs.[5] With proper alignment and support, such programs are well positioned to deliver transitions of care for patients other than admissions or readmissions of marginal value.[10] Health plans can also be expected to add value and protect their own profitability by sharing risk with contracted providers or by directly employing providers. United Healthcare, for example, is beginning to acquire physician groups for more exclusive managed covered services.

Hospital systems. Lack of integration and misalignments of financial incentives between providers, payers, and hospitals are significant drivers of ED utilization for less urgent complaints. Recent years have seen rapid growth in the number and scope of ambulatory care clinics for unscheduled care. Hospitals have been active in this sector, sometimes to address crowding in their own EDs, but more frequently to attract well-insured patients from their competitors. While some have argued that the marginal cost of ambulatory care for less complex episodes is low, the opportunity cost to hospitals that fail to promote wider access to urgent care in their communities is high.[9] The evidence from the KP model suggests that ED demand and capacity should be strategically managed and integrated for the subset of patients who represent the highest cost and risk within the population.

Physicians. Regardless of specialty, physicians in most provider groups remain incentivized to be individually productive under fee-for-service systems. This inherently leads to misalignment of incentives and competing priorities with hospitals and health plans. Most primary care providers balance professional lifestyle and payment by seeing patients in fully scheduled blocks, and increasingly defer to hospital-based providers for inpatient and after-hour care. Studies have confirmed the common refrain of patients: primary care providers are seldom available for unscheduled urgent care.[22] Most demand models suggest that the US healthcare system will require tens of thousands more physicians and allied providers than are currently being produced by our postgraduate medical education system. The KP acute care model suggests that medical homes are not the optimal location for all forms of acute or episodic care. Data and experience from KP suggest that patients with complex medical problems who become unstable despite community-based case management or individuals with new, undifferentiated complaints that may be emergency medical conditions should be rapidly evaluated in or near the ED, the crucial interface between community and hospital settings. Integration between providers across settings and time also allows for smooth transitions and optimal outcomes for patients.

In summary, KP's integration and shared financial risk between the payer (health plan), providers (the Permanente Medical Groups), and hospitals (KFH) allow for the coordinated delivery of health care for large populations in a diverse geographical setting. Cross subsidies between entities abound and are critical for success. Plan and provider revenue based on a prepayment methodology are facilitators, but may not be essential. Examples exist of a few successful systems that are not capitated, but they are a rarity and require extraordinary commitment and collaboration among all entities. Furthermore, KP has been successful in some parts of the country where it does not own and operate its own KFH hospitals. We believe the shift from fee-for-service to value-based models is also a key element of financially accountable organizations and critical to promoting population health. Recognizing the critical value of EDs and providing the resources for them to effectively carry out multiple roles will also be essential for developing health systems. Financial alignment and system integration are key to this evolution.

References

1. Consolidated Omnibus Budget Reconciliation Act of 1985 (COBRA). PL 99-272. Title IX, Section 9121, 100 Stat 167 (1986).

2. Pitts SR, Carrier ER, Rich EC, Kellermann AL. Where Americans get acute care: increasingly, it's not at their doctor's office. *Health Affairs (Millwood)*. 2010;29 (9):1620–1629.

3. Tang N, Stein J, Hsia RY, Maselli JH, Gonzales R. Trends and characteristics of US emergency department visits, 1997–2007. *JAMA*. 2010 Aug 11;304 (6):664–670.

4. Pines JM, Mullins PM, Cooper JK, Feng LB, Roth KE. National trends in emergency department use, care patterns, and quality of care of older adults in the United States. Journal of the American Geriatrics Society. 2013 Jan;61(1):12–17.

5. Gonzalez Morganti K, Bauhoff S, Blanchard JC, Abir M, Iyer N, Smith A, Vesely JV, Okeke EN, Kellermann AL. *The Evolving Role of Emergency Departments in*

the United States. Santa Monica, CA: RAND Corporation, 2013. Available at www.rand.org/pubs/research_reports/RR280. Accessed June 10, 2013.

6. Massachusetts Division of Health Care Finance and Policy. Non-emergency and preventable ED visits. *Analysis in Brief*, vol. 2004. 2004.

7. Lochner KA, Goodman RA, Posner S, Parekh A. Multiple chronic conditions among Medicare beneficiaries: state-level variations in prevalence, utilization, and cost, 2011. *Medicare Medicaid Res Rev.* 2013 Jul 23;3(3):eCollection2013. www.dor.kaiser.org/external/comparison_kaiser_vs_nonKaiser_adults_kpnc/.

8. Williams, RM. The costs of visits to the emergency department. *The New England Journal of Medicine* 1996;334:642–646.

9. Smulowitz PB, Honigman L, Landon BE. A novel approach to identifying targets for cost reduction in the emergency department. *Annals of Emergency Medicine.* 2013 Mar;61(3):293–300.

10. Taubman SL, Allen, HL, Wright BJ, Baicker K, Finkelstien AN. Medicaid increases emergency-department use: evidence from Oregon's health insurance experiment. *Science.* 2014;343(6168):263–268.

11. Selevan J, Kindermann D, Pines JM, and Fields WW. What accountable care organizations can learn from Kaiser Permanente California's acute care strategy. *Population Health Management.* 2015 Aug;18(4):233–236.

12. Gordon NP. *How Does the Adult Kaiser Permanente Membership in Northern California Compare with the Larger Community?* Oakland, CA: Kaiser Permanente Division of Research, June 2006. Available at www.dor.kaiser.org/external/comparison_kaiser_vs_nonKaiser_adults_kpnc/. Accessed May 5, 2013.

13. December 2011 Kaiser Permanente California Membership. Prepared by Kaiser Permanente Management Information and Analysis Membership Monthly Growth Report (MMGR), December 2011.

14. About Kaiser Permanente: Kaiser Permanente HealthConnect® Electronic Health Record. Available at http://xnet.kp.org/newscenter/aboutkp/healthconnect/. Accessed June 4, 2013.

15. Reed M, Huang J, Brand R, Graetz I, Neugebauer R, Fireman B, Jaffe M, Ballard DW, Hsu J. Implementation of an outpatient electronic health record and emergency department visits, hospitalizations, and office visits among patients with diabetes. *JAMA.* 2013 Sep 11;310(10):1060–1065.

16. Zhou YY, Kanter MH, Wang JJ, Garrido T. Improved quality at Kaiser Permanente through e-mail between physicians and patients. *Health Affairs (Millwood).* 2010 Jul;29(7):1370–1375.

17. Selevan JS, Fields WW, Chen W, Petitti DB, Wolde-Tsadik G. Critical care transport: outcome evaluation after interfacility transfer and hospitalization. *Annals of Emergency Medicine.* 1999 Jan;33(1):33–43.

18. Internal KP data systems used for quality and data analysis.

19. Mogranti KG, Bauhoff S, Blanchard JC, Abir M, Neema I, Smith AC, Vesely JV, Okeke EN, and Kellermann AL. The evolving role of emergency departments in the United States. RAND Corporation. 2013.

20. HCUP National Emergency Department Databases (NEDS). *Healthcare Cost and Utilization Project (HCUP).* Rockville, MD: Agency for Healthcare Research and Quality. Available at www.hcup-us.ahrq.gov/nedsoverview.jsp; 2011.

21. California Office of Statewide Health Planning and Development. Healthcare Information Division. Emergency Department Discharges, Public Data Set and Patient Discharges, Public Data Set, 2008–2011.

22. O'Malley A. After-hours access to primary care practices linked with lower emergency department use and less unmet medical need. *Health Affairs (Millwood).* 2016 Feb;35(2):175–183.

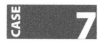

7 Urgent Care Centers

An Alternative to Unscheduled Primary Care and Emergency Department Care

Judd E. Hollander and Jesse M. Pines

Introduction

The concept of "urgent care" is commonly defined as walk-in care for acute, non-life-threatening illnesses and injuries. Urgent care centers are traditionally open for at least 12 hours per day and commonly on weekends. Some are open as early as 7 AM and close as late as 12 AM. As compared with traditional primary care, urgent care centers can also provide several additional services such as onsite plain radiography, intravenous fluids and medications, laceration repairs, basic orthopedic care, and treatment of abscesses. Many urgent care centers also provide urine- and blood-based diagnostic testing such as strep tests, urinalysis, complete blood counts, and basic metabolic panels.

Staffing consists of physicians and advanced practitioners (nurse practitioners or physician assistants) able to treat all age groups for a very wide range of illnesses and injuries, which cross all specialties of care, including orthopedics, pulmonary, cardiology, dermatology, surgery, obstetrics and gynecology, psychiatry, and more. Urgent care is intended to complement primary care practices by providing services to patients when primary care is not accessible due to scheduling constraints, or for problems that require skills or resources not commonly provided by primary care providers such as minor procedures, radiography, and laboratory testing. In addition, it has been estimated that 27 percent of US emergency department (ED) visits could be handled in urgent care centers.[1]

At one extreme, urgent care centers are operated by large corporations that have multiple sites in multiple states and operate as for-profit ventures. There are several local and regional multisite operations and a few national players. Many of the multisite practices are backed by institutional investors or owned by an insurance company. There are some few regional players that were founded by physicians and then emerged as leaders by taking on capital to scale their model. At the other end of the spectrum, sites are run by health systems as a strategy to increase access, even if they do not generate standalone profits.

The concept of an urgent care center started in the 1970s with physicians opening clinics to meet patient needs. Urgent care centers peaked in the mid-1980s, then experienced a precipitous decline, primarily because the clinics were staffed by physicians who did not have adequate training to care for the spectrum of acute, unscheduled care.

However, since the mid-1980s, there has been an increase in urgent care centers across the United States, primarily designed as a way to fill the shortage of primary care providers and to provide after-hours care when primary care providers' offices are closed. In addition, the comparative cost of an urgent care center visit relative to an ED visit has caused insurance plans and employers to actually assist patients in finding urgent care centers rather than going to the ED. Below we describe two models of urgent care centers in the United States.

PhysicianOne Urgent Care

PhysicianOne Urgent Care (www.physicianoneurgentcare.com) is one of regional leaders in the industry. It was founded by three emergency physicians in Connecticut. PhysicianOne's competitive distinction comes from achieving a consistently exceptional customer journey, whether the patient is seen on a Monday at 10 AM or Thanksgiving afternoon at 2, and by providing care on par with an ED for non-life-threatening illnesses and injuries. By focusing on the end-to-end experience of each patient, PhysicianOne has built a loyal following of patients as demonstrated by over 50 percent of the patients returning for subsequent care.

PhysicianOne's team is key to its success. In addition to a competitive benefit package and opportunities for continuous learning, the team is rewarded for obtaining customer feedback, being sensitive to a patient's time, and ensuring their experience is exceptional. PhysicianOne has built a successful business that will help hundreds of thousands of patients in Connecticut, New York, and Massachusetts in more 25 communities by the end of 2016.

In the for-profit arena, urgent care business success is defined as four-wall earnings before interest, tax, depreciation, and amortization (EBITDA) margins of over 30 percent. The key to achieving a profitable business is building a loyal customer following and controlling staffing costs. However, urgent care is a tough business since most facilities are open 75–80 hours each week, and the patients tend to come in waves. PhysicianOne urgent care focuses on controlling costs by making sure its teams are well trained and work effectively as a team to ensure that the stress of peak volumes is transparent to the patient customers.

Jefferson Urgent Care

In contrast to the for-profit model, Jefferson Health has incorporated urgent care into its access strategy (http://hospitals.jefferson.edu/departments-and-services/urgent-care). In this model the goal is not to maximize EBIDTA, but rather to create a unique patient-focused access point and to acquire new life-long customers. For that reason, many of the urgent care centers are located in close proximity to the hospital. Currently, five urgent care centers are opened or being opened, four within a mile of the main hospital in downtown Philadelphia. One of the sites is three blocks from the ED. Despite this, ED volume has continued to grow at the same pace, even though the urgent care center was seeing 40 patients per day shortly after opening. The majority of the patients did not identify a primary care provider either within or outside Jefferson, providing Jefferson Health an opportunity to provide care to this unique group of patients.

As this model is heavily focused on customer acquisition, it is of paramount importance to have an integrated electronic health record with the parent organization. Providers in the urgent care centers can view the inpatient, ambulatory, and ED records of the patients known to Jefferson. Likewise, physicians in these other locations must be able to view the records of the urgent care visits.

Best Practices

The best practices used by successful Urgent Care companies are listed below.

Site selection: Retail location of 3,000–4,000 square feet with great signage and visibility to more than 20,000 people/cars per day. Ideally in location with a daily anchor (such as a grocery store, pharmacy, or superstore). One simple way to do a preliminary assessment of location is to see if there is a Starbucks, Lowes, or major bank at the location.

Population:	>30,000 commercially insured people within a 10–15 minute drive time radius
Household income:	>$50,000 per/year
Staffing:	Physicians and/or advanced practitioners with experience in emergency medicine or family medicine with procedural experience.
	Other staffing includes radiologic technician, medical assistant or emergency medical technician, patient services associate. The key to a successful bottom line is adding incremental staff based on volume and focusing as much on teamwork as the number of full-time employees. Most centers start with three full-time employees per day and add an MA when they reach an average of >35 patients per day. An additional provider is usually not added until a clinic consistently is caring for more than four patients per hour. As allowed by state laws, highly experienced advanced practitioners are utilized by many urgent care practices. Many leading urgent care companies including PhysicianOne employ 50–75 percent advanced practitioners.
Hours:	Extended hours Monday to Friday; weekend and holiday hours
Services offered:	Basic point-of-care laboratories, radiography, standardized processes, and clinical pathways.
Efficiency:	Improving access and intake speed through same-day on-line scheduling and preregistration can help decrease door-to-doctor times.
Service levels:	Follow Net Promoter System and focus on door-to-Discharge time <50 minutes.
Marketing:	Robust digital strategy, grass roots, and developing promoters. Marketing needs to be prioritized, placing the advertisement in front of the patients who need the service.
Costs:	Capital costs and operating losses. Most successful operations will cost $600,000–800,000 to open and cover 3–6 months of operating losses.

Most brands in urgent care are located in the suburbs or urban areas populated by high incomes and distinguished by number of locations and little else. There are a few players who have overcome this distinction by ensuring they are seamlessly integrated into the care system. For example, both PhysicianOne Urgent Care and Jefferson Urgent Care ensure that patient treatment plans are shared with the patient's primary care provider. They also facilitate transitions in care either by ensuring that the patient's follow-up care is directed by the primary care provider or, if needed, by coordinating care with an appropriate specialist. All patients are contacted to confirm understanding of treatment plan and follow-up.

Consumer-centric care is on the rise and urgent care provides patients with the right care at the right time at the right price. As the payment model moves from fee-for-service to value-based care, urgent care centers are leading the way. Most urgent care centers already receive bundled reimbursement, meaning that higher value, lower cost care with fewer unnecessary tests is already being incentivized.

Urgent care is a sustainable business model that creates a local and personal health care encounter, while creating cost savings in the health system. Urgent care is one of the few innovations in healthcare that saves time and money for everyone.

Discussion

According to the Urgent Care Association of America (UCAOA), there are more than 7,100 urgent care centers in the United States.[2] The success has been attributed to providing an alternative to long waits for primary care appointments and crowded EDs, as well as providing accessible care and after-hours appointments.

While urgent care centers were historically independently owned and stand-alone facilities, the landscape of urgent care centers has changed. Now, there are large urgent care centers chains like PhysicianOne Urgent Care in many regions. In addition, hospital systems like Jefferson Health are getting into the urgent care business, using the centers to expand their service area and increase referrals. In addition, health insurers are in favor of the increase in urgent care centers with the goal of shifting higher cost ED care to these lower cost facilities.

As described above, the economics of urgent care must fit into the local marketplace, and urgent care centers are traditionally established in higher income, more populated areas. Specifically, urgent care centers are commonly placed in affluent areas with high concentrations of employer-sponsored health insurance and a young population. According to the UCAOA, 35 percent of urgent care centers are owned by physician groups, 30 percent by corporations, 25 percent by hospitals, and about 10 percent by other groups (i.e., nonphysicians and franchisors).[2] However, this balance differs considerably by community.

Yet despite the increasing popularity of urgent care centers, their impact on overall costs is not entirely clear. Urgent care centers were originally designed to keep people out of the ED, but it is unclear whether urgent care really substitutes for any considerable portion of ED care, or whether the visits substitute more for primary care visits. In addition, while urgent care centers do fill an access gap by providing walk-in care, they generally serve those who are privately insured or have Medicare insurance. In addition, unlike hospital-based EDs, urgent care centers are not subject to the Emergency Medical Treatment and Active Labor Act (EMTALA), a federal law that requires EDs to provide medical screening examinations regardless of whether patients can pay. But in some cases, urgent care centers that operate under a hospital's license may be subject to EMTALA. Many urgent care centers do not participate in Medicaid because of low payment rates. In addition, urgent care centers typically will not serve the uninsured without requiring an up-front payment.

There is also concern that urgent care centers disrupt care coordination particularly with primary care providers, because care is often handled in isolation of other ongoing healthcare needs, and urgent care centers frequently do not have access to patient medical records. However, an alternative argument is that urgent care centers are designed to deliver episodic care for isolated problems where access to broader electronic medical records and more complex cases or those requiring more advanced services are referred to EDs or back to their primary care physicians. While many urgent care centers today do not play a major role in care coordination, this may evolve in the future as more urgent care centers are affiliated with hospitals and health systems, and payment models change to payment bundles and capitated payments.

In the future, with an increased focus on value in healthcare payments in the United States, it is likely that the urgent care center model will continue grow. Particularly as more people gain coverage through the Affordable Care Act and the population ages in the context of primary care shortages, urgent care centers will fill an important gap in low-acuity but urgent care needs of the population. In addition, urgent care centers may be a viable alternative for people who have trouble establishing a relationship with a primary care physician. However, the potential for urgent care centers to offer cost savings could be expanded even more by increasing the accessibility of urgent care centers to more low-income patients, such as those with Medicaid and the uninsured, who often have no other alternative but to use hospital-based EDs. While there may be little incentive for independent urgent care centers to expand their business to the underserved in a solely fee-for-service model, hospitals and other groups that are participating in alternative payment models such as accountable care organizations that can receive shared savings may find urgent care centers as a way to substitute for some low-acuity ED use in a cost-effective manner. Urgent care centers may also be able to justify higher payments, particularly from Medicaid managed care plans, if they are able to reduce higher-cost ED use.

Ultimately, as more and more urgent care centers are owned by hospitals and health systems, as in the case of Jefferson Health, it is likely that urgent care centers will play a greater role in care coordination. This may change the role that urgent care centers play in the future, as they may be able to expand service offerings and treat more complex conditions in coordination with primary care.

References

1. Weinick RM, Burns RM, Mehrotra A. Many emergency department visits could be managed at urgent care centers and retail clinics. *Health Affairs (Millwood)*. 2010 Sep;29(9):1630–1636.

2. Urgent Care Association of America. Available at www.ucaoa.org/?page= IndustryFAQs.

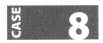

8   The "No-Wait" Emergency Department

Christopher McStay and Jody Crane

The Holy Grail of flow in the emergency department is the "no-wait" emergency department (ED), where there is, *literally*, no waiting throughout the patient journey. Everything that is value-added occurs as planned, when and where it is supposed to happen. The patient is seen and evaluated, receives the necessary diagnostic and treatment interventions in a reliable fashion, and is discharged in a timely, predictable manner.

The analogy to the Holy Grail is not a casual one. Due to the operational complexities of the ED, most would agree that creating an ED without waiting is challenging, if not impossible. This is because it is difficult to control the variation in the system.[1] The variation in arrivals is maximal due to the fact that acute patient illness follows a Poisson distribution.[2] The variation in the ability to serve patients is also extreme due to the variable nature of patient clinical presentations and the complex nature of healthcare delivery, which has yet to find all of the answers, much less the diagnostic tools to find these answers. Perhaps the greatest impact on our ability to care for patients in the ED is the fact that it is the common endpoint for all healthcare system dysfunction. The end symptom of almost every breakdown in healthcare is a dysfunctional ED. Whether we have hospital crowding, nurse shortages, a lack of specialists or primary care physicians in the community, or a natural or terrorist epidemic, all of these crises ultimately impact the emergency department, thus aptly referred to as the "safety net."

Much work has been done over the past decade or more on creating ED flow perfection. Important foundations have been laid by pioneers across the country: Mary Washington Healthcare in Virginia, with "RATED-ER" and "Super Track"; Ochsner in Louisiana, with "Q-Track"; Penn State Hershey in Pennsylvania, with "Physician Directed Queuing" (PDQ); Banner in Arizona, with "Split Flow"; Innova Fairfax in Virginia, with "Team Triage"; and California Emergency Physicians (now CEP America), with a comprehensive deployment of "Rapid Medical Evaluation" across all of their more than 100 sites.[3,4,5,6,7,8]

These innovators, along with many others, have contributed important new knowledge about the science of flow to emergency medicine. The importance of lean management and reducing waste has been well described in the literature and is now widely applied to the ED. Previously, it was thought by some that lean principles would not work in a service operations environment as complex as the ED. Queuing theory, the impact of reducing variation and matching capacity to demand, has become common vernacular, whereas 10 years ago few in emergency medicine had even been exposed to this critical aspect of operations management.[9] Finally, the theory of constraints and the understanding that systems behave as a network of interconnected queues, all of which must be optimized in order to achieve lean flow, while a common language in business schools across the country, has only recently been applied in emergency medicine.[10]

Thus, there is a new age of ED flow: the age when there is no longer fear or uncertainty about the value or impact of addressing ED flow problems; the age when the knowledge and approach is better documented than ever before; the age when physicians, nurses, and administrators are all in agreement that the flow must be perfected and are continually striving to create the "No-Wait" ED, to improve throughput, quality, and the patient experience. We are excited about the new wave of innovation that builds on previous accomplishments while blazing new paths in the true spirit of improvement.

Innovation: The University of Colorado Hospital Intake Model

The University of Colorado Hospital (UCHealth) opened its new ED in April 2013. Coincident with the opening, the hospital also opened a new inpatient tower, dramatically increasing the number of inpatient beds. The old ED suffered from a number of operational challenges stemming from architectural constraints and inpatient boarding. ED door-to-provider times were 38 minutes and the left-without-being-seen rate was 3.5 percent but as high as 8 percent. The average length of stay was 854 minutes for admitted patients and 239 minutes for discharged patients, far worse than national benchmarks. The new department chair charged the physician and nursing leaders to work with the process improvement team to create a best-in-class ED and redesign care that improved operational metrics and the overall patient experience. Using a novel rapid process optimization methodology, the multidisciplinary care design team implemented a "provider in intake" model, eliminating nursing triage altogether.[11,12] Fortunately the team had the luxury of a newly built and separate ED, as well as an urgent desire for change.

Patients arriving via ambulance are directly roomed via the emergency medical services entrance and immediately met by a multidisciplinary care team. Otherwise, all ambulatory patients go through d "Pivot," which is open 24/7, and "Intake," which is open from 9 AM to 1 AM daily. From 1 AM to 9 AM when intake is closed, patients are immediately roomed in the main ED. On arrival at pivot, patients are greeted by security staff and undergo rapid screening to ensure they do not possess dangerous objects. They are then greeted by both a Care Team Associate (registrar) and a Pivot Tech Lead to acquire demographics for electronic health record (EHR) (Epic) registration as well as a chief complaint and vital signs. The Pivot Lead rapidly (15 seconds) makes one of two decisions about patient acuity using a "bypass" tool to sort patients. "Red patient" criteria include high-risk conditions such as stroke-like symptoms, high suspicion for myocardial infarction, compromised airway, and patients who need immediate life- or limb-saving treatment. These patients skip the Intake process and are immediately roomed into the main ED by a Runner Tech. In the event that Intake is saturated (defined as eight or more waiting patients), individual patients are "bypassed" into open Main area ED beds. Non-English-speaking patients are also bypassed directly into the Main ED. The vast majority of patients from 9 AM to 1 AM do not meet "red patient" or "bypass" criteria and are roomed in Intake where a Vitals Tech enters vital signs into the medical record. The Lead Pivot Tech may order an electrocardiogram (EKG) for patients meeting specific criteria to screen for ST-elevation myocardial infarctions. The EKG will be performed in the intake rooms by a dedicated EKG technician and reviewed by the Intake attending physician. No other testing is performed in Pivot or Intake.

Patients are moved into one of four intake rooms that have two doors on opposite walls, one facing the ED walk-in (Pivot) area and the other facing toward the main ED. As patients are roomed and waiting, a visible call light system alerts the Intake physician that a patient is roomed and ready to be seen. The Intake physician and scribe, who has a workstation on wheels, evaluate the patients who have been placed into a reclining chair. Visitors are seated in adjacent chairs. Otoscopes and ophthalmoscopes are in each room in addition to basic supplies such as tape, tongue depressors, and gauze. Urine specimen containers are available to give to patients if urine samples are required as they move through the process. Gel foam dispensers are positioned outside the doorway, and there is a sink in each room. The

Intake physician makes one of the following three decisions during the course of the evaluation:

1. The patient can be fully evaluated, treated, and discharged from Intake.

   a. The scribe completes a full note and the attending physician completes discharge instructions and prescriptions.

   b. The patient is moved to an internal waiting room and discharged by a technician or a nurse.

   c. A 24/7 outpatient pharmacy is available for patients to fill their prescriptions, alleviating the need for ED administration of medications (e.g., first-dose antibiotics or pain medications).

2. The patient requires additional simple testing (radiographic or laboratory) or a procedure and may be treated in the lower/middle acuity Supertrack.

   a. The scribe completes a full note.

   b. The Intake physician orders testing and/or communicates the need for procedures via Epic.

   c. An advanced practice provider (APP) evaluates the patient and documents the encounter.

   d. The patient is then dispositioned as above.

3. The patient requires consultation, admission, further complex/comprehensive evaluation, and treatment in the Main ED.

   a. The scribe completes a basic subjective, objective, assessment, and plan (SOAP) note to communicate to the main ED providers.

   b. The Intake physician orders basic laboratory/radiographic tests as well as interventions including medications and intravenous fluids as necessary.

   c. The patient is moved to the Main ED and care continues.

The Intake physician then signals their disposition decision to rest of the care team using the call light system, electronic record dashboard, and white board in the Intake room. The Intake physician, who is always an attending physician, works in a sequential order, going to room to room with the scribe, evaluating patients. After the implementation of this process, our median door-to-provider time was consistently 8 minutes and the left-without-being-seen rate dropped to 0.26 percent. Overall ED discharge length of stay was approximately 149 minutes and admitted length of stay 307 minutes. The Intake physician sees on average 85 patients per shift and discharges approximately 20 percent of patients directly after the Intake encounter. An additional 20 percent of patients are cared for by the APP in Supertrack where most (>95 percent) are eventually discharged. At peak velocity the Intake physician can see approximately 14 patients per hour. In the event that Intake becomes saturated and no beds in the main ED are available for Bypass, a physician and scribe from the main ED may be briefly deployed to assist for 15 minutes.

Discussion

This innovation from UCHealth embodies many best practices in the front end to rapidly screen the patient for acute life- or limb-threatening disease, stream the patient to the best treatment location, and immediately discharge the patient, when appropriate. The process involves enhanced provider efficiency and innovations around the traditional concept of patient triage. Operational metrics highlight the process's early successes, which, most certainly, will be followed by satisfaction improvements, which always lag improvements in process.

The first step in optimizing flow in the ED is implementing a streamlined front end. This entails efficient, rapid identification of sick patients. In order to do this effectively, the system design must define the patient service families that will be segmented in the operational flow paradigm. The most efficient framework for this is the "Sick, Easy, Complicated" paradigm.[13] The first step is "Sick/Not Sick," followed by "Easy/Not Easy." In this model there are separate, distinct pathways for these three patient types that have very different diagnostic and treatment needs. Perfect execution at this step in the process requires an agreed-on set of patient demographics (age and chief complaint) and signs (abnormal vital signs and appearance).

In this case study, the initial sort here is accomplished by a standardized tool allowing for the rapid identification of "Red" patients. These "Red" patients are immediately placed in a Main ED bed, thereby allowing the treating nurse and physician immediate access to begin their diagnostic and stabilizing efforts. This streamlined approach reduces waste in the form of a complete triage encounter by a nurse in the front of the ED who will never see or interact with that patient again. It also reduces delays in door-to-physician times, which are critical for this patient population for safety, quality, and flow.

The next step is sorting the "Easy" patients from the "Complicated." While this is also best achieved by a well-defined, standardized approach, there is some "gray" area between what is considered easy or complicated. This is often a result of many factors, including years of experience, training background, risk tolerance, and knowledge of the evidence. While tools are necessary, flexibility in the form of clinical judgment may play a larger role at this stage.

In the case study from UCHealth, this second sort is achieved by a physician and scribe supported by medical technicians. Intriguingly, there are no staff nurses involved in the process. This is the first case demonstrated of a triage system that does not include nursing. While this may seem to be a deviation from the standard of care, the Centers for Medicare and Medicaid Services (CMS) does not weigh in at all on nurse triage as a vital part of the process. While CMS does clearly require a medical screening exam to meet the Emergency Medical Treatment and Labor Act (EMTALA) requirements,[14] the hospital defines who is qualified to perform this exam, and this role is almost exclusively left to physicians or APPs. It is also the hospital's responsibility to define the parameters around the nursing assessment. Most organizations have a requirement that a nursing assessment is performed and documented within 24 hours of the patient arrival. The regulatory requirements at the federal, state (with some exceptions), and organizational levels are surprisingly silent with respect to the activity of triage. This should be refreshing to know, as the act of triaging the patient, as this case study demonstrates, is a wasteful one. Anything more than the identification of sick patients, and the streaming of the others, should be considered waste.

The effective front-end process also involves contingencies for fluctuations in demand. On any given day, due to the variation in patient presentations, one area of the department may get overwhelmed while another has a light demand. Effective systems will have built-in, well-defined contingencies for these instances in order to maintain productivity and flow in the context of these changing environmental variables. In UCHealth's system, saturation of the four intake rooms with another patient waiting per room (four additional, eight total) would activate a direct bedding of the sickest patients to a Main ED bed. While this is an effective contingency plan, the team must ensure that this does not hide problems in the intake process. For instance, if the Intake process is not capacitated properly (too few physicians, technicians, rooms, or scribes), diverting patients during busy times could mask the root cause of the problem. It is important in any case of a contingency activation to document the activation and the presumed root cause and to work to minimize the frequency of contingency activations. This will allow for continuous improvement of the overloaded subprocess.

Workplace organization, commonly referred to as "5S" in lean management, is crucial to sustain a high-performing process. In Intake, this involves intelligent, comprehensive organization and replenishment of supplies and solid visual management principles. While many may feel that electronic dashboards and EHRs have eliminated the need for visual management at the source of the patient experience, those deeply involved in process improvement and flow in the ED ironically realize that the computer actually hides critical flow signals. Thus, these signals must be established in an effective manner where the work occurs, even if the solutions appear to be "old-school." UCHealth's visual light signaling the patient status as waiting to be seen is an excellent example of this. Another example used in the ED today includes visual wayfinding so patients can direct themselves to laboratory or diagnostic imaging. This can be as simple as a colored line on the wall or as creative as a pair of small feet and a cartoon of an x-ray in the case of radiology wayfinding in a pediatric ED. In the case of supplies, great care should be used to make sure that everything needed to care for the patient is in the room (frequently used supplies) and in a cart outside the room (infrequently used supplies). This will reduce the need to leave the area to find or replenish supplies. Equally important is the need to ensure that accountability is designed into the process relative to who is responsible for replenishing supplies and how often this is done.

Proper alignment of resources is another important component of designing an ED flow without waiting. In service operations, this entails calculating the "takt time" (how much time you have) and the cycle time (how much time it takes).[15] The takt time represents how much time you have as dictated by the patient demand over a defined period of time. For example, if 10 patients are arriving per hour, the takt time would be defined by 60 minutes divided by 10 patients, the result being 6 minutes. This defines how much time a single provider would have in order to perform that particular step in the process. The cycle time represents how much time it currently takes as defined by the process design and through direct observation.

For instance, if a physician Intake assessment takes 8 minutes, and the takt time is 6 minutes, the process is not designed to meet patient demand and thus waiting will occur. The improvement team must find a way to reduce the waste in physician activities to get the cycle time down to 5 minutes to account for variation and provide buffer capacity for surges in demand. This process is repeated for every step along the patient journey to ensure that at each step, the nursing, physician, and treatment space capacities can accommodate the demands placed on them. Searching for the step in the process with the highest utilization (greatest demand relative to capacity) and fixing that activity as previously described is the most efficient way to approach operational improvement and is known as the theory of constraints, as outlined by Eli Goldratt more than 30 years ago. The essence of this scientific method is the repeated quest for the most constrained resource in the system, implementing methods to offload the constraint, and then looking for the next constraint. By following this very simple methodology, the improvement team will sustain a consistent movement toward perfection in the most efficient manner possible.

In this case study, it is reported that the physician can evaluate 14 patients per hour. This means the physician cycle time from the start of one patient to the start of the next is 60/14, or 4.3 minutes per patient. The theory of constraints likely led the team early on to conclude that the physician would be the constraint, thus, adding a scribe to offload some of the physician's activities would serve to increase physician productivity and thus capacity for throughput. This is an excellent example of the application of the theory of constraints. In fact, scribes have been proven in multiple studies to improve physicians' productivity by up to 0.8 patients per hour, relieving them of the up to 43 percent workload burden and average of 4,000 clicks charting imposes on the already inundated physician during a typical shift.[16,17]

Many patients can be discharged directly from Intake after a brief physician encounter, which solves the immediate needs of the patient. There are different configurations of intake that involve nurses, techs, medications, and even point of care diagnostics such as I-Stat, Sonosite, and other portable imaging modalities. Again, the exact configuration of Intake will vary from organization to organization based on a number of factors, including patient acuity, resource constraints, level of care desired, and physical space available.

A benefit of nurse involvement is the ability to readily perform a nurse assessment on and give basic medications to low acuity patients who can be discharged directly from Intake. A downside of having multiple, different types of providers present in the process is that it can lead to working silos and will subject the entire process to the availability of each staff member on any given day. For instance, if both nurses and physicians are part of the process and there is a nurse or physician illness, the process will be adversely affected. However, in the example of UCHealth, there are no nurses; therefore, a nurse callout will not affect the ability of patients to be evaluated in the Intake system. Obviously, this is a more robust system that will provide more reliable performance, but this must be weighed against the trade-offs of limited treatment options for patients and against local politics of discharging a subgroup of patients by the Intake team without a nursing assessment. Most would agree that the latter is more of a sacred cow than a true quality gap; however, this battle will likely be fought at every institution that considers this option.

Patients in whom the diagnosis is not readily clear based on the initial assessment ("complicated" patients) will require ancillary testing to arrive at a presumptive or definitive diagnosis. This group can be further subdivided into those requiring a bed ("horizontal" patients) and those not requiring a bed ("vertical" patients). Perhaps the most common flaw during this phase of the system design is pushing patients to the destination before they are "in-process." Contrary to current dogma, the most important aspect of the front end is not the "door-to-doctor" interval but the "door-to-in-process" interval.[15] (Crane 2015). While most EDs send patients to the appropriate destination, they fail to get their diagnostics and therapeutics started at this stage. The art of the front-end execution is equally dependent on getting the patient in front of the doctor as much as getting what the doctor is thinking started. The patient being completely "in-process" (red fluids, yellow fluids, diagnostic imaging, and treatment) means the ED has done everything that is completely under its control and the patient is on their way toward being discharged. Thus, the most reliable systems will have the specimen collection and basic treatments available in Intake or immediately after Intake prior to moving on to the next step in the process. Thus, "horizontal, complicated" patients will have labs drawn and basic treatment started prior to heading to a Main ED treatment space, and, "vertical" patients will have them done prior to moving to the "results waiting" (i.e., an internal waiting area) or further evaluation by an APP.

In the case of UCHealth, there is a trade-off of not having nurse treatment capacity in Intake; however, there are ample technicians to get the ancillary testing started, including the always-elusive urine collection. If the patient needs a nursing intervention, such as an oral pain medication or antibiotics, the patient must be pushed to that area and may experience some additional queueing. In the ideal system, patients who need nursing interventions will have them available when and where they are needed or the appropriate substitute will be available (the physician or APP will administer the medications). Ingeniously, for those patients discharged from UCHealth Intake, a 24/7 outpatient pharmacy is available for the patient to pick up and take their first dose of medications literally on the way out the door. This eliminates the need for a nurse, an automated medication dispensing system, and the need to observe the patient for an allergic reaction.

As previously mentioned, each subsequent step in the patient's journey is as important as Intake. Each requires similar standardization in terms of who is eligible (e.g., to wait in recliners for test results), which services are available, and contingency plans for the unexpected occurrences. Likewise, each area must be properly capacitated, have the right supplies in the right locations with accountable restocking processes, and have reliable signals clearly indicating when the patient is ready for the next activity.

Due to the very nature of emergencies, the "no-wait" ED will prove to be an elusive Holy Grail as we can never completely eliminate variation in the timing or nature of patient presentations and will face persistent future pressures to reduce cost and thus resources. However, we remain optimistic about the future of ED flow innovations as our emergency medicine physician scientists continue to develop new and unique ways of reducing waste, increasing efficiency, and enhancing the patient experience. This case study at UCHealth is an excellent example of what can be achieved: 79 percent reduction in door-to-physician times, 93 percent reduction in left-without-being-seen times, and a 48 percent reduction in discharged length of stay. Each of these accomplishments would be considered admirable in its own right, but the three together is truly astonishing and can be accomplished only through application of these scientific principles and leadership with the will to follow the lead of others, knowing they will end up looking back on a path never before taken.

References

1. Noon CE. Understanding the impact of variation in the delivery of healthcare services. *Journal of Healthcare Management*. 2003;48(2):83–98.

2. Poisson SE. *Probabilité des jugements en matière criminelle et en matière civile, précédées des règles générales du calcul des probabilités*. Bachelier. 1837, 206.

3. Crane J, Noon CE. *The Definitive Guide to Emergency Department Operational Improvement: Employing Lean Principles with Current Best Practices to Create the "No-Wait" Department*. Boca Raton, FL: CRC Press, 2011.

4. Guarisco J, et al. qTrack reengineering emergency department workflow. Institute for Industrial Engineering. https://webcache.googleusercontent.com/search?q=cache:FF6yV9iPG3IJ;www.iienet2.org/uploadedfiles/SHS_Community/Membership/qTRACK%2520-%2520Re-engineering%2520ED%2520Workflow.pdf+&cd=1&hl=en&ct=clnk&gl=us.

5. Deflitch C, et al. Physician-directed queuing (PDQ) improves healthcare delivery in the ED: early results. *Annals of Emergency Medicine*. 2007;50(3):S125–S126.

6. Cochran JK, Roche KT. A multi-class queuing network analysis methodology for improving hospital emergency department performance. *Computers and Operations Research*. 2009;6(50):1497–1512.

7. Mayer T. Innovations: initiating early patient care through team triage and

treatment. Urgent Matters. 2013. Available at http://smhs.gwu.edu/urgentmatters/news/innovations-initiating-early-patient-care-through-team-triage-and-treatment. Accessed December 15, 2015.

8. McDonnell M. CEP's rapid medical evaluation program revolutionizes treatment process in emergency departments. *Business Wire.* 2006. Available at www.businesswire.com/news/home/20060309005072/en/CEPs-Rapid-Medical-Evaluation-Program-Revolutionizes-Treatment. Accessed December 15, 2015.

9. Erlang AK. The theory of probabilities and telephone conversations. *Nyt Tidsskrift for Matematik.* 1909:20(B).

10. Goldratt EM, Cox J. *The Goal: A Process of Ongoing Improvement.* Great Barrington, MA: North River Press, 1984.

11. Wiler JL, Bookman K, Birznieks DB, et al. Rapid process optimization: a novel process improvement methodology to innovate health care delivery. *American Journal of Medical Quality.* 2016. pii: 1062860616637683. [Epub ahead of print].

12. Wiler JL, Ozkaynak M, Bookman K, et al. Elimination of triage: implementation of an innovative process redesign in an urban academic emergency department. *Journal of the Joint Commission on Quality and Patient Safety.* 2016 Jun;42(6):271–280.

13. Crane JT, Jensen KJ. Size matters. ACEP Scientific Assembly. 2014. Available at http://virtual.acep.org/common/tracks.aspx/11. Accessed on December 15, 2015.

14. Joint Commission Resources. Comprehensive accreditation manual. 2016. Available at www.jcrinc.com/2016-comprehensive-accreditation-manuals/. Accessed December 15, 2015.

15. Crane JT, Jensen KJ. The effective physician. ACEP Scientific Assembly. 2015. Available at http://virtual.acep.org/common/tracks.aspx/11. Accessed December 15, 2015.

16. Arya, R. Impact of scribes on performance indicators in the emergency department. *Academic Emergency Medicine* 2010;17:490–494.

17. Hill, R, Sears, LM, Melanson SW. 4,000 clicks: a productivity analysis of electronic medical records in a community hospital ED. *American Journal of Emergency Medicine.* 2013;31(11):1591–1594.

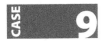

9 Transforming Care Delivery through Telemedicine

Judd E. Hollander and Brendan G. Carr

Introduction

The last decade has seen an explosion in the use of telehealth and telemedicine in both the health and the healthcare sector. From wearable devices, smartphone apps, and home monitoring equipment to Health Insurance Portability and Accountability Act (HIPAA) compliant video chat capabilities – specifically where data are kept private and secure – and remote capable robotics, technology and healthcare have collided over the last decade to dramatically transform the way that we deliver healthcare. In truth, however, this is part of a much bigger societal shift in how we shop, communicate, travel, socialize, and eat. Technology is ever present in our lives and healthcare has actually been slower to adopt change than many other industries. Most (95%) Americans have SMS-capable cellphones and computers (84%), about half (45%) have smartphones, two-thirds (67%) use social media, and 90 percent are interested in technology-based platforms to improve health.[1,2] The global market for mHealth healthcare-related technology has more than quintupled over the last 5 years from 4.5 billion in 2013 to a projected 23 billion in 2017.[3]

There isn't a single definition of telehealth or telemedicine, in part because since the early days of use cases only for space travel and military medicine, the landscape has been (and is) in perpetual flux. The World Health Organization defines telehealth as "the delivery of health care services, where distance is a critical factor, by all health care professionals using information and communication technologies for the exchange of valid information for diagnosis, treatment and prevention of disease and injuries, research and evaluation, and for the continuing education of health care providers, all in the interests of advancing the health of individuals and their communities."[4] The Health Resources and Service Administration (HRSA), home to the US government's Office for the Advancement of Telehealth (OAT), defines telehealth as "the use of electronic information and telecommunications technologies to support long-distance clinical health care, patient and professional health-related education, public health and health administration. Technologies include videoconferencing, the internet, store-and-forward imaging, streaming media, and terrestrial and wireless communications."[5] HRSA also makes a distinction between telehealth and telemedicine, defining the latter as referring "specifically to remote clinical services." For the purposes of payment, the Centers for Medicare and Medicaid Policy explain that "telemedicine seeks to improve a patient's health by permitting two-way, real-time interactive communication between the patient, and the physician or practitioner at the distant site. This electronic communication means the use of interactive telecommunications equipment that includes, at a minimum, audio and video equipment."[6]

Definitions aside, it is critical that telehealth and telemedicine be thought of as a means to an end. They are tools that can be used to bring care to the patient when and where they need it. And this frame – that the user experience is important in healthcare – is also a part of a bigger societal shift. As consumer culture has changed and evolved, so has the approach to medicine and healthcare delivery. Patient-centeredness, satisfaction, and a buyer's market in healthcare have created market forces that reward not just high-quality care but highly convenient care. Although formal definitions exist for quality, in remarks to the Senate

Finance committee, the director of the Agency for Healthcare Research and Quality (AHRQ) summed up what quality means in healthcare by explaining, "Simply put, health care quality is getting the right care to the right patient at the right time – every time."[7] As the definition of quality is increasingly inclusive of patient preferences, health systems will need to become increasingly nimble in meeting the needs of patients to consume their healthcare in the flexible manner in which they consume every other consumer good. We describe below the use of telemedicine as a part of transforming our health system into a connected and patient-centered care delivery experience.

Case Example 1

Frances is a 63-year-old retired teacher with mild to moderate heart failure. She notices one morning that she is a little more winded than usual and texts her doctor's office. The office responds with a text link to 10 different time slots for a video visit later that day. She selects one and later that day has a 10-minute video chat with her doctor, who suggests some alterations to her medications. She feels reassured and goes to bed but awakens in the middle of the night with shortness of breath, gets frightened, and touches the JeffConnect app (described further below) on her phone where she is connected with an emergency physician within minutes. They chat, the emergency physician is reassured by her respiratory rate and the patient is reassured by being "seen" by a physician. She takes an additional dose of diuretic and the On-Demand doctor schedules an early-morning visit by the community paramedicine team, who check her blood pressure, heart rate, oxygenation, and weight, and then participate in a 5-minute check-in to review her medication plan with her primary care provider. They leave her a Bluetooth scale that communicates with the office of her primary medical doctor (PMD) and they discuss a plan for diuresis to achieve a 5-pound weight loss over the next few days.

Case Example 2

Bill presents hypotensive and febrile to a community emergency department where he is met by an emergency physician who recognizes that he is septic. He orders several tests including laboratory blood tests, blood cultures, and a chest x-ray; establishes large-bore intravenous access; orders a fluid bolus and antibiotics; and then asks the nurse to have the virtual resuscitation service engaged so that they can maximize Bill's resuscitation while the single coverage provider maintains control over the rest of the busy department. After about an hour, Bill's condition worsens despite aggressive resuscitation and is started on vasopressors by the resuscitation service. The two physicians agree on a plan to intubate Bill and transfer him to the referral center. The resuscitation expert travels virtually with Bill and smoothly transitions his care into the intensive care unit at the receiving hospital by giving a virtual face-to-face report to the receiving team.

Case Example 3

After suffering from chronic knee pain for years, Mike finally decides to have the bilateral knee replacement his doctor recommended. The local providers suggest that because of his comorbid conditions the procedure should be performed by the orthopedic team at the downtown referral center. He is reluctant to travel downtown but calls the orthopedic team to ask about logistics. They report that his primary medical doctor can do the blood and stress tests, that the anesthesia team will interview him using a video chat, and that he can have a virtual postoperative visit from his home so that he can show off how well he is doing after his physical therapy. Going downtown to the referral facility for only one visit rather than the many that he expected makes the decision easy for him to move forward with the surgery.

Innovation

Patients have demonstrated their priorities and preferences with their feet and their wallets. Convenient, rapid access to care, and nimble connected capabilities are important preferences driving healthcare decisions. Jefferson Health made a commitment to creating a patient-centered health system with the goal of bringing care to the patients rather than bringing patients to an urban hospital setting. One component of the Jefferson Health strategy was to grow a robust telemedicine program that was voted by our employees to be named JeffConnect.

Vision Development

Following a series of meetings between Jefferson leadership, key stakeholders, and industry executives, our healthcare team conducted a series of interviews, conference calls, and divisional meetings with more than 30 patients, physicians, and administrators in order to identify areas of medical practice and education that were most likely to be positively impacted through the use of telehealth.

Four key domains where telehealth could be optimally utilized were identified: (1) outpatient care, (2) during care transitions into and out of the hospital, (3) in the inpatient setting, and (4) in the creation of the premier research and education center for telehealth.

Prioritization of Initiatives

When we launched our health system transformation, we prioritized some use cases for early implementation and others for delayed implementation. The financially lowest risk *early telehealth opportunities* were those focused on covered employees (e.g., on-demand sick visits at no cost), conditions with bundled payments (e.g., postoperative visits for surgical procedures), or conditions with incentives in place to decrease readmissions or revisits (e.g., heart failure). Replacing visits with convenient telehealth encounters provides patients with a more user-friendly and convenient experience that is at the same time more efficient for providers and lower cost to payers.

More transformative opportunities included expanding Jefferson's well-established infrastructure for neurologic and neurosurgical emergency consultations to include broader critical care and resuscitation service lines (e.g., sepsis, out-of-hospital cardiac arrest) and redefining acute care delivery by creating a virtual emergency department model where acute unscheduled care is expedited outside the traditional four walls of the hospital (Figure CS9.1).

JeffConnect Program

The JeffConnect program is based in the philosophy that, in an ideal world, medical advice and healthcare would be available whenever and wherever patients are sick, injured, or scared. JeffConnect services help accomplish the triple aim of improving the experience of

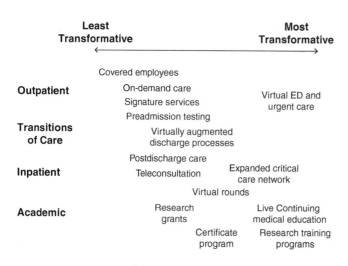

Figure CS9.1 Initial plan for JeffConnect telemedicine program including four domains of care along the continuum of transformation.

care, improving the health of populations, and reducing per capita costs while simultaneously better engaging patients in their own healthcare. The program is focused on developing patient-centered solutions throughout the whole JeffConnect care continuum (Figure CS9.2).

Many institutions have focused primarily on the areas that are high cost for payers, but not necessarily the most stressful for patients. This is represented in the JeffConnect care continuum, where most interventions (reduction in admissions, creation of observation care, reduction of readmissions) are on the right side of Figure CS9.2. The left side of Figure CS9.2, focused on meeting the preferences of patients during their time of need, has the potential to make a larger impact on both day-to-day life and the overall healthcare experience of most Americans. JeffConnect goes beyond traditional patient-

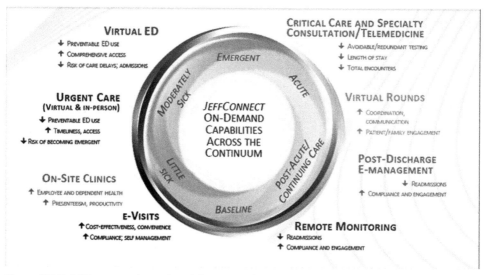

Figure CS9.2 JeffConnect on-demand capabilities across the continuum.

centered medical home models by connecting patients with healthcare providers across the care continuum, from maintaining the well-being of healthy patients and offering consultations for episodes of acute care to managing postdischarge care.

Patients Who Are a "Little Sick"

In the JeffConnect model, most individuals are usually at their baseline (bottom of Figure CS9.2). Patients who fall off their baseline, as illustrated by Frances in Case Example 1, and become a "little sick" can be treated either by their own provider through asynchronous communication, telephone consultation, and scheduled e-visit or by an on-demand physician who is available 24/7 to provide virtual care. To avoid fragmenting care, these emergency physicians function as "available-ists" and coordinate care with the patients and other providers. Patients who utilize the emergency department because they desire the convenience of providers, laboratories, testing, and medications all in one place might choose less costly options if they were as convenient. In the future, creating a virtual urgent care or emergency department by adding imaging and laboratory testing onto on-demand video visits could meet patient needs and improve the patient experience. The associated cost reduction becomes almost a secondary goal but nevertheless aligns patient and payer goals. We believe that easy availability of evidence-based expert care when patients want to engage is more likely to shift patient behavior than increased focus on financial disincentives for health systems.

Emergency Department Care

Despite innovation in the approach to caring for those who are a "little sick," some patients will have acute exacerbations of their chronic conditions or suffer an acute illness or injury and will require treatment in an emergency department. For the majority of patients who do not require admission, JeffConnect will provide the tools to help coordinate outpatient care and to improve transition plans. Patients who understand their discharge instructions and are connected to outpatient services are more likely to return to their baseline. Ultimately, we hope that regional care coordination exchanges, in which networks connect patients to needed resources across health systems (think OpenTable for visiting nurses) can assist patients who require follow-up care to ensure smooth transitions home.[4] Mobile integrated healthcare can provide home visits to encourage medication compliance and behavior change after a visit and link patients back to their usual source of care, as illustrated in Case Example 1.

Some acutely ill or injured patients will need highly specialized care, as was the case for Bill in Case Example 2 above. When critical care capabilities are not available at the hospital closest to the patient, provider-to-provider (physician–nurse team) telemedicine consultation and remote monitoring creates efficiencies, spreads best practices, and enables more patients to stay in their communities. Jefferson Expert Teleconsulting allows Jefferson providers to collaborate with partnering hospitals and to participate in provider-to-provider remote consults.

Hospital-Based Care and Transitions Home

In the acute care setting, patients can benefit from improved engagement of their families and caregivers. The timing of physician rounds may not be conducive to having family members physically present. "Virtual rounds," which connect caregivers and family members with patients and their providers in real time through a secure video platform, increases patient and family engagement while also increasing care coordination and communication.

A logical extension of virtual rounds is the use of group visits at the end of an acute hospitalization to improve patients' transition home. JeffConnect communication options include videoconferencing with all inpatient providers, the patient, their family, and even the primary care provider, who will be charged with continuing the course of care in the outpatient setting at the time of discharge. Utilization of telemedicine by transition of care coordinators prior to scheduled outpatient visits creates comfort with the home-based use of similar platforms and opens the door to many different soft-touch mechanisms to enhance understanding and compliance with discharge recommendations and to ensure convenient follow-up care, as was illustrated by Mike's postoperative visit in Case Example 3 above.

Remote Second Opinions and Streamlined Intake Processes

As a quaternary referral center, many patients seek the perspective of experts in the field or multidisciplinary teams, as was illustrated by Mike's referral to the orthopedic experts in Case Example 3. In his example, he not only was able to discuss his case and determine an operative plan but was able to interact with the anesthesiologist responsible for his preoperative clearance and coordinate any testing that needed to be completed prior to his trip downtown to the referral center.

When Not a Patient

Last, of course, we need to empower people to take care of their own health during the time that they aren't "patients."[5] Mobile apps and on-demand virtual consults can enhance medication compliance, behavior change, and health and wellness.

Creation of the National Academic Center for Telehealth

As telehealth represents the future of medicine, it represents an area ripe for investigation and development of educational programs. As a premiere academic medical center, Jefferson is combining entrepreneurial and academic initiatives to develop an innovative National Academic Center for Telehealth (NACT). In addition to offering coursework to emerging health professionals, the NACT is researching telehealth solutions to inform evidence-based practices. Key goals include establishing training programs required to build a telehealth workforce of the future, identifying and answering key research questions related to the practice of telehealth, and establishing best practices and quality benchmarks for the use of innovative technology to deliver high-quality healthcare.

Developing the First Generation of Telehealth Researchers

Developing a center that has a cadre of researchers who have been successful in obtaining federal and industry funding would provide the foundation to grow the world's largest academic center for telehealth. Investigations would include optimal methods of health services delivery, ideal patient-centered telehealth solutions, injury and illness surveillance, and big data analysis.

Telehealth Training Certificate Program

This program would train providers and staff who support the telehealth initiative in all phases of telehealth program implementation and maintenance. This would include items such as operational guidelines for staff and providers, care pathways and protocol development, provider skills including presentation techniques, simulation center development, interaction/video review, and quality improvement. The program will be developed and trialed with Jefferson providers and then expanded to help train other institutions/providers developing telehealth programs. Using a combination of professionals with sales force training, executive presentation skills, and medical knowledge, this program would make Jefferson the "go-to" site for training telehealth professionals.

Live Continuing Medical Education for Providers during the Telehealth Referral

Most current continuing medical education (CME) programs are traditional lectures or interactive case discussions. By granting CME to providers who partner with Jefferson telehealth physicians, we would bring a value-added program to our referring physicians. This program would dovetail live telehealth management of the patient with a structured educational opportunity in critical care areas (stroke, sepsis, resuscitation) and would leave the provider with additional educational materials and an opportunity to earn CME. "Live CME" changes the future of medical education by providing real-time coaching and bedside teaching beyond the residency training period. It can also be used to expand resident education and supervision outside daytime hours.

Discussion

The case examples and narratives above provide an overview of the efforts that Jefferson has taken over the last year to markedly transform care delivery. Instead of emphasizing the technical aspects, legal challenges, and financial complexities associated with this change, we have focused on what we have learned from patients and providers about what they want care delivery to look like. Essential to this transformation has been a strong leadership commitment to this mission and a clear management strategy focused on change management. These issues are beyond the scope of this chapter but their importance cannot be underemphasized. Patient-centered care delivery is first and foremost about the patient. Technology is an amazing adjunct to our ability to deliver high-quality care, but adoption of a high-quality telemedicine program is only secondarily about the technology. Where we once applied Osler's advice to the diagnosis, we now apply it to the delivery system, but in both cases they could not be more true: "Listen to the patient, he is telling you the diagnosis."

References

1. Rainie L, Cohn D. Census: computer ownership, internet connection varies widely across U.S. 2014. Available at www.pewresearch.org/fact-tank/2014/09/19/census-computer-ownership-internet-connection-varies-widely-across-u-s/.

2. Ranney ML, Choo EK, Wang Y, Baum A, Clark MA, Mello MJ. Emergency department patients' preferences for technology-based behavioral interventions. *Annals of Emergency Medicine*. 2012;60(2):218–227.

3. Emerging mHealth Report. 2014. Available at www.pwc.com/gx/en/healthcare/

mhealth/assets/pwc-emerging-mhealth-full.pdf.

4. World Health Organization. Telemedicine: opportunities and developments in member states: report on the Second Global Health Survey on eHealth. 2010. Available at www.who.int/goe/publications/goe_telemedicine_2010.pdf.

5. What is telehealth? How is telehealth different from telemedicine? *HealthIT.gov*.

Available at www.healthit.gov/providers-professionals/faqs/what-telehealth-how-telehealth-different-telemedicine.

6. Telemedicine. *Medicaid.gov*. Available at www.medicaid.gov/Medicaid-CHIP-Program-Information/By-Topics/Delivery-Systems/Telemedicine.html.

7. What is health care quality and who decides? 2009. Available at www.hhs.gov/asl/testify/2009/03/t20090318b.html.

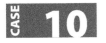

Coordinating Emergency Care through Telemedicine

Sarah A. Sterling, Kristi Henderson, and Alan E. Jones

Introduction

Telehealth was born out of necessity. Patients living in rural, remote areas have always had diminished access to healthcare. Those with the means could travel great distances, and those who were unable to travel often received inadequate care, if any at all. Even now in the twenty-first century, many patients in rural areas are still unable to see a specialist or get necessary medical treatment without traveling long distances or waiting long periods for an appointment. While the physician shortage is partially responsible, perhaps a more important factor is the inefficient use of our existing healthcare workforce coupled with limited access points to the healthcare system. A more efficient use of existing resources could occur through better patient and physician scheduling, reduced travel times, and sharing patient volume across the entire medical staff regardless of location. With telehealth, many of these goals can be realized, as a clinician's practice setting can be extended to underserved locations and populations. Though telehealth has the potential to improve access for many different healthcare services in rural areas, it is particularly applicable to emergent care, where rapid patient assessment and stabilization are necessary for improved patient outcomes.

Innovation

Timely, appropriate care may improve outcomes in many emergent conditions.[1,2,3] However, rural areas have dramatically reduced access to timely, high-quality emergency care, potentially compromising the care that is provided.[4] Mississippi, in particular, is a state with large rural populations separating urban areas and a centrally located single, academic, tertiary care hospital that serves as the state's only Level I trauma center. According to recent census results, more than half of Mississippi's population resides in rural areas (1.6 million people of 3 million people) with 32 of the 99 hospitals in the state classified as critical access hospitals.[5,6] Naturally, these large rural populations translate into substantial challenges to accessing specialized care for rural populations.[5] One study found that average transportation times to a certified neurocritical care unit in Mississippi exceeded 90 minutes, despite air ambulance use.[7] Similarly, another study found significantly longer transport times for traumatically injured patients in rural areas, with an average transport time of nearly 45 minutes.[8] Further compounding the logistical complications of coordinating emergency care and specialist evaluation in a state with such a large rural area geographically and by population is the difficulty of recruiting and retaining physicians in rural areas.[9,10,11]

Despite evidence suggesting improved outcomes when emergency care is provided by emergency medicine–trained and board-certified physicians,[12,13] practical limitations such as finding qualified emergency clinical providers prevent their use in many rural emergency departments (EDs). This trend is only expected to increase as the demand for emergency medicine–trained and board-certified physicians continues to outstrip the supply.[14] To improve access to high-quality, specialized emergency care in rural areas, our telemedicine program, TelEmergency, was developed in 2003 using a dual nurse practitioner and physician model.[15,16]

Improving Access in Rural Populations

Emergency medicine leadership at the University of Mississippi Medical Center (UMMC) recognized the healthcare disparities that existed between urban and rural EDs. Definitive and quality care was delayed often in patients transferred from rural areas, due to a combination of limited resources, limited subspecialist availability, and prolonged transport times to better equipped facilities. Noting this, the chairman of the department of emergency medicine and the clinical director of nursing began monitoring numerous metrics reflective of operations and quality of care. It was clear that patients from rural areas had lower quality care and that change needed to occur.

Unsuccessful Efforts to Improve Access

In an effort to remedy this challenge, multiple efforts were deployed to minimize disparities and improve outcomes for patients with emergencies in rural settings. One of the first attempts to improve care was through a rural scholars program designed to place new emergency physicians in rural, community EDs. This program was combined with emergency medicine continuing medical education courses for nonemergency physicians. However, neither effort was particularly impactful. Participation was poor, and for those who did participate, the impact was short lived. New physicians recruited to rural areas often remained in the rural area only to fulfill the time commitment required of the program. Further, physicians often did not reside in the rural area of their practice, but instead commuted to the rural hospital for their clinical shifts. Feedback from patient satisfaction surveys indicated rural communities wanted a healthcare provider who lived in their community and had a vested interest in the health of the people locally.

A Revised Strategy

With little success from the new physician and continuing education programs, leadership reevaluated how to improve rural access to timely emergency care. The ideal goal was to design an intervention to facilitate access to board-certified emergency medicine physicians. In order to better understand who was already staffing these rural EDs, an assessment was done of the critical access hospitals across the state. This survey found that the existing healthcare workforce in rural communities was largely comprised of family medicine physicians and family nurse practitioners. To address the emergency medicine physician workforce shortage, a novel approach was necessary to improve access to specialized care.

From the survey results, a telemedicine program was designed, TelEmergency. This system used the existing healthcare providers in a new way by recognizing that rural communities did not have board-certified emergency medicine physicians nor would they be likely to recruit or retain an emergency medicine–trained workforce. Instead, the revised objective was to improve access through the use of the existing nurse practitioner infrastructure and to provide enhanced training in clinical knowledge and procedural knowledge appropriate for emergency conditions. Using a dual nurse practitioner/physician model not only could address access issues, but also could help relieve staffing constraints facing rural EDs.[9,10] Combined with augmented clinical training in emergency care for nurse practitioners, telemedicine could provide a bridge to connect rural EDs with emergency medicine physicians, who could provide guidance and, if necessary, co-management of patients.

The TelEmergency dual nurse practitioner/physician model consisted of on-site, specially trained nurse practitioners in rural EDs collaborating with a remote emergency medicine–trained and board-certified physician located at UMMC, with nurse practitioners consulting the TelEmergency physician as needed.

The Development of the Nurse Practitioner Clinical Residency Training Program

As part of the TelEmergency program, we developed an educational curriculum, or "clinical residency," tailored to nurse practitioners. This clinical residency in emergency medicine included 8 weeks of didactics and 135 clinical hours in a trauma center working with emergency medicine physicians. The program focused on key concepts and skills necessary to practice in an emergency care setting, including the recognition of emergent conditions, generation of treatment plans, and emergent procedures.

Lectures, targeted readings, cadaver labs, simulation, and telesimulation laboratories were used to enhance the knowledge and skills of the nurse practitioners in these rural EDs. For the on-site clinical provider, emergency procedural skills were vital to the successful implementation of this program. Therefore, this program was particularly focused on procedural skills. Beyond improving the skills and knowledge of the rural workforce, this program facilitated access to the knowledge and clinical expertise at the tertiary medical center through telehealth technology.

Assessment of Readiness and Staffing Rural EDs

Following the completion of the clinical residency, nurse practitioners were tested to assess their readiness to practice in an emergency care setting. Four written examinations studied the content of their knowledge and competency. Additionally, clinical evaluations were conducted on completion of the clinical residency. During these, the nurse practitioner was given three different complex case scenarios and was evaluated on ability to conduct a complete history and physical examination, order and interpret diagnostic tests, and generate an appropriate diagnosis, treatment plan, and disposition.

Clinical evaluations also assessed key procedural skills through a skills evaluation. Examples of procedures include endotracheal intubation (for all ages), layered suturing, and fracture reduction and splinting. Following successful completion of the didactic and clinical training, the nurse practitioner was eligible to staff a TelEmergency ED.

The initial TelEmergency nurse practitioner training class included 30 nurse practitioners. Though this was a large initial class, a class of this size was necessary to provide adequate coverage to staff three rural hospitals 24 hours per day. Subsequent training programs ranged from three to five nurse practitioners each semester. Completion time for the program averaged 6 months.

Preparation to Implement the TelEmergency Program

While the training of nurse practitioners was necessary to provide competent staff in rural EDs, additional efforts were needed to implement information technology and to ensure that state medical licensure boards encompassed this new expanded scope of practice and that these services would be financially viable.

To allow for two-way audio-video connections between the rural hospital and the academic medical center, hardware, software, and a secure broadband connection were required. An initial information technology assessment was conducted by UMMC to determine the needs of each hospital. None of the critical access hospitals was found to have the required equipment or connection to ensure that the quality of the connection was sufficient, dependable, and secure. Therefore, a new, secure T1 line was installed for this program, and the necessary equipment was provided. Every rural hospital received identical set-ups including the hard-wiring of the ED's trauma room and a mobile telemedicine cart that could be moved to the location of the patient in the event of simultaneous TelEmergency patient consults. Both types of technology configurations allowed for two-way audio and video communication through a secure and private telecommunication line.

At the onset of the program in 2003, electronic medical records were not available at any of the rural hospitals, so UMMC provided access to its own electronic medical records. However, as more hospitals implemented electronic medical records, providers electronically documented clinical notes in their facility's native information systems with data sharing occurring between systems. This provided a way to share records for continuity of care, the review of outcomes, and to track the impact and success of the program. Radiology images were viewed through UMMC's picture archiving and communication system (PACS), and all rural hospitals contributed their images. The TelEmergency physician at UMMC could then view the image and consult the radiology department if a final interpretation was needed. Laboratory results were not shared by the rural hospitals. These results either were reported verbally by the nurse practitioner or were faxed to UMMC for TelEmergency physician review.

Finally, neither public nor private insurance companies in Mississippi reimbursed for telehealth at the onset of the program. Medicare provided limited reimbursement, but isolated reimbursement was not a feasible way to sustain the program. Initially, funding was obtained through a combination of grant funding and contract fees paid by the rural hospitals for the TelEmergency service. Knowing that the future of the program depended on a more reliable funding model than grant funding or limited reimbursement, UMMC led advocacy work to change the telehealth reimbursement climate in Mississippi as well as at the national level. A grassroots lobbying effort united the Mississippi state legislature around the importance of improving rural emergency care via telehealth. This effort resulted in the passage of legislation requiring public and private reimbursement for telehealth in Mississippi. Additionally, the outcomes from the TelEmergency program were used by the US Congress to advocate for the Centers for Medicare and Medicaid Services (CMS) to expand telehealth reimbursement. CMS has expanded its reimbursement for telehealth annually, and legislation has been submitted every year to introduce new payment models that could further expand the use of telehealth.

Implementation of the TelEmergency Program

The initial implementation of the TelEmergency Program began with three hospitals in October 2003. These three hospitals were part of an initial pilot program for 1 year before additional hospitals were added. The pilot program was required by the Mississippi state medical board to prove feasibility and quality of the TelEmergency program prior to approving new regulations that would allow the practice of medicine utilizing telehealth technology. The Mississippi state medical board required quarterly progress reports noting the activity and overall success of the program. During the pilot phase, every patient presenting to the rural ED was co-managed by the local, rural nurse practitioner and UMMC TelEmergency physician. This reflected the heightened concern to ensure quality care in addition to the heightened monitoring of the program by the State medical and nursing board in its infancy.

Throughout the pilot year, patient outcomes were monitored and 100 percent of the charts were reviewed. Satisfaction of providers, patients, and administrators was evaluated. Assessment of the pilot project showed that provider, administrative, and, most important, patient satisfaction with the program was high. Additionally, the pilot provided feedback on ways to improve the program, including modification of the requirement that every patient presenting to the rural ED be co-managed with a UMMC TelEmergency physician.

Noting that TelEmergency consultation was burdensome and unnecessary in some lower-acuity situations, consultation guidelines were created to ensure quality while recognizing that the nurse practitioner was able to care for low-acuity patients independently. The guidelines never prohibited TelEmergency consultation but did recommend TelEmergency consultation based on certain indicators such as specific high-risk symptoms, patient age, and specific vital sign parameters. Collaboration and co-management was encouraged. The consultation with the UMMC TelEmergency physician rates remained around 50 percent after implementation of the consultation guidelines, indicating continued collaboration and high utilization of the system.

New rural hospitals were added based on their request and availability of grant funding to support the infrastructure needs of the program. The number of hospitals gradually grew from three original hospitals to 19 hospitals over 12 years. This included four hospitals that terminated their contract over that period, leaving 15 active hospitals in the program. The four rural hospitals that terminated their contracts included one hospital that closed, two that were purchased by another health system, and one that went bankrupt and was unable to meet the minimum requirements necessary to be a participating hospital.

Telehealth Process

The TelEmergency consultation process requires excellent collaboration and coordination of care between the nurse practitioner and the TelEmergency, emergency medicine physician for the process to occur quickly and efficiently. This is especially true when the nurse practitioner is faced with a critically ill patient in a rural ED with limited resources. The TelEmergency process and coordination needed are best demonstrated through the example of trauma patients who require care at UMMC, the state's lone Level I trauma center. The workflow in Figure CS10.1 shows how a TelEmergency patient is managed in this program.

Consult Initiation

When notified of an anticipated critical patient, or when a patient with traumatic injuries is identified during clinical evaluation, the on-site nurse practitioner at the rural ED calls the central communication center for UMMC and for the state of Mississippi, Mississippi MED-COM. Mississippi MED-COM was established in 2008 following Hurricane Katrina with the aim of improving communication and coordinated care across the state of Mississippi. MED-COM is staffed by experienced paramedics and emergency medical technicians who help coordinate emergency care for referring hospitals and pre-hospital personnel. MED-COM operates under a series of protocols to help determine appropriate transfers to UMMC, though they involve the in-house emergency medicine physicians whenever indicated or requested by the transferring physician. MED-COM also helps

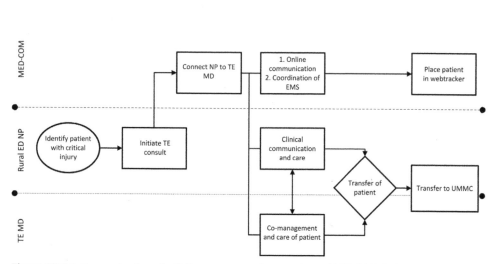

Figure CS10.1 Emergent pathway for TelEmergency consult generation and MED-COM. EMS: emergency medical services; MD: medical doctor; NP: nurse practitioner; TE: TelEmergency.

coordinate online medical control for pre-hospital personnel throughout the state and TelEmergency consults as they are generated.

Consult Management

When notified of a critical TelEmergency consult by the on-site nurse practitioner, MED-COM notifies the TelEmergency physician, an attending emergency medicine physician in the ED at UMMC, that an incoming critical patient is expected at one of the TelEmergency sites. Simultaneously, the patient's demographics are sent to UMMC from the remote site for generation of an official TelEmergency consult, and a record is created in the electronic medical record for the TelEmergency physician located at UMMC. The TelEmergency physician is then connected to the nurse practitioner via recorded phone call, while MED-COM is still online. While discussing the details of the patient and patient location, the TelEmergency physician pulls up the consult by video conferencing on a secure, closed circuit.

The TelEmergency physician and the nurse practitioner in the rural ED evaluate the patient and collaborate via audio-video teleconferencing. This allows the emergency medicine physician to be involved and participate in the patient's physical exam and evaluation, without interfering with the nurse practitioner's evaluation and management, delaying care, or introducing unnecessary repetition and communication of clinical data. Additionally, for critically ill patients requiring resources that outstrip the rural hospital's abilities, such as an unstable trauma patient requiring surgical intervention, the TelEmergency physician and MED-COM coordinate air or ground medical transport and establish a receiving facility while the nurse practitioner manages the patient's initial evaluation and stabilization.

Though all TelEmergency sites do not use TelEmergency coverage continually, TelEmergency coverage/consultation is available through the University of Mississippi Medical

Center, with an attending emergency medicine physician providing TelEmergency consultations 7 days per week, 24 hours per day.

Critical Interventions

For the unstable patient requiring interventions, the on-site nurse practitioner can perform procedures such as endotracheal intubation or needle decompression and can obtain vascular access through intraosseous or central line placement with the simultaneous supervision and real-time support of the remote TelEmergency physician. The nurse practitioner and TelEmergency physician can further communicate to decide on the resuscitation plan, need for interventions, and the patient's plan for admission or discharge.

While the patient is being actively resuscitated by the nurse practitioner and TelEmergency physician, MED-COM is behind the scenes arranging the transport to UMMC. Since UMMC is the only Level I trauma center in the state, transfer destinations are simplified for multisystem trauma patients.

Coordinating Care during Transfer

MED-COM communicates about the patient's status with the air (or ground) critical care transport team. Through MED-COM, the TelEmergency physician can communicate important information to the transport team about the patient, tailoring the transport to the patient's needs. Therefore, additional medications or blood products that are anticipated can be brought and administered as needed with the TelEmergency physician's verbal order, reducing administration times.

Once the patient is en route with the appropriate transportation and crew, the TelEmergency physician who evaluated the patient by TelEmergency consult can notify the receiving emergency medicine physician and trauma team in the ED at UMMC. This allows for more accurate preparation and early mobilization of appropriate resources and specialists at the trauma center. The TelEmergency physician also provides online medical control for paramedics across the state with the assistance of MED-COM, so while the patient is in transport, the TelEmergency physician can provide assistance to the transport team, continue necessary medication orders, and, importantly, update the receiving team in the ED to changes in the patient's condition or status.

Quality Assessment and Review

All video and audio TelEmergency consults are recorded for quality-improvement purposes and for targeted education should the consult be flagged for review by the TelEmergency physician, the nurse practitioner, or MED-COM personnel. Further, a portion of each TelEmergency nurse practitioner's charts are randomly selected and reviewed by the emergency medicine attending physicians at UMMC to assure quality and standard of care. Focused education and feedback is provided to individual nurse practitioners as indicated.

Analysis of the effects of TelEmergency implementation on nine rural hospital ED operations found that admissions to the same rural hospital, transfer to another facility, and patients discharged against medical advice statistically increased in the year after TelEmergency implementation, suggesting improved identification of high-risk patients that were previously unrecognized. Additionally, our analysis of nearly 4,200 patients at 14 rural hospitals over 3 years with a documented TelEmergency consult found that the top diagnoses in patients receiving a TelEmergency consult were chest pain (11 percent), blunt trauma (7 percent), and abdominal pain (6 percent). Further, 23 percent of patients were admitted to the local, rural hospital and 34 percent of patients required transfer to another facility. These results suggest TelEmergency is utilized both for high-risk complaints and by potentially high-risk patients.

Research assessing outcomes of the TelEmergency program provides evidence of its benefit. Noting historically disparate outcomes in cardiac arrests managed in rural hospitals, one study assessed the effect of TelEmergency on the survivability of cardiac arrests presenting to rural hospitals. In that study, cardiac arrest patients who presented to rural hospitals utilizing TelEmergency consultation had similar survival rates to an urban, academic medical center.[17] Though initial assessment of outcomes is reassuring, further research assessing outcomes is needed and is currently under way.

Discussion

Physician shortages and long transport times make timely access to high-quality emergency care in rural areas quite challenging. However, as part of the TelEmergency program, 65 nurse practitioners were trained to staff rural, TelEmergency hospitals. TelEmergency, with its dual nurse practitioner/emergency medicine physician model, provides a potential solution to this challenge by improving access to quality emergency care, which otherwise may not be possible.[15,16] In a decentralized system with limited resources and diminished access to specialized care services, a telemergency system enhances communication and coordination of care to allow patients with critical illnesses access to appropriate, high-quality emergency care regardless of where they are.

Designing and implementing a telehealth program should focus on improving access to high-quality healthcare and provide sustainable staffing for rural EDs. Though quality of clinical care is essential, sustaining a telehealth program requires much more. An appropriate financial, policy, and regulatory environment is necessary to build a program that is adopted, supported, and financially sustainable. Many existing healthcare and financial policies and licensure regulations were written prior to telehealth utilization, and therefore unintentionally prohibit its use. The work required to allow for a broad-scale telehealth program is multifactorial. It requires the education of stakeholders, the commitment to provide well-trained, current clinical staff, and the dissemination of program outcomes in order to garner the support needed to sustain this new, more efficient method of healthcare delivery.

References

1. Newgard CD, Meier EN, Bulger EM, et al. Revisiting the "golden hour": an evaluation of out-of-hospital time in shock and traumatic brain injury. *Annals of Emergency Medicine.* 2015;66(1):30–41.

2. Marler JR, Tilley BC, Lu M, et al. Early stroke treatment associated with better outcome: the NINDS rt-PA stroke study. *Neurology.* 2000;55(11):1649–1655.

3. De LG, Suryapranata H, Ottervanger JP, et al. Time delay to treatment and mortality in primary angioplasty for acute myocardial infarction: every minute of delay counts. *Circulation.* 2004;109 (10):1223–1225.

4. Carr BG, Branas CC, Metlay JP, et al. Access to emergency care in the United States. *Annals of Emergency Medicine.* 2009;54(2):261–269.

5. Mississippi Office of Rural Health. Rural Health Information Hub for Mississippi. Available at www.raconline.org/states/ mississippi. Accessed November 16, 2015.

6. Parker T. State fact sheets. USDA. Available at www.ers.usda.gov/data-products/state-

fact-sheets/state-data.aspx?StateFIPS=28&
StateName=Mississippi. Accessed
November 16, 2015.

7. Ward MJ, Shutter LA, Branas CC, et al.
Geographic access to US neurocritical care
units registered with the neurocritical care
society. *Neurocritical Care.* 2012;16
(2):232–240.

8. Carr BG, Caplan JM, Pryor JP, et al.
A meta-analysis of prehospital care times
for trauma. *Prehospital Emergency Care.*
2006;10(2):198–206.

9. Williams JM, Ehrlich PF, Prescott JE.
Emergency medical care in rural America.
Annals of Emergency Medicine. 2001;38
(3):323–327.

10. Peterson LE, Dodoo M, Bennett KJ, et al.
Nonemergency medicine-trained physician
coverage in rural emergency departments.
Journal of Rural Health. 2008;24
(2):183–188.

11. van Dis DJ. Where we live: health care in
rural vs urban America. *JAMA.* 2002;287
(1):108.

12. Jones JH, Weaver CS, Rusyniak DE, et al.
Impact of emergency medicine faculty and
an airway protocol on airway management.
Academic Emergency Medicine. 2002;9
(12):1452–1456.

13. Weaver CS, Avery SJ, Brizendine EJ, et al.
Impact of emergency medicine faculty on
door to thrombolytic time. *Journal of
Emergency Medicine.* 2004;26(3):279–283.

14. Camargo CA Jr, Ginde AA, Singer AH,
et al. Assessment of emergency physician
workforce needs in the United States, 2005.
Academic Emergency Medicine. 2008;15
(12):1317–1320.

15. Galli R, Keith JC, McKenzie K, et al.
TelEmergency: a novel system for
delivering emergency care to rural
hospitals. *Annals of Emergency Medicine.*
2008;51(3):275–284.

16. Summers RL, Henderson K, Isom KC, et al.
The anniversary of TelEmergency. *Journal
of Mississippi State Medical Association.*
2013;54(12):340–341.

17. Henderson K, Isom K, Summers RL.
Relative survivability of cardiopulmonary
arrest in rural emergency departments
utilizing telemedicine. *Journal of Rural
Emergency Medicine.* 2014;1(1):9–12.

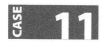

Bringing Diagnostic Testing to the Bedside

Point of Care Testing

Benjamin Easter and Kelly Bookman

Introduction

Point of care testing (POCT) is defined as any diagnostic test administered outside the central laboratory and near the patient. POCT is facilitated by advances in sensor technology and biomarker development that have allowed laboratory testing to be moved out of the central laboratory and closer to the bedside.[1] Key requirements for POCT include that the device be simple to use and affordable, that the reagents and consumables are robust in storage and usage as well as safe, and that the results are concordant with an established laboratory method including being sensitive, specific, and precise.[2]

Although technology has decreased turnaround times (TAT) for actual sample analysis in central laboratories, POCT allows for faster overall TAT than conventional central laboratory testing by decreasing both preanalytical and postanalytical time in addition to faster sample processing.[1] Preanalytical time includes sample transport and preparation (i.e., walking the sample to the laboratory or using pneumatic tubes, centrifugation), and postanalytical time includes data entry and forwarding. Thus, POCT can decrease the "brain to brain" time, which is the time between when a physician orders a test and when the physician interprets and acts on the result.[3]

This chapter will focus on the implementation of a POCT program at a large, academic emergency department (ED) and use its experience to discuss the benefits and challenges of such an innovation.

Innovation

The University of Colorado Hospital (UCH) ED is an academic, tertiary care facility located in the city of Aurora, approximately 8 miles from downtown Denver. It has an annual census of about 100,000 visits. The hospital is a referral center for the entire Rocky Mountain region and is the primary training site for the University of Colorado School of Medicine and for graduate medical education in virtually every specialty.

Coincident with a move to a new ED in 2013, UCH expanded its ED POCT program. Basic metabolic panel (BMP), hemoglobin (Hgb), arterial blood gas (ABG), venous blood gas (VBG), and rapid strep were added, and troponin (cTnI), pregnancy, and breathalyzer alcohol testing were continued. These tests were selected based on frequency of ordering, ease of use, and cost. After discussion with the central laboratory, certain tests that the i-STAT system could perform, such as lactate, D-dimer, and prothrombin time and international normalized ratio (PT/INR), would continue to be performed by the hospital's central laboratory. This decision was based on concerns about quality of POCT, cartridge costs, and difficulty of quality assurance. The idea was to consider a later expansion of the program if the initial phase was successful.

Results

Adoption of POCT resulted in significant time savings. TAT for POCT tests decreased 17–38 minutes compared with their respective laboratory-performed tests. Data for two of

Table CS11.1

Test Name	Annualized volume	Laboratory turnaround time (minutes)	POCT turnaround times (minutes)	Aggregate time saved (hours)
BMP	52,452	35	3	27,974
cTnI	12,456	45	7	7,889

the most commonly performed POCT, BMP and cTnI, are depicted in Table CS11.1. With the average patient in the UCH ED having 2.1 tests ordered (either POCT, laboratory, or both), in aggregate, POCT resulted in thousands of hours of decreased waiting time for results.

Since the implementation of POCT was done in concert with a complete process improvement effort, the effect of this decreased TAT from POCT on ED throughput measures is confounded by the other workflow changes that were simultaneously put into place. However, conservatively, if even 10 percent of the saved time were recovered, the drop in length of stay would be sufficient to sustain a 4 percent increase in patient volume with no need for increased staffing.

Challenges

POCT, as with all laboratory testing, requires rigorous quality control (QC). At UCH, the POCT process allows for all 200 staff nurses and technicians to perform bedside POCT as part of their primary clinical workload while on shift. All staff performing the tests must pass written tests and demonstrate proficiency with using the machines. In addition, the POCT machines must undergo QC checks at least monthly and with each new shipment of testing cartridges, so all machines are taken offline together and the QC process lasts 2–4 hours if all are operating normally. Since the machines are used at high volume in the UCH ED, the machines have been found to require replacement more frequently than recommended by the manufacturer. To manage the necessary QC, the POCT program eventually hired a laboratory-assigned representative specifically to assist the ED personnel, as there were episodes of noncompliance that could have led to cessation of the program.

Even with adequate QC in place, the POCT Hgb test was insufficiently precise to allow continued, safe usage. Review revealed that for accurate results, the blood sample must be shaken prior to placement in the device for analysis. Without agitation, the machine frequently reported a Hgb value that was incorrect. Values could be either too high or too low, but were not consistently off in a systematic fashion. Despite attempts at education, imprecise Hgb values continued to be obtained, and as a result, after approximately 5 months of use, the POCT Hgb test was discontinued.

Discussion

The use of POCT is steadily increasing in the United States, with growth rates expected to average >15 percent in the coming years.[4] As EDs nationally try to improve or maintain high-quality care despite crowding issues, many have turned to employing POCT. POCT has been found to decrease the ED length of stay (LOS) for discharged patients and expedite triage of patients who need urgent care, both of which increase throughput.[5] Further, it has been well established that the survival rate of critically ill patients is improved by early recognition and treatment, which POCT can impact by decreasing delays to treatment initiation. One of the issues that ED leadership has control over that may mitigate the impact of crowding is increasing the efficiency of front-end operations. Establishing protocols that include using POCT as a way to screen patients for high acuity and to triage sicker patients more quickly can both decrease delays in treatment and more rapidly identify low-risk and nonemergent patients.

Rapid TATs for test results are most beneficial in cases in which delays in treatment of at least 1 hour can have significant effects on outcomes and are the primary determining factor delaying patient management decisions. Acute coronary syndrome is one example of a disease that has improved outcomes based on rapid decision-making. It has been recommended that troponin I results should be available within 30 minutes to avoid increased adverse outcomes. Most POCT platform troponin testing can provide results within 20 minutes and some as quickly as 7 minutes,[6,7] and studies have shown that time to percutaneous and other interventions is decreased using POCT.[8,9] Another example of decreased delay in treatment is using POCT lactate for early initiation of resuscitation in septic patients. One study demonstrated a more than 2-hour decrease in time to results when POCT lactates are sent at triage versus being ordered by provider discretion,[10] and since improved outcomes are based on initiating therapy in the first 3–6 hours, this can translate into improved quality of care for these patients. For patients with stroke, rapid assessment of a patient's coagulation status is vital to starting thrombolysis in appropriate candidates. There are several POCT products on the market that have rapid TAT for INR, platelets, and Hgb. Venous thromboembolism can be rapidly ruled out using POCT, thus decreasing ED LOS for unaffected patients. POCT D-dimer can have negative predictive values of up to 98 percent and can decrease ED LOS for discharged patients by more than 1 hour.[11,12] Revenue savings can also be realized in the prevention of workflow delays such as decreasing wait times for computed tomography imaging by using POCT creatinine.[13] Elimination of such delays can create the space for more studies to be performed. In order for EDs to truly avail themselves of these types of improved outcomes, standardized pathways or clinical decision-making protocols may need to be developed or revamped.

Although there are many clear benefits of POCT in the ED, there are many challenges. Discussions with the central laboratory and hospital administration need to occur about the clinical context to describe the return on the investment in terms of increased ED throughput and improved clinical outcomes. The direct cost per analysis by POCT is greater than the cost per analysis performed in central laboratories. However, when combined with the numerous steps required to transport the samples to the laboratory and return them consecutively, POCT can potentially save on costs.[5] Another consideration is quality control and regulatory issues. Most POCT are run by ED staff with limited technical background when compared with the technicians in central laboratories. This means that central laboratory cooperation and oversight is necessary to assure quality as well regulatory compliance. In addition, ED staff must receive training and ongoing annual or semi-annual certification that they are competent to perform the tests.[14,15]

Probably the most important element for assuring quality in POCT is to establish an effective POCT management program focused on quality of testing, regulatory compliance, and efficient management of resources.[16] This team should include a POCT coordinator, laboratory medical director, and representatives from ED nursing and physician leadership and be responsible for oversight, new product implementation, and training/education of staff performing the tests. The importance of a skilled program coordinator cannot be overemphasized, and there is even a certificate program available.[16] The program coordinator is primarily responsible for creating the education program around good laboratory practice and orientation to all POCT devices, maintaining and optimizing documentation of POCT-related materials, and developing and enforcing QC.[13]

Training materials should include standard operating procedures for all devices, and users must verify competency. Some bedside devices require that users input their identification before they can be used; this allows POCT coordinators to track users and even lock out certain staff if they are not certified.[13] Proper documentation including all test results and testing materials, patient identification (full name, date of birth, sex), information identifying the requesting physician, test administrator, reagent batch number, and internal QC results should be documented for each test. POCT results should be distinguished in the medical record from those results obtained from the central laboratory.

Regarding QC, there are both internal QC and external quality assessment methods used for all laboratory testing, both POCT and centralized testing. These methods are designed to alert the operator of any change in the stability of the test over time. Internal QC uses a control sample to analyze accuracy and consistency across POCT machines. External quality assessment uses a sample of unknown quantity usually provided from an external source such as the manufacturer or another accredited resource.[5] As the use of POCT increases, the laboratory-trained professionals who understand the principles of quality assessment are best positioned to set guidelines for POCT application. Currently, minimum guidelines for nonlaboratory trained staff in the process of being written.[17] These minimum guidelines include internal and external QC whenever there is a new shipment, a new lot number, a result that is not consistent with clinical expectations, or when a repair has been performed on the machine.

These QC activities are usually the responsibility of the already busy ED staff for POCT. This increased manpower needed for QC has to be weighed in comparison to the potential increased efficiencies allowed by the use of POCT in terms of more rapid patient throughput and potentially fewer deteriorating patients since they are receiving intervention earlier in their course due to improved TAT of critical laboratory results. That said, there has been much work by device manufacturers to incorporate QC internally to the device to make the instruments user friendly for nonlaboratory personnel.[17] One way that some facilities try to unburden the ED staff from QC activities is to have a POCT coordinator or laboratory staff member perform them, but best practice is to have the personnel who are doing the POCT rotate through the QC process. Another example of efforts to improve quality of POCT results is to reduce postanalytical errors. Thus, most POCT machines are now able to wirelessly transmit the results to a central data management system, which avoids human transcription mistakes.[16,17]

The UCH experience exemplifies most of the benefits and challenges seen throughout the literature on POCT. As described and shown in Table CS11.1, it reaped the benefits of decreased TAT. However, because POCT implementation was concurrent with a full process redesign, there was no clear, direct attribution to decreased ED LOS. UCH experienced the difficulties associated with a large nonlaboratory staff performing POCT in that they had trouble with the education of all their staff to adequately agitate the specimens, which led to inaccurate Hgb results and loss of use of that POCT. In addition, UCH encountered the difficulty of having the central laboratory not be willing to grant a broad enough menu of POCT to allow for gaining the biggest benefits of POCT, which are decreased delays in time-sensitive interventions such as in the case of sepsis (using POCT lactate) and stroke (using POCT INR) and increased speed of diagnoses that can be rapidly triaged as negative and the patients dispositioned, such as in the case of venous thromboembolism (using POCT D-dimer). Further, they did not initially establish a POCT management program and ultimately had to organize one to avoid losing the program due to regulatory and QC noncompliance.

In conclusion, POCT when thoughtfully implemented can be a way to reduce crowding by decreasing LOS, which increases patient throughput. It is also an excellent way to rapidly separate nonemergent patients from urgent/emergent patients, allowing for decreased delays in time-sensitive interventions for critically ill patients as well as allowing for rapid disposition of patients with potentially dangerous complaints who can be ruled out with quick POCT. There are many challenges, such as cost and time-consuming QC, but the overall benefit of increased efficiencies in terms of both patient care and throughput can outweigh the negatives in a well-constructed POCT program.

References

1. Quinn A, Dixon D, Meenan B. Barriers to hospital-based clinical adoption of point-of-care testing (POCT): a systematic narrative review. *Critical Reviews in Clinical Laboratory Sciences.* 2016;53:1:1-12.

2. St John A, Price C. Existing and emerging technologies for point-of-care testing. *Clinical Biochemistry Reviews.* 2014;35 (3):155–167.

3. Bingisser R, Cairns C, Christ M, Hausfater P, Lindahl B, Mair J, Panteghini M, Price C, Venge P. Cardiac troponin: a critical review of the case for point-of-care testing in the ED. *American Journal of Emergency Medicine.* 2012;30:1639–1649.

4. Scalise D. Poised for growth: point-of-care testing. *Hospitals & Health Networks.* 2006;80:77–83.

5. Rooney K, Schilling U. Point-of-care testing in the overcrowded emergency department: can it make a difference? *Critical Care.* 2014; 18:692.

6. Chan C, Mak W, Cheung K, Sin K, Yu C, Rainer T, Renneberg R. Evidence-based point-of-care diagnostics: current status and emerging technologies. *Annual Review of Analytical Chemistry (Palo Alto Calif).* 2013;6:191–211.

7. Yang Z, Min Zhou D. Cardiac markers and their point-of-care testing for diagnosis of acute myocardial infarction. *Clinical Biochemistry.* 2006, 39:771–780.

8. Storrow A, Lyon J, Porter M. A systematic review of emergency department point-of-care cardiac markers and efficiency measures. *Point Care.* 2009;8:121–125.

9. Renaud B, Maison P, Ngako A, Cunin P, Santin A, Herve J, Salloum M, Calmettes MJ, Boraud C, Lemiale V, Grego JC, Debacker M, Hemery F, Roupie E. Impact of point-of-care testing in the emergency department evaluation and treatment of patients with suspected acute coronary syndromes. *Academic Emergency Medicine.* 2008;15:216–224.

10. Goyal M, Pines J, Drumheller B, Gaieski D. Point-of-care testing at triage decreases time to lactate level in septic patients. *Journal of Emergency Medicine.* 2010;38:578–581.

11. Geersing G, Janssen K, Oudega R, Bax L, Hoes A, Reitsma J, Moons K. Excluding venous thromboembolism using point of care D-dimer tests in outpatients: a diagnostic meta-analysis. *British Medical Journal.* 2009;339: 2990.

12. Lee-Lewandrowski E, Nichols J, Van Cott E, Grisson R, Louissaint A, Benzer T,

Lewandrowski K. Implementation of a rapid whole blood D-dimer test in the emergency department of an urban academic medical center: impact on ED length of stay and ancillary test utilization. *American Journal of Clinical Pathology.* 2009;132:326–331.

13. Larsson A, Greig-Pylypczuk R, Huisman A. The state of point-of-care testing: a European perspective. *Upsala Journal of Medical Sciences.* 2015;120:1–10.

14. Briggs C, Kimber S, Green L. Where are we at with point-of-care testing in haematology? *British Journal of Haematology.* 2012;158:679–690.

15. Briggs C, Longair I, Kumar P, Singh D, Machin SJ. Performance evaluation of the Sysmex haematology XN modular system. *Journal of Clinical Pathology.* 2012;65:1024–1030.

16. Lewandrowski K, Gregory K, Macmillan D. Assuring quality in point-of-care testing evolution of technologies, informatics, and program management. *Archives of Pathology & Laboratory Medicine.* 2011 Nov;135:1405–1414.

17. Gill J, Shephard M. The conduct of quality control and quality assurance testing for PoCT outside the laboratory. *Clinical Biochemist Reviews.* 2010 Aug;31:85–88.

Regionalization of Care

M. Kit Delgado, Fred Lin, and Brendan G. Carr

Introduction

Emergency medicine has dramatically evolved over the last half-century in response to the public's expectation of high-quality, accessible, and timely acute care. Outcomes for patients experiencing severe trauma, cardiac arrest, myocardial infarction, stroke, and burns have improved significantly.[1,2,3,4,5] Much of this progress has been a result of substantial scientific and clinical discovery, but improvement of the delivery system has also played an important role.

The goal of high-quality emergency care is to get the right resources to the right patient in the right place at the right time.[6] Classically, regionalization efforts focused on getting the sickest patients from smaller facilities with fewer resources to larger specialty care centers with more experienced staff and specialized resources. This model of care runs the risk of over- or under-triaging, where patients may be either transported or transferred to facilities with greater resources than they require or not transferred to specialty centers that might provide life- or limb-saving intervention during their time of need.

In the past decade, the Institute of Medicine (IOM) has recognized the positive impact of regional care delivery models for specific conditions, but there remains a significant challenge in the ability to appropriately match patients with high-quality care system-wide. Contributing factors include a lack of specialists, delays in care, hospital crowding, poor regional coordination resulting in fragmentation, and variation of care among providers and hospitals. The IOM recommended the development of coordinated, regionalized, and accountable emergency care systems in the United States.[6,7]

The challenge moving forward will be to discover novel ways to capitalize on the free flow of information, the ready access to technology, and the increasing role of patient preferences in the delivery of care. Although the concept of high-value care has permeated much of the house of medicine, there is no clear sense of how value will be defined in emergency care. The development of shared ownership of outcomes within a region across healthcare stakeholders could serve to align incentives and allow for innovation in the delivery of more patient-centered care not only for specific acute conditions, but for all patients presenting to emergency departments (EDs).

Case Presentation

Mike Smith is a 54-year-old police officer who tripped and fell down four steps on a Saturday afternoon while carrying some boxes of books for his daughter, who just returned from college. His daughter heard him fall, rushed downstairs, found him unconscious, lying on the basement floor, and called 911. Emergency medical technicians (EMTs) from the local fire department arrived 7 minutes later. They found the patient sitting up on the basement floor with a visible forehead hematoma and a small laceration oozing blood. He could not remember what happened and was a little groggy with a Glasgow coma scale (GCS) of 13, but was clearly breathing comfortably and protecting his airway. His only past medical history was hypertension, for which he was taking hydrochlorothiazide. The EMTs bandaged his wound, applied a cervical collar, and loaded him on a backboard. They made the decision to transport him to his local community hospital 4 miles away rather than call for air medical evacuation to the local trauma center downtown, 27 miles away (approximately a 40-minute drive).

On arrival at the local community hospital ED, he was immediately placed in a room and evaluated by an emergency physician. At the time of examination, Mr. Smith's mental status was back to normal (GCS of 15). No signs of trauma other than the hematoma noted by the EMTs were found on physical examination, and his cervical collar was removed using a clinical decision rule to justify its removal. He was cleared from the backboard and expeditiously transported to receive a computed tomography (CT) scan of the head. The CT scan revealed a 2 mm frontal subdural hematoma without midline shift. As the local community hospital did not have an on-call neurosurgeon, the emergency physician called the transfer center phone number of the closest trauma center. This trauma center notified the transferring physician that their hospital did not have any open beds in the intensive care unit. The transferring physician called the other trauma center downtown, which accepted the patient for transfer. The emergency physician called the local helicopter emergency medical services (EMS) crew, who arrived within 15 minutes and flew the patient to the trauma center. The patient was brought from the trauma center helipad to the trauma area within the ED where the multidisciplinary trauma team was awaiting his arrival. As the CT scan image was unavailable from the community hospital, the trauma team ordered a repeat head CT as well as a cervical spine CT, which revealed the stable appearance of the hematoma and no cervical spine injury. The patient was placed in the ED observation unit. In the morning, his clinical status remained the same with a normal GCS, and Mr. Smith was discharged home with his daughter.

Ongoing Challenges in Emergency Care Regionalization and Recent Innovations

Mr. Smith received medically appropriate emergency care in a state with an established regionalized trauma system. Nevertheless, this case illustrates multiple challenges to achieving the ultimate goal of regionalization: *to deliver the right resources to the right patient in the right place in the right time.* By adopting recent innovations, Mr. Smith's care could have been much more efficient, cost effective, and patient centered. Key ongoing challenges in emergency care regionalization and examples of innovations that have overcome these challenges include the following.

Challenge #1: Determining the Need for Time-Sensitive Critical Care Interventions

Developing more efficient and cost-effective emergency care requires (1) determining what resources are needed to care for the patient and (2) matching patients to facilities that are capable of caring for them. *Overtriage* refers to sending patients to a higher level of care than is required for their illness or injury, and *undertriage* refers to sending patients to facilities without the resources required to optimally care for them. The first potential opportunity to determine the needs of the patient is at the point of EMS dispatch based on information gathered on the 911 call. However, there are relatively few conditions, such as cardiac arrest or gunshot wounds to the chest, for which an EMS dispatcher can definitively determine the need for critical care resources with information obtained from an untrained caller. As a result, EMS providers make the vast majority of initial triage decisions after arrival at the patient's side.

To ensure that severely injured patients are taken to centers with the resources to care for them, the American College of Surgeons Committee on Trauma (ACSCOT) developed the Field Triage Decision Scheme in 1987. The scheme is regularly updated with a goal of reducing the proportion of severely injured patients transported to nontrauma centers (undertriaged) to less than 5 percent while maintaining the proportion of patients without serious injuries transported to trauma centers (overtriaged) to less than 50–75 percent.[8] Similar prehospital triage criteria have been developed for other time-sensitive conditions that benefit from regionalized care, such as acute ischemic stroke.[9,10] In general, these decision aids are primarily focused on minimizing undertriage, and this has direct implications for the value proposition of care regionalization.

In the case of Mr. Smith, application of the most recent version of the ACSCOT Field Triage Decision Scheme would have resulted in the recommendation to transport him to a trauma center due to a GCS of 13). The EMS personnel decided to transport him to his local hospital given their suspicion that he would not require any emergent life- or limb-saving interventions. Most patients with a story like Mr. Smith's do not have an intracranial bleed, and for them, this choice would have increased cost-effectiveness, but a small minority of patients with GCS 13 deteriorate clinically, and for them, the decision might have resulted in a worse outcome. There is evidence that compliance with existing field triage criteria would improve outcomes while safely reducing costs related to overtriage at more expensive trauma centers.[11] However, strict adherence to the criteria would result in an undertriage rate of 15–20 percent of severely injured patients going to nontrauma centers and an overtriage rate of more than 50 percent of patients who do not need trauma center resources going to trauma centers. These evidence-based triage criteria developed over the last 25 years demonstrate the complex trade-off between sensitivity and specificity – key drivers of cost-effectiveness. To further advance the accuracy of field triage, additional data points are needed. For example, ongoing investigations will determine whether point-of-care lactate could be useful in predicting traumatic hemorrhage in the setting of higher blood pressure thresholds, or whether novel biomarkers for brain injury could be useful if measured at the point of care.[12,13]

Even with these potential innovations, field triage will never be perfect, and emergency physicians working in hospitals without specialty coverage will always have to determine whether each patient they treat potentially needs a higher level of care. In the case of Mr. Smith, after obtaining the CT scan in relatively rapid fashion, the emergency physician had obtained all the diagnostic information needed to make a disposition decision. Based on the patient's age, CT scan findings, lack of significant comorbidities or other injuries, and not taking anticoagulants, Mr. Smith was at very low risk of clinical deterioration. Studies have shown that the likelihood of requiring a neurosurgical intervention in these situations is remote (less than 1–2 percent), and either a brief period of observation or a normal repeat CT scan in 6–12 hours is enough to safely discharge these patients home.[14,15]

However, for a number of reasons (including medicolegal reasons), the vast majority of emergency physicians would not feel comfortable making this disposition decision without consulting with a neurosurgeon. On-call specialists at trauma centers are often connected to emergency physicians calling from outside hospitals via its hospital transfer center. The default goal of the conversation is rarely to determine whether the patient needs transfer or not but to initiate the transfer process and establish a provider-to-provider transition of care. Given the relatively limited amount of information that can be relayed over a phone conversation and the difficulties associated with reimbursement and liability for decision-making done at facilities where they are not on staff, trauma center specialists will almost always recommend patient transfer.

Innovation #1: Teleradiology- and Telemedicine-Facilitated Consultation to Determine the Need for Transfer and to Provide Treatment Recommendations

The real-time electronic sharing of radiographic images in addition to phone consultation with a trauma center specialist is one of the most promising ways of improving interhospital transfer decision-making. This brings the cognitive expertise of trauma center specialists to the patient rather than transferring all patients to a trauma center.

The University of New Mexico Hospital (UNMH) implemented one of the first regionalized systems in the United States to use teleradiology for guiding transfer decisions from outlying hospitals. This hospital is the only Level I trauma center in the entire state and as such received the transfers from great distances of hundreds of patients with minor traumatic brain injury who ended up being discharged on arrival. In 2007, the hospital launched a secure web-based platform onto which radiology images collected from outside hospitals could be uploaded and viewed at the time of the UNMH transfer center phone conversation with the on-call UNMH neurosurgeon. With seven outlying community hospitals, 66 consultations took place in the first year of implementation. For consultations that would have resulted in transfer based on the phone conversation, 44 percent of transfers were avoided after review of the images.[16] Furthermore, among those that were not transferred, viewing the images resulted in management recommendation changes in 56 percent of patients.[16]

Comparable systems were implemented in Israel for patients similar to Mr. Smith with a GCS of 13–15 and low-risk intracranial bleeds (e.g., subdural hematoma <5 mm). Only 3 percent of patients who were not transferred and who were observed at the facility without a neurosurgeon required a delayed transfer.[17] None of these patients required a delayed neurosurgical procedure.[17] To address the challenge of surgical specialists not always being able to access a computer at the time of phone consultation, other trauma centers are pilot testing the use of sharing radiographic images over mobile phones.[18,19] Furthermore, although more resource intensive, the sharing of radiographic images can be augmented by real-time video consultation and coaching of care. This has been shown to be particularly successful for general trauma care for hospitals in rural areas; consultation to determine need for transfer for burn, maxillofacial, and hand injuries; and management of acute ischemic stroke.[20,21,22,23,24]

The availability of teleradiology- or telemedicine-facilitated consultation in Mr. Smith's case likely would have made a transfer to the trauma center avoidable. This would have spared the insurance and out-of-pocket costs of transport, trauma team activation, and additional costs from a second hospital encounter, and would have spared his family the burden of coming to the trauma center only to see him discharged shortly after arrival. Additional potential benefits to the healthcare system include not contributing to ED crowding at the trauma center by sparing the opportunity costs of staff and imaging resources, enabling them to focus on other patients in need of care. Many barriers remain to implementing such a workflow, including reimbursement for consultation services and finding a provider (e.g., general surgeon or hospitalist) at the local hospital willing to admit, observe, and make the ultimate disposition decision for the patient.

Challenge #2: Determining Optimal Transport Destination and Transport Mode

As described above, once the potential need for a critical care intervention is established in the field or in an ED, the patient needs to be matched to a destination hospital with the capability and availability to deliver the required care. As illustrated in the case of Mr. Smith, transfer to another hospital may require multiple phone calls to locate a hospital with the capacity to accept the patient. This challenge is magnified in mass casualty events when multiple patients have different clinical needs. Once the destination hospital is selected, the choice between helicopter and ground EMS transportation needs to be made. Helicopter EMS transport results in faster transport times if the expected ground transport time is at least 30 minutes. However, since helicopter transport costs 5 to 15 times as much as ground transport, the use of helicopter EMS would be considered cost-effective for trauma transport only if there is at least a modest survival benefit (a least an average absolute risk reduction in mortality of 1.3 percent) or some sustained improvement in disability outcomes.[25] Therefore, the decision to use a helicopter is complex and needs to take into account the ready availability and capabilities of both ground and helicopter EMS options, the expected ground transport time, and an assessment of the likely reduction in morbidity or mortality.

Innovation # 2: Dispatch and Regional Network Communications Systems

The Birmingham Regional Emergency Medical Services System (BREMSS) was established by the University of Alabama in 1996 to coordinate and improve prehospital medical emergency response for a seven-county area in central Alabama. The system has since expanded statewide. If patients meet trauma, stroke, or ST-elevation myocardial infarction (STEMI) criteria, EMS contacts the communication center, which is staffed 24/7 by paramedics. Every hospital in the region that is designated as a trauma, stroke, and STEMI hospital reports their real-time status to the communications center through an intranet computer system. The paramedic at the communications center makes the decision for hospital destination based on hospital availability, transport time (ground or helicopter), and patient condition. The goal of the system is to match patients to the right hospital and prevent patients from being sent to hospitals that may not have the capability or capacity to treat the patients, necessitating further transfers. The system was also designed to be scaled up to respond in the event of a mass casualty event. Since implementation of the system, the relative mortality risk for trauma has decreased by 11 percent.[26] Based on its success and the ability to scale up for mass casualty events, in July 2006, BREMSS was given the Homeland Security Award from Mitretek Systems and the John F. Kennedy School of Government at Harvard University.

A regional network communication system can also use expensive air medical resources more efficiently. Maryland instituted the first statewide EMS and air medical transport system in the early 1970s under the pioneering vision of trauma surgeon R. Adams Cowley. As opposed to most other regions in the country, a central entity, the Maryland State Police

Aviation Command, dispatches all helicopter EMS scene flights. Since implementing a rule that helicopters would be dispatched only if the expected ground transport time was more than 30 minutes for trauma patients, there was a 49 percent decrease in helicopter transports, while still maintaining system-level improvement in mortality over time.[27] In the case of Mr. Smith, a regional network communication system may have prevented the need for multiple phone calls to find a trauma center that could accept his transfer.

Challenge # 3:   Lack of Data and Motivation to Improve Population-Level Acute Care Outcomes

One of the biggest challenges to the efficient delivery of regionalized emergency care is the lack of actionable population-level data. Prospective studies to investigate how often transfer scenarios like Mr. Smith's occur on a regional level would be logistically challenging due to the need to collect data from both community hospitals, not typically involved in research, and the tertiary care hospitals that receive patients as transfers. Most state trauma registries collect data only from designated trauma centers, and although ED and inpatient administrative claims data can provide a more thorough portrait of acute care within a state, only a handful of states permit the linkage of acute care transfers between hospitals. In addition, administrative data have significant limitations due to the lack of key prehospital, physiologic, clinical, and laboratory data. This creates significant challenges for adjusting outcomes for severity of illness or injury.

Although logistical challenges of using data to understand the performance of the trauma system from the regional perspective exist, the lack of shared incentive to improve the injury outcomes of a community further complicates matters. At present, hospital performance is benchmarked individually, and in the fee-for-service environment, redundancies in care are frequently rewarded, potentially creating inefficient incentives. A more innovative approach would align incentives for hospitals within a region to work collaboratively to improve system-level efficiency and population-level outcomes.

Innovation # 3:   Creation of Statewide Population-Level Datasets and Quality Improvement Program

In 2005, the North Carolina Chapter of the American College of Cardiology sponsored the Reperfusion in Acute Myocardial Infarction in North Carolina Emergency departments (RACE) project, a statewide initiative to identify and overcome barriers to rapid myocardial reperfusion by establishing optimal regional systems of care with parallels to existing trauma systems.[28] One of the first steps was identifying the current state of STEMI care in each facility using a standard survey form as well as a prospective data collection form on 10 consecutive acute myocardial infarction and STEMI patients treated at participating hospitals without percutaneous coronary intervention (PCI), and all STEMI patients treated at participating PCI centers. After this initial baseline data collection period, a multilevel intervention was implemented involving streamlining EMS triage and transport protocols, non-PCI ED transfer protocols, interhospital communications, and cardiac catheterization laboratory performance benchmarks.

After implementation, median reperfusion times significantly improved according to first door-to-device (presenting to PCI hospital 85 to 74 minutes, P.001; transferred to PCI hospital 165 to 128 minutes, P.001), door-to-needle in non-PCI hospitals (35 to 29 minutes,

P = 0.002), and door-in to door-out for patients transferred from non-PCI hospitals (120 to 71 minutes, P 0.001). Nonreperfusion rates were unchanged (15 percent) in non-PCI hospitals and decreased from 23 percent to 11 percent in the PCI hospitals.[28] Further analyses of vulnerable populations, including women, minorities, and the elderly, which traditionally suffered longer treatment times, demonstrated significant reductions in these populations that were comparable to middle-aged white male patients. In women, the men versus women door-to-electrocardiogram (ECG) time disparity fell from a baseline of 4.3 minutes (95 percent CI, 0.8 to 7.3) to 0.1 minutes (95 percent CI, –2.4 to 2.0), making an overall reduction of 4.4 minutes (95 percent CI, 8.1 to 0.4).[29] Among patients presenting to or transferred to PCI hospitals, clinical outcomes including death, cardiac arrest, and cardiogenic shock did not significantly change following the intervention.[28] However, patients treated within guideline goals had a mortality of 2.2 percent compared with 5.7 percent for those exceeding guideline recommendations (P 0.001).[30] Significant challenges to broader implementation remain as approximately 80 percent of patients requiring transfer out of non-PCI hospitals still had door-in door-out exceeding recommended benchmarks of 30 minutes or less, despite an improvement in the median time from 97 minutes preimplementation to 58 minutes postimplementation.[31]

Another excellent example of systemic data collection leading to the design of an effective regionalized system of care comes from the state of Arizona. The Save Hearts in Arizona Registry and Education, established in 2004 by the Arizona Bureau of Emergency Medical Services and Trauma System (BEMSTS), was intended to be a centralized data collection, reporting, and quality improvement/education program for out-of-hospital cardiac arrests in the state of Arizona. Data reporting in 2005 consisted of voluntary submissions containing patient prehospital care reports from 30 EMS systems for anyone receiving cardiopulmonary resuscitation (CPR), defibrillation, or epinephrine, all subjects having had no vital signs on EMS arrival. Those data were then manually extracted by the SHARE Program Research and Quality Improvement Director, entered into an enhanced Utstein database, and combined with additional measures such as survival to hospital discharge stratified by presence of bystander CPR, mean EMS response time, initial cardiac rhythm, return of spontaneous circulation (ROSC), and neurological/functional status. These data suggested that out-of-hospital cardiac arrest patients had a 3.4 percent overall survival rate, with up to 8.6 percent survival for those with initial rhythm of ventricular fibrillation/ventricular tachycardia.[32]

The data demonstrated a low incidence of layperson CPR, indicating public education on this lifesaving skill was necessary.[33] The data also demonstrated that survival was not significantly impacted by transport interval. This suggested that a modest increase in transport interval associated with bypassing the closest hospital en route to specialized care is safe and warrants further investigation.[34] In 2007, criteria were established for a statewide network of specialized cardiac receiving centers with the ability to provide therapeutic hypothermia, prompt PCI, and guideline-based postarrest critical care. Further EMS protocols were established in 2008 to help transport patients directly to these cardiac receiving centers.[35]

Implementation of bypass protocols to cardiac arrest receiving centers was associated with major improvements in outcomes. Of the potentially eligible patients who achieved ROSC, provision of therapeutic hypothermia increased from 0 percent to 44.0 percent and the rate of PCI increased from 11.7 percent to 30.7 percent. All-rhythm survival increased from 8.9 to 14.4 percent. Survival with favorable neurologic outcome increased from 5.9

percent to 8.9 percent. For witnessed, shockable rhythms, survival increased from 21.4 percent to 39.2 percent, and favorable neurologic outcome increased from 19.4 percent to 29.8 percent.[35]

Conclusion

Over the last several years, dramatic changes have taken place in healthcare delivery. At the same time, there has been an increased emphasis on understanding the connection between health and healthcare and on improving community and population health outcomes. Stories such as Mr. Smith's clearly illustrate the connection between communities and the healthcare systems that serve them. In order to optimally match patients in need of life- and limb-saving treatment to facilities with the capabilities and capacity to care for them, appropriate data systems and incentives will need to be developed. Although not yet a reality, an innovation whose time has come is the development of population-based payment modifiers based on regional performance. In order for facilities to have a shared interest in improving the emergency care outcomes of the communities they serve, the manner in which the community uses emergency care resources needs to be empirically defined, and then incentives to improve care for the community need to be developed for the system as a whole. This sort of community-based incentive has the potential to align the interests of the many unaffiliated stakeholders within a community.

References

1. Sise RG, Calvo RY, Spain DA, et al. The epidemiology of trauma-related mortality in the United States from 2002 to 2010. *Journal of Trauma and Acute Care Surgery.* 2014;76(4):913–920.

2. Fox CS, Evans JC, Larson MC, et al. Temporal trends in coronary heart disease mortality and sudden cardiac death from 1950 to 1999 the Framingham Heart Study. *Circulation.* 2004;110:522–527.

3. Rosamond WG, Chambless LG, Folsom AR, et al. Trends in the incidence of myocardial infarction and in mortality due to coronary heart disease, 1987 to 1994. *New England Journal of Medicine.* 1998;339 (13):861–867.

4. Lackland DT, Roccella EJ, Deutsch AF, et al. Factors influencing the decline in stroke mortality: a statement from the American Heart Association/American Stroke Association. *Stroke.* 2014;45(1):315– 353.

5. Ryan CM, Schoenfeld DA, Thorpe WP, et al. Objective estimates of the probability of death from burn injuries. *New England Journal of Medicine.* 1998;338(6):362–366.

6. Institute of Medicine. *Hospital-Based Emergency Care: At the Breaking Point.* National Academies Press, 2006.

7. Carr BG, Asplin BR. Regionalization and emergency care: the Institute of Medicine reports and a federal government update. *Academic Emergency Medicine.* 2010;17 (2):1351–1353.

8. Sasser SM, Hunt RC, Faul M, et al. Guidelines for field triage of injured patients: recommendations of the National Expert Panel on Field Triage. *MMWR Recommendations and Reports.* 2009;58:1–35.

9. Kothari RU, Pancioli A, Liu T, et al. Cincinnati Prehospital Stroke Scale: reproducibility and validity. *Annals of Emergency Medicine.* 1999;33(4):373–378.

10. Kidwell CS, Starkman S, Eckstein M, et al. Identifying stroke in the field prospective validation of the Los Angeles Prehospital Stroke Screen (LAPSS). *Stroke.* 2000;31 (1):71–76.

11. Faul M, Wald MM, Sullivent EE, et al. Large cost savings realized from the 2006 Field Triage Guideline: reduction in overtriage in US trauma centers.

Prehospital Emergency Care. 2012 Apr–Jun;16(22):222–229.

12. Guyette FX, Meier EN, Newgard C, et al. A comparison of prehospital lactate and systolic blood pressure for predicting the need for resuscitative care in trauma transported by ground. *Journal of Trauma and Acute Care Surgery.* 2015;78(3):600–606.

13. Caswell SV, Cortes N, Mitchell K, et al. Development of nanoparticle-enabled protein biomarker discovery: implementation for saliva-based traumatic brain injury detection. *Advances in Salivary Diagnostics.* 2015:121–129.

14. Carlson AP, Ramirez P, Kennedy G, et al. Low rate of delayed deterioration requiring surgical treatment in patients transferred to a tertiary care center for mild traumatic brain injury. *Neurosurgical Focus.* 2010;29 (5):E3.

15. Washington CW, Grubb RL Jr. Are routine repeat imaging and intensive care unit admission necessary in mild traumatic brain injury? *Journal of Neurosurgery.* 2007;298(20):2371–2380.

16. Moya M, Valdez J, Yonas H, et al. The impact of a telehealth web-based solution on neurosurgery triage and consultation. *Journal of Telemedicine and e-Health.* 2010;16(9):945–949.

17. Klein Y, Donchik V, Jaffe D, et al. Management of patients with traumatic intracranial injury in hospitals without neurosurgical service. *Journal of Trauma and Acute Care Surgery.* 2010;69(3):544–548.

18. Bullard TB, Rosenberg MS, Ladde J, et al. Digital images taken with a mobile phone can assist in the triage of neurosurgical patients to a level 1 trauma centre. *Journal of Telemedicine and Telecare.* 2010;69 (3):544–548.

19. Plant M, Novak C, McCabe S, et al. Use of digital images to aid in the decision-making for acute upper extremity trauma referral. *Journal of Hand Surgery (European Volume).* 2015:1753193415620177.

20. Duchesne JC, Kyle A, Simmons J, et al. Impact of telemedicine upon rural trauma care. *Journal of Trauma and Acute Care Surgery.* 2008;64(1):92–98.

21. Saffle JR, Edelman L, Theurer L, et al. Telemedicine evaluation of acute burns is accurate and cost-effective. *Journal of Trauma and Acute Care Surgery.* 2009;67 (2):358–365.

22. Roccia F, Spada MC, Milani B, et al. Telemedicine in maxillofacial trauma: a 2-year clinical experience. *Journal of Oral and Maxillofacial Surgery.* 2005;70(3):295–301.

23. Wallace D, Jones S, Milroy C, et al. Telemedicine for acute plastic surgical trauma and burns. *Journal of Plastic, Reconstructive & Aesthetic Surgery.* 2008;61 (1):31–36.

24. Silva GS, Farrell S, Shandra E, et al. The status of telestroke in the United States: a survey of currently active stroke telemedicine programs. *Stroke.* 2012;43 (8):2078–2085.

25. Delgado MK, Staudenmayer KL, Wang NE, et al. Cost-effectiveness of helicopter versus ground emergency medical services for trauma scene transport in the United States. *Annals of Emergency Medicine.* 2013;62(4):351–364.

26. Abernathy JH III, McGwin G Jr, Acker JE III, et al. Impact of a voluntary trauma system on mortality, length of stay, and cost at a level I trauma center. *The American Surgeon.* 2002;68(2):182–192.

27. Hirshon JM, Galvagno SM, Comer A, et al. Maryland's helicopter emergency medical services experience from 2001 to 2011: system improvements and patients' outcomes. *Annals of Emergency Medicine.* 2015;76(3):332–340.

28. Jollis JG, Roettig ML, Aluko AO, et al. Implementation of a statewide system for coronary reperfusion for ST-segment elevation myocardial infarction. *JAMA.* 2007;298(20):2371–2380.

29. Glickman SW, Granger CB, Ou FS, et al. Impact of a statewide ST-segment-elevation myocardial infarction regionalization program on treatment times for women, minorities, and the elderly. *Circulation Cardiovascular Quality and Outcomes.* 2010;3:514–521.

30. Jollis JG, Al-Khalidi HR, Monk L, et al. Expansion of a regional ST-segment-elevation myocardial infarction system to an entire state. *Circulation.* 2012;126:189–195.

31. Wang TY, Nallamothu BK, Krumholz HM, et al. Association of door-in to door-out time with reperfusion delays and outcomes among patients transferred for primary percutaneous coronary intervention. *JAMA.* 2011;305 (24):2540–2547.

32. Bobrow BJ, Vadeboncoeur TF, Clark L, et al. Establishing Arizona's statewide cardiac arrest reporting and educational network. *Prehospital Emergency Care.* 2008;12(3):381–387.

33. Vadeboncoeur T,F Bobrow BJ, Clark L, et al. The Save Hearts in Arizona Registry and Education (SHARE) program: who is performing CPR and where are they doing it? *Resuscitation.* 2007;75(1):68–75.

34. Spaite DW, Bobrow BJ, Vadeboncoeur TF, et al. The impact of prehospital transport interval on survival in out-of-hospital cardiac arrest: implications for regionalization of post-resuscitation care. *Resuscitation.* 2008;79:61–66.

35. Spaite DW, Bobrow BJ, Stolz U, et al. Statewide regionalization of post arrest care for out-of-hospital cardiac arrest: association with survival and neurologic outcome. *Annals of Emergency Medicine.* 2014;64(5):496–506.

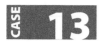

13 Clinical Decision Support Tools

Kelly Bookman and Ali S. Raja

Introduction

Given the wide variety of patients who present to the emergency department (ED) for care, it is not surprising that there is considerable evidence for providers to sift through when determining appropriate clinical pathways for diagnosis and treatment. The American College of Emergency Physicians (ACEP), similar to a number of other national and international professional societies, has developed evidence-based guidelines that recommend best practices. However, keeping up with them and incorporating them into daily practice is a Sisyphean task.

In order to facilitate the delivery of high-quality clinical care, computerized clinical decision support (CDS) systems were developed to guide ED clinicians using electronic health records (EHRs) and computerized order entry (CPOE) as to best practices, based on patient characteristics, tests or medications under consideration, and diagnoses suspected.

These CDS systems are not unique to the ED. In fact, the first CDS system was developed more than 50 years ago at Kaiser Permanente and involved patients sorting punchcards of symptoms into "yes" or "no" piles. These were then combined with electrocardiogram, phonocardiogram, and ballistocardiogram data, as well as vital capacity, visual acuity, height, and weight, to populate a differential diagnosis list for the patients' physicians.[1] Over the ensuing decades, CDS has evolved. Since then it has been successfully used to provide recommendations for medication ordering and dosing, appropriate laboratory and imaging utilization, and adherence to best practice guidelines. It has also become integrated into electronic clinical systems, allowing both the automated population of data fields (saving data-entry work for providers and other healthcare personnel) and automated ordering of tests (based on CDS recommendations).

In the ED, a number of homegrown and commercial CDS systems exist, and many of them are regularly updated with new content as current guidelines, best practices, and decision rules are published. However, not all CDS systems are created equal. The optimal characteristics of a CDS system are well established; the best designed must be:

- Fast: Significant effort should be spent to ensure that the number of clicks is minimized, so as to minimize the time that clinicians must spend with the CDS system.
- Anticipatory: The CDS system should be able to determine clinicians' needs in real time, presenting them with information as soon as – or even before – they need it.
- Integrated: If a CDS system is able to pull data in from an integrated EHR, it can obviate the need for clinicians to enter data themselves.
- Nonobtrusive: A great CDS system does not have unnecessary hard stops (which prevent moving forward without appropriate data entry). This also minimizes the change of false or inaccurate data entry in order to just move past CDS (often seen in poorly designed CDS systems).
- Redirecting: Ideally, CDS should suggest and facilitate the correct ordering of tests and medications rather than simply preventing incorrect ordering. If the wrong antibiotic dose is ordered, for example, the correct dose should pop up as a suggestion.

- Able to allow for monitoring and feedback: Clinicians respond to comparative data, especially when it is local. Feedback regarding variations in practice based on data gathered from CDS has been demonstrated to improve adherence to evidence-based guidelines, and good CDS should allow for this.
- Up to date: Keeping track of all of the recent literature and evidence is a full-time task, but clinicians expect this when they work with CDS systems. Commercial vendors often have teams to do this, and smaller or homegrown systems can rely on free, publicly available, curated libraries such as the Harvard Medical School eLibrary of Evidence.[2] Out-of-date guidelines are often worse than no guidelines at all.

CDS can productively inform a number of decisions in the ED. However, a significant portion of CDS development to date has focused only on use in imaging. The ACEP Choosing Wisely list, a multidisciplinary collaborative led by the American Board of Internal Medicine Foundation, which includes tests that patients and their clinicians should discuss and potentially not use, includes five imaging tests among 10 total tests. Many of these recommendations are similar to international recommendations as well (e.g., the European Society of Cardiology's guidelines for imaging use for patients with suspected pulmonary embolism). Given this, the remainder of this chapter focuses on imaging CDS, but the innovation and evidence discussed apply to other CDS systems as well.

Innovation

At the University of Colorado Health (UCHealth), we implemented embedded CDS into the ED workflow of the EHR for the ordering of high-cost imaging studies. UCHealth has four main campuses, three of which are community based and one an academic facility, providing a combined 324,000-plus ED visits annually. The academic facility and two of the community sites are Level II trauma centers; the third community site is a Level III trauma center. The entire system shares an integrated EHR (Epic), which has been in use at the academic facility for more than 4 years and at the community sites for a little over a year. Workflows are essentially the same across all of the EDs. This similarity in workflows and a collaborative ED service line leadership allows us to institute and study the effects of EHR optimizations on a system-wide level.

Recently, a Top 5 list was published in the Journal of the American Medical Association aimed at improving the value of emergency care.[3] Three of the five (computed tomography for pulmonary embolism [CT PE], CT of the brain for trauma, and CT of the cervical spine) were high-cost imaging studies that were deemed to have a low impact on patient care. All have previously validated, widely accepted scoring systems that can be used to drive medical decision-making.[4,5,6,7] At UCHealth, we embedded the Pulmonary Embolism Rule-Out Criteria (PERC), Wells score, National Emergency X-Radiography Utilization Study (NEXUS) cervical spine criteria, and Canadian CT Head Rules directly into the image ordering workflow to facilitate the use of these tools with a goal of decreasing variability in practice across providers. The philosophy was that as an integrated part of the usual work-flow, CDS will help providers use the tools more frequently and optimize evidence-based decision-making about when to order high-cost, potentially low-impact imaging studies.

At UCHealth EDs, when a provider places an order for one of the aforementioned imaging studies, the CPOE system prompts them via an interruptive alert to use the scoring tool and takes them with one "click" directly to the tool, which is built into the EHR. The alert is designed to fire only if the patient fits the clinical criteria and the system also pulls in patient-specific data already in the EHR to transparently demonstrate to the provider what criteria the algorithm is using. For example, when a CT PE is ordered, the patient must be older than 18, not pregnant, and have a normal heart rate and pulse oximetry in order for the alert to fire and drive the provider to use the PERC criteria.[8] The provider is then automatically brought to a window displaying an interactive version of the rest of the PERC criteria. Once the provider answers the remaining questions that are part of PERC, if there is no indication for the CT PE, the order is automatically removed from the orders section with another alert explaining that the patient "PERCs out" and therefore no imaging or D-dimer testing is necessary. Similarly, if the patient has a positive PERC screening, the tool instantly opens a palette of questions that represents the Wells score. Again, once the Wells score is calculated, an alert shows the score and performs the appropriate action, that is, recommends ordering a D-dimer for score less than 4, or continuing with the CT PE order if the score is greater than 4. Each alert brings the provider back into the orders activity so that the entire CDS experience is conducted within the usual provider workflow. All of the embedded scoring tools function in a similar fashion.

Getting these scoring tools embedded into the EHR required collaboration between the Epic analysts and subject matter experts. At UCHealth, we have developed an Epic physician builder team, which is comprised of inpatient, ambulatory, and emergency medicine physicians. The emergency medicine physician builder was able to build these interruptive alerts and then have them tested by the analyst rather than requiring dedicated Epic analyst resources. This significantly expedited getting this design feature into the EHR. This embedded CDS workflow was presented at the Epic annual user group meeting in 2015 as one of the first of its kind.

A large part of the implementation of this process was the collaboration across the health system to engage stakeholders and help explain the goal of the CDS in order to increase acceptance and usage of the new tools. First, we engaged both formal and informal leaders at each hospital site to help develop the tools. We then collected preimplementation data about variability in practice as a tool to describe the need for CDS assistance. The local leadership team led this initiative and described the preimplementation "burning platform" before the new functionality was implemented, as a way to gain broader acceptance, decrease change resistance, and improve utilization. In this way, we were able to drive adoption of the new workflow based on frontline provider understanding of the reasons for it as well as leadership approval of the process. Involving both frontline and local leadership is paramount to being able to get providers to accept this kind of workflow change. The implementation was successful in our system. Across the five participating sites, the rate of brain CT acquisition was significantly lower (10 percent, 95 percent CI [7 percent, 13 percent]; $p < 0.0001$), as was the acquisition of cervical spine CT imaging (6 percent, 95 percent CI [0 percent, 11 percent]; $p = 0.0464$), after our novel CDS implementation. At the largest facility ($>100,000$ visits per year), the rate of brain CT acquisition was significantly lower (16 percent, 95 percent CI [12 percent, 21 percent]; $p < 0.0001$); the rate of chest CT acquisition was also significantly 19 percent lower (19 percent, 95 percent CI [8 percent, 28 percent]; $p = 0.0016$); and the rate of spine CT acquisition was significantly lower (7 percent, 95 percent CI [2 percent, 18 percent]; $p = 0.0155$).

Discussion

CDS for imaging in the ED is exceptionally relevant. In April 2014, President Obama signed into law the Protecting Access to Medicare Act (PAMA).[9] It includes a provision for CDS based on appropriate use criteria for the use of advanced imaging (CT, magnetic resonance imaging, and nuclear medicine) in outpatient settings, including the ED. The Centers for Medicare and Medicaid have mandated adoption of PAMA-compliant CDS, the January 2017 implementation date has been pushed back but a new date has yet to be announced. This mandated adoption of CDS, if rolled out well and with significant input from ordering clinicians, should help curb some of the significant variation in imaging currently seen in the ED.[10,11]

UCHealth's implementation of CDS is a fantastic example of a successful integration led by emergency physician and radiology partners and champions. Other similarly successful implementations of CDS for imaging have been seen in EDs across the country.[12,13] However, other sites have seen CDS implementations go badly, primarily for the following two main reasons:

- CDS with low-quality evidence:[14] Clinicians generally understand evidence and can differentiate between high-quality evidence-based CDS and that based on consensus opinion. CDS should present only well-validated high-quality evidence-based decision support; anything less will likely result in pushback from and noncompliance by clinicians. In fact, PAMA requires a transparent and validated grading process for evidence to be adopted into CDS. Fortunately, for anyone looking for unbiased evidence to adopt into CDS, the emergency physician co-led Harvard Medical School eLibrary of Evidence offers it, freely available.[3]
- CDS implemented with a "top-down" approach: In order to gain provider acceptance, the implementation of CDS must be led by a clinician champion. The authors of this chapter both serve as the clinical leaders and champions for CDS at their respective sites, which allows other emergency clinicians to see that their input, through their champions, is valued. At least one (and likely more) CDS implementation has failed because of an outside mandate (often by radiology departments) without the approval of ordering providers.[15]

When poorly designed or implemented CDS is put into place, there may be legitimate concerns about providers "gaming" the data entry in order to bypass excessively obtrusive or inappropriate CDS. However, when CDS is implemented well and presents evidence-based recommendations, this "gaming" is minimal.[16]

The use of CDS is not limited to workstations. A multinational European group from France and Switzerland successfully evaluated the use of handheld devices to improve the appropriateness of imaging for patients with suspected PE; they found that the handheld device CDS not only improved the appropriate use of testing but did so more effectively than a paper guideline with the same information.[17] This reiterates the fact that evidence-based guideline development and promulgation are not enough – there needs to be real-time, provider-facing CDS to help guide adherence to these guidelines.

Once CDS has been put into place and adopted by providers, the next step is feedback reporting. A well-established quality improvement intervention in other contexts, the practice of feedback reporting is often time intensive and requires manual chart review for determination of appropriateness. However, CDS allows for automated data capture and, when integrated with algorithms to determine appropriateness, can improve adherence to evidence-based guidelines beyond that obtained by CDS alone.[18]

As the specialty of emergency medicine continues to develop evidence-based quality metrics to help measure and guide the care of patients in the ED, we have the unique opportunity to build paired CDS, designed to also capture data on quality metric adherence.

If CDS and quality metrics are developed and integrated together, we can obviate the need for intensive retrospective data capture and allow for widespread adoption of quality measure reporting.[19,20]

While PAMA has mandated clinician-focused CDS, the next step will be the development of patient-oriented CDS for the ED. With it, we hope to determine patient preferences and risk tolerances, discuss evidence-based recommendations for testing and imaging, and present patient-specific prevalences for injury given individual patient signs and symptoms.[21,22]

Beyond this next step, CDS will continue to develop over the coming years. As it becomes more seamlessly integrated into EHRs, it should actively pull not only historical factors from patients' charts, but also the information from the current examination as soon as it is entered, providing guidance to physicians as data are entered in real time. The next steps will involve patient-specific test suggestions to guide patient–provider shared decision-making, with the goal of improving the utilization of resources for all patients seen in the ED.

References

1. Collen MF, Rubin L, Neyman J, et al. Automated multiphasic screening and diagnosis. *American Journal of Public Health and the Nation's Health.* 1964;54:741–750.

2. Harvard Library of Evidence. Available at http://libraryofevidence.med.harvard.edu/. Accessed February 15, 2016.

3. Schuur JD, Carney DP, Lyn ET, et al. A top-five list for emergency medicine: a pilot project to improve the value of emergency care. *JAMA Internal Medicine.* 2014;174(4):509–515.

4. Wells PS, Anderson DR, Rodger M, et al. Derivation of a simple clinical model to categorize patient's probability of pulmonary embolism: increasing the models utility with the SimpliRED D-dimer. *Journal of Thrombosis and Haemostasis.* 2000;83(3):416–420.

5. Hoffman JR, Mower WR, Wolfson AB, et al., for the National Emergency X-Radiography Utilization Study Group. Validity of a set of clinical criteria to rule out injury to the cervical spine in patients with blunt trauma. *New England Journal of Medicine.* 2000;343(2):94–99.

6. Stiell IG, Wells GA, Vandemheen KL, et al. The Canadian C-spine rule for radiography in alert and stable trauma patients. *JAMA.* 2001;286(15):1841–1848.

7. Stiell IG, Wells GA, Vandemheen K, et al. The Canadian CT head rule for patients with minor head injury. *The Lancet.* 2001;357(9266):1391–1396.

8. Raja AS, Greenberg JO, Qaseem A, et al. Evaluation of patients with suspected acute pulmonary embolism: best practice advice from the Clinical Guidelines Committee of the American College of Physicians. *Annals of Internal Medicine.* 2015;162(9):701–711.

9. Pitts JR. H.R.4302 - 113th Congress (2013–2014): Protecting access to Medicare Act of 2014. Available at www.congress.gov/bill/113th-congress/house-bill/4302. Accessed May 28, 2015.

10. Andruchow JE, Raja AS, Prevedello LM, et al. Variation in head computed tomography use for emergency department trauma patients and physician risk tolerance. *Archives of Internal Medicine.* 2012;172(8):660–661.

11. Prevedello LM, Raja AS, Zane RD, et al. Variation in use of head computed tomography by emergency physicians. *American Journal of Medicine.* 2012;125(4):356–364.

12. Raja AS, Ip IK, Prevedello LM, et al. Effect of computerized clinical decision support on the use and yield of CT pulmonary angiography in the emergency department. *Radiology.* 2012;262(2):468–474.

13. Ip IK, Raja AS, Gupta A, et al. Impact of clinical decision support on head computed

tomography use in patients with mild traumatic brain injury in the ED. *American Journal of Emergency Medicine.* 2015;33 (3):320–325.

14. Hussey PS, Timbie JW, Burgette LF, et al. Appropriateness of advanced diagnostic imaging ordering before and after implementation of clinical decision support systems. *JAMA.* 2015;313(21):2181–2182.

15. Drescher FS, Chandrika S, Weir ID, et al. Effectiveness and acceptability of a computerized decision support system using modified Wells criteria for evaluation of suspected pulmonary embolism. *Annals of Emergency Medicine.* 2011;57 (6):613–621.

16. Gupta A, Raja AS, Khorasani R. Examining clinical decision support integrity: is clinician self-reported data entry accurate? *JAMA.* 2014;21:23–26.

17. Roy P-M, Durieux P, Gillaizeau F, et al. A computerized handheld decision-support system to improve pulmonary embolism diagnosis. *Annals of Internal Medicine.* 2009;151(10):677–686.

18. Raja AS, Ip IK, Dunne RM, et al. Effects of performance feedback reports on adherence to evidence-based guidelines in use of CT for evaluation of pulmonary embolism in the emergency department: a randomized trial. *American Journal of Roentgenology.* 2015 Nov;205(5):936–40.

19. Gupta A, Ip IK, Raja AS, et al. Effect of clinical decision support on documented guideline adherence for head CT in emergency department patients with mild traumatic brain injury. *JAMIA.* 2014;21:347–351.

20. Raja AS, Gupta A, Ip IK, et al. The use of decision support to measure documented adherence to a national imaging quality measure. *Academic Radiology.* 2014;21 (3):378–383.

21. Raja AS, Lanning J, Gower A, et al. Prevalence of chest injury with the presence of NEXUS chest criteria: data to inform shared decision making about imaging use. *Annals of Emergency Medicine.* 2016 Aug;68(2):222–226.

22. Hess EP, Grudzen CR, Thomson R, et al. Shared decision-making in the emergency department: respecting patient autonomy when seconds count. *Academic Emergency Medicine.* 2015;22(7):856–864.

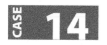

Automated Patient Follow-Up Program

Tom Scaletta, Kristin L. Rising, and MeganRanney

Introduction

As early as the 1980s, physicians and hospital systems have made efforts to track, characterize, and reduce poor outcomes for patients after emergency department (ED) discharge.[1,2,3,4] Since implementation of the Centers for Medicaid and Medicare Service's 30-day hospital readmission quality measure, identifying patients at risk of a poor post-hospitalization outcome has become even more of a focus. Despite more than 40 years of research on how to most safely treat and discharge patients from the ED, some studies report a 30-day ED return visit rate over 20 percent.[5] This high rate of return suggests that patients have ongoing needs after ED discharge.

Many departments have employed telephonic human outreach programs ("callbacks") in attempt to improve outcomes for patients post ED discharge. Although these efforts have been effective in improving patient-reported outcomes and satisfaction, most use clinical personnel to contact discharged patients, which is extremely time and resource intensive.[6,7,8] When using clerical staff to reach out by telephone, the cost is approximately $2.00 per patient, assuming two attempts to reach each patient; this cost doubles if the staff caller is a nurse.[9]

Technology-based follow-up for patients discharged from the ED offers numerous potential advantages. If designed correctly, technology-based outreach can be automated, 24/7, multilingual, low cost, and highly scalable. In addition, this type of follow-up can incorporate patients' preferences for contact modality, allowing patients to choose methods (such as text messages or e-mail) that may be less interruptive than phone calls and more timely than mailed paper surveys.[10,11]

The following case study describes a low-cost, electronic contact system designed to identify discharged ED patients at risk of adverse outcomes. EffectiveResponse (Taylor Healthcare) was praised in 2013 by the Robert Wood Johnson Foundation as a best practice and received distinguished recognition in 2014 by Urgent Matters as an emergency care innovation.

Innovation

For the last two decades, one of the authors (Tom Scaletta) has overseen programs to call back discharged ED patients in order to assess patient well-being and satisfaction with service. He has an undergraduate degree in math and computer science and used to do Fortran programming for an actuarial firm before his medical training. In 2004, he resurrected these skills and used FileMaker Pro to facilitate a database to manage ED callbacks at Edward Hospital ED, a 70,000-visit comprehensive, suburban ED in Naperville, IL. This database functioned as a workflow tool for a callback clerk. Edward Hospital remained in the top decile (for every quarter, according to Press-Ganey Associates) since the callback program was implemented in 2004. However, callback positions were expensive and required significant management-led training due to high personnel turnover, and there were additional costs related to equipment and space.

As mobile phone use became ubiquitous across most sociodemographic groups, Dr. Scaletta theorized that electronic postdischarge contact would reduce facility costs and increase reach. He founded a technology company (Smart-ER) to devise an e-survey methodology called EffectiveResponse. In 2013 he introduced this innovation to the Edward Hospital ED, as well as to a 30,000-visit freestanding ED in Plainfield, IL. These sites are part of Edward-Elmhurst Health, a highly regarded Chicago area healthcare system that consistently achieves 99th percentile in patient satisfaction each quarter according to Press Ganey Associates.

The Edward-Elmhurst information technology (IT) department has been integral to the program's success. It created a process by which a 26-element data extract of all ED patients from the prior day is uploaded to the cloud server every day at 7 AM. EffectiveResponse then automatically sends an e-survey link (see Figure CS14.1) by e-mail and text message at 9 AM to every patient discharged from the ED for whom there is contact information, both that day and again the subsequent day (total of two contacts).

There is an option to move the data back into the EHR. The health system IT governance team vetted the process to ensure personal health information security protection, and the ED leadership team approved the five-question e-survey.

Adult patients (and parents of pediatric patients) can use their smartphones, laptops, or tablets to enter the e-survey portal via a link in the invitation text or e-mail message. Responses to questions that warrant concern are flagged and result in automated triggers that generate alerts for appropriate ED personnel. For instance, the first survey question ("How are you feeling today as compared to when you were seen?" [Answers: better, worse, same]) is used to determine if a discharged patient is maintaining the proper medical trajectory. Clicking "worse" triggers a fax alert that is sent to the on-duty charge nurse, who then determines if the patient requires reassurance, education, aftercare modification, or return to the ED. Whenever possible, alerts are dovetailed into existing workflows. For instance, the charge nurse already receives actionable microbiology results by fax. Thus, when a patient reports feeling worse after discharge, a fax notification is sent to the charge nurse, who then determines whether the patient requires aftercare notification or a return visit. The rate of this event averages one notification per charge nurse shift.

The second question consolidates aftercare issues. Any issues identified by a patient trigger a pop-up box for the on-duty ED case manager. The case manager position is staffed 10 hours per day in the Edward Hospital ED, with issues being sent to a work queue in off hours. The case manager can respond to the patient within an "active issues management

Figure CS14.1 Smart-ER automatic e-survey link.

From: **Smart-ER** <do-not-reply@smart-er.net>
Date: Wed, Apr 20, 2016 at 10:45 PM
Subject: Edward Hospital wants to hear how you are doing today!
To: JohnQPatient@gmail.com

Please **CLICK HERE** to let the staff at Edward Hospital know how you are doing today.

Thank you!

This is an automated message, so please do not reply to this email. You may click here to unsubscribe.

(AIM) module" (see below). Patients who reported both feeling worse and an aftercare issue receive attention from both a charge nurse and case manager.

Question three asks the patient to rank the provider by "level of concern shown." A top performance rate is calculated with a group average of 60 percent. Since the reach rate of discharged patients is one-third, a statistically valid number of responses is obtained for providers each month. "Low" and "very low" responses result in a pop-up prompting an explanation and send this information to the medical director. Patients can view physician profiles and view qualifications and personal characteristics.

Question four requests a nurse ranking on "level of concern shown." Any issues pertaining to the nurses are referred to nurse management. The last question ("Would you like to add anything else about your patient experience?") serves as a broad, catch-all for any other service issues. ED leaders review these comments and respond to patients using the AIM module. When areas outside the purview of the ED are mentioned, the system can relay a notification to the external department supervisor. The final page of the survey offers a URL to the hospital portal, which is Epic MyChart. This linkage has resulted in EffectiveResponse being the top referrer to MyChart and has helped us achieve our meaningful use goal of over 25 percent portal adoption.

The AIM module routes alerts to the appropriate clinical staff. Users who are assigned to reconcile a particular question log in and see a list of active issues. Clicking a case shows a dashboard of information and the patient response (see Figure CS14.2).

Categorization of the issue invokes a predesigned template that can be modified by the user (Figure CS14.3). Messages are sent to patients in the same manner in which the e-survey was completed, by either text or e-mail.

Monthly reports to hospital and department leadership include patient demographics and survey statistics (Figure CS14.4).

Aggregate comments can be viewed for each response. Monthly provider reports offer individualized information including patients per hour, average length of stay for discharged patients, and the percentage of all discharged patients who were contacted.

Figure CS14.2 AIM module dashboard.

DOS:March 04, 2016

To: (630)

Subject: Re: Your Recent Feedback

Message:

Thank you very much for sharing information about your recent visit to Edward Hospital.

I recommend that you change the bandage once a day. You can remove it, take a bath or shower, and then replace it for the rest of the day.

We value your trust and will continue to strive to offer our community the very best health care.

Sincerely,

Tom Scaletta MD
ED Chairperson

| Send | C | Cancel |

Figure CS14.3 AIM patient messages.

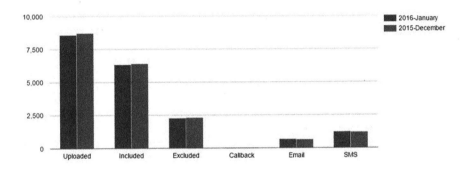

All Locations

Uploaded		8582	
	Excluded	2259	(26.3%)
	Included	6323	(73.7%)
	Contact Method		
	Callback	0	(0%)
	SMS	1221	(19.3%)
	Email	696	(11%)

Total contacted: 1917 (30.3%)

Figure CS14.4 AIM monthly report.

Experience with Implementation

In 2015, patients treated at Edward Hospital were 96 percent English speaking (2 percent Spanish, 1 percent other, 1 percent unknown), 57 percent privately insured (21 percent Medicaid, 16 percent Medicare, 5 percent uninsured), and 50 percent age 21–60 years (34 percent age < 20 years, 61 percent age 61–80 years, 7 percent > 80 years). From November 2014 through October 2015 we evaluated 97,395 ED visits. Of these, 23,757 (24.4 percent) were excluded from receiving postdischarge notifications because they were admitted, transferred,, or had an ED care plan. E-mail addresses were acquired from 65 percent and cell phone numbers were obtained from 90 percent of patients discharged home. Those patients who shared both an e-mail address and a cell phone number received the survey by both platforms (30 percent of population were sent both text and e-mail link); however, only one response to each e-survey was permitted.

Patient acceptance of follow-up by electronic contact was high. The delivery rate of e-mails was 94 percent, half were opened, and less than 1 percent of patients unsubscribed. The delivery rate of text messages was 78 percent, and less than 0.5 percent opted out. Overall, 35.1 percent of patients who received a notification responded. We found that patients connected via the text link twice as often as by the e-mail link.

A total of 808 patients (3.9 percent of respondents) reported feeling worse, and 961 patients (4.7 percent of respondents) reported an aftercare issue. Finally, 584 patients (2.9 percent of respondents) reported a physician complaint, each of which was reported to a medical director. We have received about five unsolicited positive comments for each negative comment. The potential benefits of this process are illustrated by the following two actual cases.

> A 35-year-old male was diagnosed by a veteran emergency physician with a "lumbar strain." The next day the patient received an EffectiveResponse e-survey and relayed that he was experiencing fever and numbness. Within minutes of completing the e-survey he received a phone call from the charge nurse, who instructed him to return to the ED, and within 2 hours of the e-survey he had a magnetic resonance scan showing an epidural abscess, and went right to surgery. He made a full recovery.

> A 7-year-old girl sustained a closed wrist fracture and was referred to the on-call orthopedic surgeon. The patient's mother completed the e-survey and reported that she called for an appointment and was informed by the receptionist that their insurance (Medicaid HMO) was "out of network." The case manager called the orthopedist's office, explained the on-call obligation, and scheduled a visit for the child. The patient's mother expressed her gratitude.

We found that EffectiveResponse allowed us to decrease cost and the hassles associated with a staff-led callback program, while being more effective in our ability to contact patients postdischarge.

Discussion

In the era of value-based care, it is important to reduce 30-day readmissions and improve patient satisfaction, as these are publicly reported measures directly linked to payment by federal payers in the United States. Although "bounce backs" (ED return visits) may not represent failures of ED management, emergency care providers are nonetheless under pressure to maximize patient outcomes while minimizing ED utilization.[12] Traditional postdischarge contact may help achieve this goal but is expensive and time consuming. Implementation of a system that automatically reaches out to all discharged patients with contact information on file, such as EffectiveResponse, has the potential to identify more patients with problems, earlier in their postdischarge course, potentially preventing costly hospitalization or other adverse outcomes.

EffectiveResponse was developed as an electronic surveillance tool to prevent near misses and adverse events for all patients discharged from the ED. This intervention demonstrates how technology can be used to meet goals that were traditionally achieved only with multiple, dedicated callback staff: it reaches many patients, improves patient satisfaction, provides real-time provider feedback for ED treat-and-release visits, and may reduce negative outcomes. By relying heavily on automated short message service (SMS, aka text-message) communication, it is an intervention that is significantly lower cost than human callbacks (approximately $1 per ED patient, as compared with $2 when using staff or $4 for nursing) and almost universally available among patients regardless of socio-economic status.[10]

Multiple studies demonstrate that postdischarge telephone calls and electronic communication improve appointment adherence after an ED visit. To our knowledge, only one study has demonstrated e-mail's efficacy in improving ED patient satisfaction, and no study has been conducted on effectiveness.[13,14,15,16] A few studies have examined the efficacy of text-messaging in changing acute disease trajectories, but only for specific diagnoses (versus this product, which is delivered across the diagnostic spectrum) and among limited ED populations.[17,18,19] A significant differentiator of EffectiveResponse from other potential competitors is its inclusion of questions about patients' clinical course and access to aftercare, which helps identify unexpected rapid disease progression or initial misdiagnoses. Although this case study was performed at a single site with a relatively nondiverse population, anecdotal evidence is emerging from other sites that confirms the ability of such programs to improve patient satisfaction scores.[20]

Despite our enthusiasm for this product, it is important to highlight potential limitations to electronic postdischarge notification programs. First, while text-messaging has been reported to be effective at improving appointment attendance among diverse populations, including among low-income primarily Spanish-speaking ED patients[16] and homeless veterans,[21] it is unknown whether lower-income or nonwhite patients will respond at higher or lower rates, nor is it known whether they will need more or fewer services postdischarge. Similarly, common sense says there may be lower uptake and acceptability among geriatric populations, who have lower rates of use of mobile phones in general, and text-messaging and e-mail in particular.[22] The usefulness of this tool in older cohorts should be explored.

A second issue with automated callback programs is the cost of initial implementation, including both technology support and workflow changes. Although an automated text-message program may save significant time and expense compared with a comprehensive callback program, autonotification programs (such as EffectiveResponse) are generally delivered as a "software as a service," with monthly subscription fees. Hospitals and departments may also choose to build their own programs, but doing so is typically expensive and requires notable technologic expertise and IT support. Additionally, staff are needed to respond to postdischarge issues when they are identified.

A third consideration is that there may be a distinct population for whom a human touch is especially important and for whom an automated callback program may not yield the same benefit.[23] Patients may not acknowledge their own deterioration or lack of appropriate follow-up plan, and it may be only through conversation with hospital personnel that their needs become apparent. Other patients may be resistant to reporting poor outcomes or feedback through an impersonal online system. Those supplemental efforts must be weighed against the cost of the personnel required to implement a limited, conventional callback effort.[24]

Finally, it is worth mentioning privacy concerns. Although electronically sending personal health information by an unencrypted text message or e-mail does not meet the US Office of Civil Rights standards for HIPAA-compliant communication, most hospital systems permit electronic contact with patients under specific conditions. Linking to a secure portal like EffectiveResponse is allowable, since the exchange of sensitive information is minimized. This requires that the signed consent for treatment list postdischarge electronic contact as a component of consent for treatment. It is important that the consent also allows patients the opportunity to opt out. More secure methods of communication can include encrypted messages, delivered through smartphone applications or e-mail. But the disadvantages to these methods are that they exclude the 30–40 percent of ED patients who do not have smartphones, and they require patients to remember additional passwords.[11] As epitomized by the lack of utilization of patient portals, such additional steps are likely to result in lower response rates.

Notable outcomes from this case study include the high delivery rate (94 percent of e-mails and 78 percent of texts, with <1 percent opting out), acceptable response rate (over one-third of patients contacted responded to the queries), and the low percentage of cases requiring human follow-up (<9 percent). The response rates are higher than those reported in a recent study of e-mail appointment reminders to discharged patients.[2] There are a number of other postdischarge communication tools (e.g., Cipher Health, Sense Health). Overall, postdischarge communication tools appear to be effective for uncovering service complaints and near-misses in near-real-time, assisting in addressing complaints and improving future service delivery.

In conclusion, this case study demonstrates the promise of technology-based, automated postdischarge follow-up for ED patients. This novel approach uses technology to automate a postdischarge patient follow-up process, with the ability to incorporate postdischarge evaluation into existing hospital workflows. It has the potential to markedly grow post–acute care contact rates, improve satisfaction, and prevent avoidable ED reevaluations or hospitalizations after ED discharge. Future work should continue to focus on integrating automated processes into current clinical care workflows in order to reduce the requirement for human contact when not inherently needed, identify ways to improve response rates, and evaluate the impact on longer term patient care outcomes.

References

1. Keith KD, Bocka JJ, Kobernick MS, et al. Emergency department revisits. *Annals of Emergency Medicine.* 1989;18(9):964–968.

2. Nuñez S, Hexdall A, Aguirre-Jaime A. Unscheduled returns to the emergency department: an outcome of medical errors? *Quality and Safety in Health Care.* 2006;15(2):102–108.

3. Hu KW, Lu YH, Lin HJ, et al. Unscheduled return visits with and without admission post emergency department discharge. *Journal of Emergency Medicine.* 2012;43(6):1110–1118.

4. Gabayan GZ, Derose SF, Asch SM, et al. Patterns and predictors of short-term death after emergency department discharge. *Annals of Emergency Medicine.* 2011;58(6):551–558.

5. Rising KL, Victor TW, Wiebe DJ, et al. Patient returns to the emergency department: the time-to-return curve. *Academic Emergency Medicine.* 2014;21(8):864–871.

6. McLean S, Gee M, Booth A, et al. Targeting the Use of Reminders and Notifications for Uptake by Populations (TURNUP): a systematic review and evidence synthesis. *Health Services and Delivery Research.* 2014;2(34):1–184.

7. Vaiva G, Vaiva G, Ducrocq F, et al. Effect of telephone contact on further suicide attempts in patients discharged from an emergency department: randomised controlled study. *BMJ.* 2006;332(7552):1241–1245.

8. Guss DA, Gray S, Castillo EM. The impact of patient telephone call after discharge on

likelihood to recommend in an academic emergency department. *Journal of Emergency Medicine.* 2014;46(4):560–566.

9. Robert Wood Johnson Foundation. Improving patient satisfaction in the emergency department (ED) with a call back clerk. 2008. Available at: www.rwjf.org/en/library/articles-and-news/2013/04/post-visit-patient-contact-improves-patient-satisfaction.html. Accessed April 16, 2016.

10. Fox S, Duggan M. Mobile Health 2012. 2012. Available at www.pewinternet.org/~/media//Files/Reports/2012/PIP_MobileHealth2012_FINAL.pdf. Accessed April 16, 2016.

11. Ranney ML, Choo EK, Wang Y, et al. Emergency department patients' preferences for technology-based behavioral interventions. *Annals of Emergency Medicine.* 2012 Aug;60(2):218–227.

12. Sabbatini AK, Kocher KE, Basu A, et al. In-hospital outcomes and costs among patients hospitalized during a return visit to the emergency department. *JAMA.* 2016;315(7):663.

13. Patel PB, Vinson DR. Physician e-mail and telephone contact after emergency department visit improves patient satisfaction: a crossover trial. *Annals of Emergency Medicine.* 2013;61(6):631–637.

14. Arora S, Burner E, Terp S, et al. Improving attendance at post-emergency department follow-up via automated text message appointment reminders: a randomized controlled trial. *Academic Emergency Medicine.* 2015;22(1):31–37.

15. Sharp B, Singal B, Pulia M, et al. You've got mail … and need follow-up: the effect and patient perception of e-mail follow-up reminders after emergency department discharge. *Academic Emergency Medicine.* 2015;22(1):47–53.

16. Biese K, Lamantia M, Shofer F, et al. A randomized trial exploring the effect of a telephone call follow-up on care plan compliance among older adults discharged home from the emergency department. *Academic Emergency Medicine.* 2014;21(2):188–195.

17. Arora S, Peters AL, Burner E, et al. Trial to examine text message-based mhealth in emergency department patients with diabetes (TExT-MED): a randomized controlled trial. *Annals of Emergency Medicine.* 2014;63(6).

18. Suffoletto B, Kristan J, Chung T, et al. An interactive text message intervention to reduce binge drinking in young adults: a randomized controlled trial with 9-month outcomes. *PLoS One.* 2015;10(11):e0142877.

19. Ranney ML, et al. A mixed methods pilot study of a depression prevention intervention for adolescents in the emergency department. *Journal of Adolescent Health.* 2016 Jun (published online).

20. Thew J. A better way to elicit patient feedback. 2015. Available at http://healthleadersmedia.com/page-1/NRS-318250/A-Better-Way-to-Elicit-Patient-Feedback.

21. McInnes DK, Petrakis BA, Gifford AL, et al. Retaining homeless veterans in outpatient care: a pilot study of mobile phone text message appointment reminders. *American Journal of Public Health.* 2014;104(Suppl. 4):S588–S594.

22. Anderson M. Technology Device Ownership: 2015. Available at www.pewinternet.org/2015/10/29/technology-device-ownership-2015/. Accessed April 16, 2016.

23. Ranney ML, Thorsen M, Patena JV, et al. You need to get them where they feel it: conflicting perspectives on how to maximize the structure of text-message psychological interventions for adolescents. Proceedings of the Annual Hawaii International Conference on System Sciences. 2015-March https://experts.umich.edu/en/publications/you-need-to-get-them-where-they-feel-it-conflicting-perspectives-

24. Irizarry T, DeVito Dabbs A, et al. Patient portals and patient engagement: a state of the science review. *Journal of Medical Internet Research.* 2015;17(6):e148.

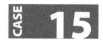

Using Data on Patient Experience to Improve Clinical Care

Seth Glickman and Abhi Mehrotra

Introduction

Measuring the patient experience usually invokes images of lengthy paper surveys mailed to patients. This typical process of paper surveys is laden with many barriers to truly understanding the patient experience and use data to improve clinical care.

Limitations include the following:

- Poor response rates: Paper-based products are typically challenged by response rates that are inadequate. This may be due to modality of surveying as well as respondent burden.
- Timeliness of response: Frequently, surveys are administered days to weeks after the delivery of care, leading to a response bias as well as a lag in reporting.
- Clinical relevance: Survey scores or comments are frequently not attributable to an individual provider, shift, or clinical situation.
- Response bias: Along with a limitation of response rates comes the bias of which cohort of patients is surveyed. Typically, only ambulatory patients are included in the potential pool, thus excluding the patients who receive the most intense care (and time) of the providers and staff.[1,2,3]

Measurement of the patient experience has been mandatory for compliance with US accreditation and hospital conditions of participation with the Centers for Medicare and Medicaid Services (CMS).[4,5] For a subset of hospitalized patients, the Hospital Consumer Assessment of Healthcare Providers and Systems (H-CAHPS) survey is mandated by administration by CMS. Most hospitals also contract with survey vendors to attain patient responses to their outpatient visits as well.[6] The CAHPS program will also be extending to Clinician and Group version (CG-CAHPS). Additionally, an emergency department (ED) survey is under development and testing (Emergency Department Patient Experiences with Care Survey [EDPECS]).[7]

However, these survey methodologies continue to be plagued by the limitations noted above. CMS is expanding survey techniques for the EDPECS testing by introducing three modalities: mail only, phone only, and mail with phone follow-up. Additionally, the EDPECS survey is planned for variable administration, encompassing both ambulatory and admitted ED patients.

In the end, all of these survey instruments subjectively measure a patient's perception of care without identifying a clinical focus of improvement to objectively influence the quality of care delivery.

Innovation

Developed by physicians for physicians, the Bivarus platform focuses on capturing the patient voice and arming physicians, nurses, and administrators with actionable data for meaningful, patient-centered interventions to improve care delivery and service operations. The approach relies on a few basic principles: (1) surveys with simple, effective interfaces,

(2) customized, dynamic surveys, and (3) near-real-time data to monitor interventions and generate advanced analytic insights.

From the patient perspective, survey interactions are very easy to use, simple and noninvasive from a time or resource point of view. Surveys, consisting of 10 measures, are delivered to adult patients via their preferred method (e-mail or text message) within 24–48 hours after a healthcare experience. Patients answer using a five-point scale for each measure, and free-text comments are also possible. The surveys are optimized for completion on personal smartphones, including on iOS, Android, and Blackberry operating systems. Typically taking less than 2 minutes to complete, the surveys place little burden on the patient.

The measurement system uses a novel sampling algorithm to determine which set of 10 measures is dynamically presented to a single patient (Patient Quality Assessment Tool, US Patent Application No. 13/530,042, patent pending). Unique to Bivarus, the item bank is fully customizable and contains 100 questions across 10 key domains, including patient safety, communication, and transitions of care. Users also have the option to create their own new measures specific for the organizational information needs. Survey items were developed after a series of interviews with key stakeholders at the University of North Carolina (UNC), including physicians, nurses, hospital administrators, and patients. Items have undergone an iterative process of development and testing to optimize content validity, reliability, and patient understanding.

This sampling algorithm takes into account both the relative importance given to measures (configurable by customers) (Figure CS15.1) and the reliability of prior observations. The primary objective of this approach is to provide an efficient estimate of the underlying quality level of service provision for a given component of service, knowing that any one-service encounter is a fallible measure of that underlying component. It is designed to provide clinical and operational leaders with two estimates: (1) the best guess of the true value quality level and (2) the uncertainty associated with this best guess. Therefore, more

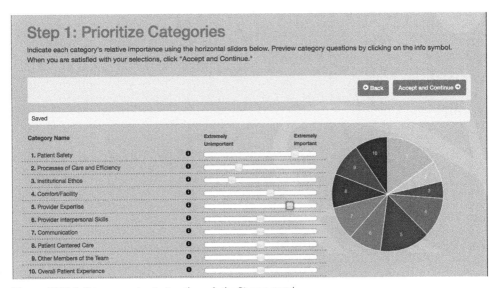

Figure CS15.1 Category customization through the Bivarus portal.

important measures are asked more frequently and question occurrence is adjusted as new observations are obtained. This unique methodology guarantees that the obtained mean response is not due to chance. So, even though our typical item bank contains 50–100 measures, a patient never has to answer more than 10 measures.

Technical specifications. The platform consists of three distinct components: the management Portal that allows users to customize surveys and see analytic reports, a survey delivery system (SDS) that sends surveys and collects results from patients, and a data integration hub (Transformer) that accepts and normalizes data uploaded by client hospitals. The Portal, SDS, and Transformer live in physically and logically discrete server environments, communicating with each other via a REST-based service-oriented architecture. Client data can be transmitted to the platform using a REST-based application program interface (API) or secure file transfer protocol (SFTP). Each component in the platform is based on a Ruby on Rails technology stack and is developed using industry-standard best practices, including a hybrid Agile project management methodology, extensive unit and integration tests, version control, and static analysis.

Security features. The platform was designed and operates under policies created by the chief privacy officer and technical staff to ensure it fully complies with HIPAA/HITECH security requirements. Each component of the platform is deployed in a payment card industry (PCI)-compliant managed private cloud environment and is protected by firewalls (application and operating system), intrusion detection systems, and an integrated logging/auditing system. Security and application performance is monitored continuously via third-party tools, and technical staff and administrators receive alerts via text message and/or e-mail if an issue is detected. All patient data are encrypted at rest and during transmission to and from the platform using industry standard AES 256 or greater encryption.

All of the patient data, including comments and responses to individual questions, are available for immediate viewing in a web-based portal by registered users. The UNC ED values the ability to review the data on a daily basis. Data are updated every 6 hours and available 24/7 through the web-based portal, providing granular feedback about every aspect of the patient experience. Trends in quantitative and qualitative feedback help identify opportunities for interventions and service recovery, which are then monitored through the same portal (Figure CS15.2). Detailed reporting and analytics, including at the individual provider level, are used to develop and implement programs designed to improve operational efficiency, quality, and patient safety.

Results

Bivarus has resulted in several key outcomes, including significantly improved response rates (25–50% depending on service area, up to five times the historical response rates), improved care delivery and service operations, increased patient safety, and actionable feedback for providers and operational leaders.

The Bivarus platform is unique regarding how the data are used in interventions and improved provider performance. For example, the UNC ED identifies and focuses on interventions through a daily data review, and a 90-day action plan is developed for each intervention. Compared with the high-level data from previous surveys, Bivarus data can be tied to an individual patient visit. The discussions are centered no longer on the accuracy of the data, but rather on how the department and/or providers can best act on the data. This philosophical change has facilitated improvements in care delivery and service operations.

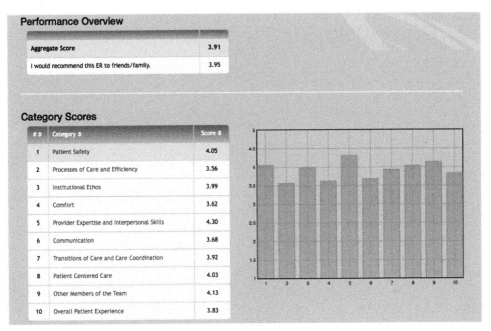

Figure CS15.2 Overview of category scores within the Bivarus portal.

Bivarus provides scientifically precise provider-specific reports, which are being used to derive provider scorecards for physicians and residents in the UNC ED (Figure CS15.3). And these report cards are making their way into resident's curricula vitae as they begin looking for full-time attending positions. Physicians at UNC have become more engaged with the data and no longer question its accuracy. In addition, physicians are requesting and using the Bivarus data for credentialing and recertification purposes. A mentoring program was recently implemented to match mentors with residents with the aim of improving their skills and ratings. The pairing is based on mentors' strengths (higher scores) and areas in which residents need to show improvement (lower scores). To date, a mentor has been identified for each of the three domains: communication, patient-centered care, and provider expertise and interpersonal skills. Providers appreciate the shift from a punitive system to one that offers the ability to directly receive patient feedback, identify areas for improvement, and monitor their performance.

The technology has also generated significant insights into patient safety. Over a 12-month period starting in the summer of 2012, the UNC ED safety team was able to identify 242 safety-related comments within the free-text comments submitted via the Bivarus platform. Of the comments reported, there were 12 adverse events, 40 near-misses, 23 errors with minimal risk of harm, and 167 general safety issues (e.g., gaps in care transitions). Of the 40 near-misses, 35 (75%) were preventable. Of the 52 adverse events or near-misses, 5 (9.6%) were also identified via an existing patient occurrence reporting system. Using Bivarus the clinical leadership group is better able to create a more complete reporting system, incorporating the patient's unique perspective, as they strengthen their safety culture.

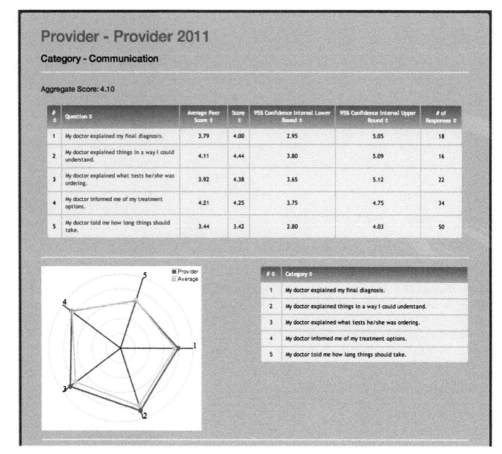

Figure CS15.3 Detailed provider reporting in the Bivarus portal.

Discussion

The patient experience will grow increasingly important in measuring and improving healthcare quality. Critics express three major concerns about patient-reported measures, particularly those assessing "patient satisfaction."[2] First, patient feedback may not be credible because patients lack formal medical training. Second, patient-experience measures may be confounded by factors not directly associated with the quality of processes. Third, patient-experience measures may reflect fulfillment of patients' a priori desires – for example, their request for a certain treatment, regardless of its benefit. However, our research supports patient-reported experiences in quality assessment. We have found that patient-reported measures not only are strongly correlated with better outcomes but also largely capture patient evaluation of care-focused communication with nurses and physicians, rather than nonclinical aspects of patient experience, such as room features and meals.[8,9] We also show that quality and patient experience are related across multiple disease conditions, indicating that patient-experience measures represent a unique dimension of quality that is otherwise difficult to measure objectively.

Although there are unresolved methodologic issues related to the measurement and interpretation of patient experiences – that is, survey content, risk adjustment, and the mode and timing of survey administration – we believe that both theory and the available evidence suggest that such measures are robust, distinctive indicators of healthcare quality. Therefore, debate should center not on whether patients can provide meaningful quality measures but on how to improve patient experiences by focusing on activities (such as care coordination and patient engagement) found to be associated with both satisfaction and outcomes, evaluate the effects of new care-delivery models on patients' experiences and outcomes, develop robust measurement approaches that provide timely and actionable information to facilitate organizational change, and improve data-collection methods and procedures to provide fair and accurate assessments of individual providers.[2]

We believe that it will also be very important to transition from simply benchmarking the patient experience to transforming clinical delivery, similar to approaches in other industries. While our knowledge of the importance of data has changed and the data have become more accessible, our understanding of *how* to use data to improve performance is still lagging significantly.

One of the most common healthcare applications of data is the idea of benchmarking performance compared with peers. The concept gained industry visibility when Xerox adopted benchmarking of its performance on the way to winning the Baldrige Award in 1989, which recognizes US business, healthcare, education, and nonprofit organizations for performance excellence. Xerox referred to the practice as "competitive benchmarking," defining the set of standards the company wanted to meet and comparing those with its competitors.[10]

Historically, benchmarking was a means of setting internal standards, not of evaluating relative performance. Competitive benchmarking was not the only analysis technique adopted by Xerox; the company adopted quality improvement as a core principle and implemented statistical process control methodology along with the competitive benchmarking effort.

Application of benchmarking in healthcare, such as that used in the CAHPS program, falls far short of this comprehensive approach to quality management. We often hear of managers touting their performance percentile relative to some benchmark data set of "peers." Benchmarking very rarely incorporates the competitive approach established by Xerox to elevate overall performance; instead, it focuses on relative rankings.

Benchmarking without performance management has a serious flaw: it tells us where we are, but not what to do or where to go. It also has unintended consequences. Patient experience (or, more commonly, "satisfaction") is often a factor in determining compensation for senior managers to the detriment of using assessment of the patient experience for improving service operations. Rather than a positive achievement, we fear we have institutionalized administrative aspects of assessment of the patient experience rather than the concept of improving service operations. In fact, the constant "strive for five" throughout the healthcare system is evidence of how measurement of patient experience has been coopted into a performance metric for senior managers.[3] Strive for five is a marketing campaign for higher scores, not a commitment to a better patient experience. Just to show how convoluted the process has become, a patient experience executive at a US hospital said that because of financial pressure, her entire focus was on raising their HCAHPS scores; however, many of those had already topped out.[11] Her plight isn't actually that surprising considering the profound "ceiling effects" of these measures (meaning most hospital scores are clustered within a very tight range at the top of the measurement scale).

In contrast, one of the most remarkable stories in the quality literature is the concept of the Toyota production system (TPS).[12] Toyota has developed a culture of performance through a system designed to eliminate manufacturing defects, improve efficiency, and provide flexibility in work processes while standardizing production. This concept of the TPS has transformed manufacturing in many industries, including the US auto industry, and is slowly transforming the healthcare delivery system as well.

TPS provides a model for a culture that is fixed on delivery of the highest quality product on a consistent basis. To achieve this goal, the model revolves around the key concepts of planning, measurement, and accountability. Planning is identifying the process so it can be optimized to reduce waste and inefficiency. Measurement is critical because it not only informs the planning process, but also serves as a tool to assess current performance against expectations. Finally, accountability provides clear lines of responsibility and authority, but not in a traditional fashion. In the TPS model, everyone is empowered to stop a process that is not working according to plan, while management and leadership are accountable for addressing the issues underlying this deviation. This intrinsic approach provides an opportunity for firms to use data to improve their structures, processes, and outcomes; in other words, their quality.

TPS stands in stark contrast to consumer assessment of automobile performance. Every year, a sample of Toyota purchasers is surveyed to assess their automobile purchase. These data are used in reports such as the J.D. Powers consumer car ratings. While these data are valuable to consumers and manufacturers, they are not used to drive the production processes at Toyota. J.D. Powers makes an extrinsic assessment of performance, not related to Toyota's internal management processes.

There are several critical insights to be gleaned from TPS by healthcare providers and systems. First, while we have made massive investments in technology to support healthcare delivery, we have invested relatively less in the critical aspects of assessing the processes of care and the use of data to improve the delivery of care. Adoption of an electronic health record technology solution is not the adoption of a Toyota production culture. The chasm between data collection and a TPS model is significant, and one that is not being discussed in many healthcare management or policy circles.

Second, policymakers are fixed on our extrinsic J.D. Powers approach to quality assessment. This type of approach was critical to a strategy of engaging providers to take ownership of their services and outcomes, but now that that message has been received, we have not been able to reconcile the continued emphasis on extrinsic performance assessments with the need for the actionable data envisioned under the TPS model.

What's missing is a means of increasing our capacity to support the intrinsic TPS model in healthcare delivery. This effort will include new models of data collection and analysis, redoubled efforts toward making available data actionable, and new cultures of performance management. In fact, it's easy to argue that the intrinsic management approach embodied by the TPS model is the only means to true business transformation in healthcare.[13]

As we learn more about the use of the Bivarus platform in clinical practice, users seem to have discovered many of the core TPS concepts. These include the opportunity for using real-time feedback from patients to inform planning and tracking, and measurement tools to foster accountability by providing an opportunity to address issues identified in the care delivery process in real time. This enables multidisciplinary work teams to solve issues and serves to make those issues more transparent to all involved – ultimately resulting in a better patient experience and improved patient outcomes.

References

1. Better methods, better numbers. *Emergency Physicians Monthly*, Aug 2013.

2. Manary MP, Boulding W, Staelin R, Glickman SW. The patient experience and health outcomes. *The New England Journal of Medicine.* 2013 Jan 17;368(3):201–203.

3. Glickman SW, Schulman KA. The mismeasure of physician performance. *American Journal of Managed Care.* 2013 Oct;19(10):782–785.

4. The Patient Protection and Affordable Care Act (Pub. L. 111–148). 2010. Section 10331 (a). See also www.ajmc.com/journals/issue/2013/2013-1-vol19-n10/the-mis-measure-of-physician-performance/P-2#sthash.5hQaiUsr.dpuf

5. Surveys and tools to advance patient care: about CAHPS. Available at http://cahps.ahrq.gov/about.htm.

6. Hospital care quality information from the consumer perspective. Available at www.hcahpsonline.org.

7. Emergency Department Patient Experiences with Care (EDPEC) Survey. Available at www.cms.gov/Research-Statistics-Data-and-Systems/Research/CAHPS/ed.html.

8. Boulding W, Glickman SW, Manary MP, Schulman KA, Staelin R. Relationship between patient satisfaction with inpatient care and hospital readmission within 30 days. *American Journal of Managed Care.* 2011;17:41–48.

9. Glickman SW, Boulding W, Manary M, et al. Patient satisfaction and its relationship with clinical quality and inpatient mortality in acute myocardial infarction. *Circulation: Cardiovascular Quality and Outcomes.* 2010;3:188–195.

10. Total Quality Management. The Evolution of Benchmarking: The Xerox Case. September 16, 2009.

11. https://healthcareitstrategy.com/2013/08/01/shift-happens-the-experience-failure-of-a-top-10-hospital/.

12. Culig MH, Kunkle RF, Frndak DC, Grunden N, Maher TD Jr, Magovern GJ Jr. Improving patient care in cardiac surgery using Toyota production system based methodology. *The Annals of Thoracic Surgery.* 2011;91:394–399.

13. Institute of Medicine of the National Academies. *Best Care at Lower Cost: The Path to Continuously Learning Health Care in America.* Washington, DC: National Academies Press, 2012.

Community Paramedicine

The Geisinger Experience

Manish N. Shah and David J. Schoenwetter

Introduction

The ambulance-based emergency medical services (EMS) system is a unique component of the overall healthcare system. It is staffed with highly trained emergency medical technicians and paramedics who traditionally provide in-home assessment, acute treatments, and transport to an emergency department (ED) immediately after a call for assistance.[1] These providers are trained to operate throughout the community, delivering care in settings with limited medical resources, such as a patient's home or a public place. This service is available to all, regardless of one's financial resources, race, or ethnicity. It is uniform throughout urban, suburban, and rural communities and is available regardless of day of week, time of day, or location. Although the type of interventions have evolved since the early days of EMS to therapies such as defibrillation and intubation, EMS providers have been rarely used in roles or settings beyond caring for patients with acute medical problems, delivering life-sustaining interventions, and then transporting patients to hospitals.

The EMS system's broader potential was recognized more than 20 years ago in a report from the National Highway Transport Safety Administration, *EMS Agenda for the Future.*[2] Isolated efforts to leverage EMS resources to enhance the community's health have existed, often within research protocols. Until recently, however, no sustained focus or efforts have taken place to integrate the EMS system with the broader community's health needs. As this role is gaining acceptance, the model of care is being called *community paramedicine* or *mobile integrated healthcare.*[3,4] The reasons for this change in approach are likely multifactorial and include the following:

1. Advocacy by EMS leaders to educate others in the community health value of the EMS system.
2. Shortage of healthcare providers, necessitating the optimal use of all healthcare resources, including the EMS system.
3. Transition of the overall healthcare system from a fee-for-service model to one that is population-based and focused on value and satisfaction, thus incentivizing health systems to optimize their care delivery systems.
4. Growing evidence demonstrating the feasibility, acceptability, and effectiveness of community paramedicine programs.

EMS providers have indicated a desire to participate in programs to promote community health.[5] Programs appear to be successful, although the evidence supporting these programs is limited, constraining the ability to definitively determine if the programs benefit the community. For example, EMS providers have successfully screened for vaccination status, depression, and impaired cognition and have worked to decrease ED use and unmet needs.[6,7,8,9,10,11] However, no randomized controlled trials and few rigorous nonrandomized trials have been performed to evaluate community paramedicine programs. Nonetheless, the skills of EMS providers, existing structure of the EMS system, and needs of communities have created an opportunity for community paramedicine programs.

Innovation

The Mobile Health Paramedic Program is an excellent example of a community paramedicine program responding to local needs and resources. Geisinger Health System, which is a national leader in population health, has its own health insurance plan, extensive primary care networks, and programs to manage its patients' health. Despite this advanced infrastructure and processes, Geisinger found that its patients have challenges that could not be addressed by the existing healthcare system. Thus, the Mobile Health Paramedic Program became an innovative solution to help Geisinger patients.

Created as a pilot program, the primary goal of the Mobile Health Paramedic Program was to develop a nimble, flexible, clinical resource that can be deployed promptly based on the needs of the patient, at the discretion of the treating provider. First implemented in March 2014, the Mobile Health Paramedic Program was staffed by EMS paramedic providers already employed through Geisinger Health System, ensuring integration into the continuum of care within the Geisinger Health System. Unlike existing in-home programs (e.g., visiting nurse services), this pilot program was designed to provide care for those who do not meet criteria for existing in-home programs and to fill existing program gaps. The goal of the pilot program was to integrate with the patient's overall healthcare plan using two-way communications between case managers, Proven Health Navigator/medical homes, and other members of the patient's treatment team, using real-time written documentation in the patient's electronic health record. The clinical interventions of the Mobile Health Paramedic Program team are determined by the paramedic's existing scope of practice, namely, acute assessment and intervention. Example skills are listed in Box 16.1. Any clinical intervention within the scope of practice, and approved by medical oversight, could be rendered to the patient if it was felt by the provider that it was indicated for the patient. The Mobile Health Paramedic Program could also provide follow-up visits for patients who received previous care, either in the home or at another location (such as a clinic or ED), but the program did not provide routine medical needs. To coordinate with other providers, the Mobile Health Paramedic Program uses standard communication resources including telephonic, remote audiovisual communication devices through portable computers, and communication tools available in the electronic health record.

Box 16.1 Example Clinical Assessment and Interventions Performed by the Mobile Health Paramedic Program

- Home assessment
  - Safety, activities of daily living, living environment compatible with health

- Patient clinical assessment
- Medication reconciliation
- Diagnostic studies
  - Point-of-care blood sugar analysis as well as phlebotomy, at the discretion of the managing provider
  - 12-lead electrocardiogram
  - Pulse oximetry, resting and ambulating

Operations

The pilot project was based out of an existing EMS asset, an EMS agency licensed within a specific service area within the Geisinger Health System. The acute care facility base for the pilot was Geisinger Wyoming Valley Medical Center. The medical center operated a Pennsylvania Department of Health, Bureau of EMS (BEMS) licensed advanced life support (ALS) quick response unit, or "ALS Squad," in which their primary service area overlaps with the medical center. In addition to the medical center for acute care and inpatient services, the region also contained a number of primary care sites that are coordinated within the Geisinger Health System under the Community Practice Service Line (CPSL). The CPSL sites share services and coordinate care using similar processes and services through a medical home model called ProvenHealth Navigator, which provides case managers to help coordinate and oversee patient care, and health navigators to help patients better manage their chronic diseases. The goal of the pilot was to ensure that the mobile health paramedics would be integrated into this team, providing the patient and the patient's treatment team with an additional clinical resource.

To be eligible for this pilot program, patients had to meet several criteria. First, they had to be within a 20-mile radius "as the crow flies" of Geisinger Wyoming Valley Medical Center. Second, the payer had to be either Medicare or a Geisinger Health Plan (GHP) patient. Finally, the patient had to be an established patient at one of five existing Geisinger Medical Groups (Kingston, Wyoming, Pittston, Moosic, or Dallas) or the Geisinger Wyoming Valley Heart Failure Clinic. If eligible, a patient's care team member would contact the Mobile Health Paramedic via pager or telephone when a specific clinical need was identified. The paramedic would go to the home, provide a patient assessment and identify clinical and related issues (e.g., lack of food in the home), communicate back to the treatment team, and coordinate additional care resources as necessary. The outcome of the encounter would be determined by the goals of the patient, the resources available in the home, and the managing provider's (e.g., family practitioner's) comfort with the care plan being safe and effective.

The goals of care were always to manage the patient outside an acute care institution. However, patient safety (combined with patient preference) was the primary driver of patient disposition. Therefore, while many patients were managed in their homes or with a proximate follow-up visit in the clinic, patients were also transported to the ED or admitted directly to the hospital if their condition warranted it.

Heart Failure: "Pilot within a Pilot"

Within this pilot project, we identified that patients with heart failure cared for by the Geisinger Wyoming Valley Medical Center could potentially benefit from the resources of the Mobile Health Paramedic Program. Heart failure is a chronic disease that requires routine care and also results in frequent acute exacerbations, necessitating ED visits and often admission.[12] The reasoning was that intervention during the acute decompensation phase of heart failure by the Mobile Health Paramedic Program paramedics could potentially have the greatest impact to prevent ED visits and hospital admissions.

During the pilot phase, in addition to the standard eligibility criteria described previously, the Mobile Health Paramedic Program would be dispatched to a patient's home if the patient's managing cardiology provider felt the paramedic's assessment and clinical skills could be of value. Interventions in the home for heart failure patients included history and

Table CS16.1 Performance Measures for the Mobile Health Paramedic Program

	Heart failure patients	Other patients	Total
Home visit encounters	149	297	446
Diuresis	132	7	139
Phone encounters	2,746	266	3,012
Total encounters*	3,027	570	3,597

*As of March 31, 2016, there are 950 unique patients.

physical examination, medication reconciliation, and evaluation of heart failure symptoms. Adjustments in the patient's medications could be coordinated with the heart failure team, which could include the combination of the nurse coordinator, the cardiologist, and a heart failure–specific pharmacist. Intravenous diuretics could be administered for patients experiencing volume overload, and laboratory studies could be obtained as ordered by the patient's managing provider. The Mobile Health paramedics worked with the nurse coordinator, and the patient's primary case manager when applicable, to arrange follow-up appointments for either heart failure or associated medical needs. As a flexible, in-home clinical resource, the number and timing of visits were tailored to the patient's needs.

Within 3 months, the Mobile Health Paramedic Program was formally implemented as a component of heart failure care for patients at the Geisinger Wyoming Valley Medical Center. Results from the heart failure pilot, along with the aggregate results from the Mobile Health Paramedic Program, are shown in Table CS16.1. The heart failure component of the pilot program continues to be one of the most active patient enrollment and integration groups.

Medical Oversight

The heart failure program did require medical oversight that was internally developed, and was externally evaluated by the Geisinger Health System. For the broader Mobile Health Paramedic Program, there are two components to the medical oversight of the program. The first is the program medical director, an emergency medicine physician who is credentialed by the Commonwealth of Pennsylvania to provide medical direction to a licensed EMS agency. The role of the medical director is to provide medical oversight to all of the clinical interventions that are offered by the program. This is to ensure that the scope of practice is adhered to in all circumstances, that the paramedics are appropriately trained for the work that they are performing, and that there is continuity in the clinical pathway between the intervention of the paramedic and the patient's global care plan.

The second component of clinical oversight is the provider responsible for the individual patient and the individual encounter. This provider was the individual who was overseeing the patient's care in their individual environment, whether through the primary care or medical home model, the ED, or the heart failure clinic. This provider would use the treatment team to integrate with the Mobile Health Paramedic Program, all documenting in the same electronic medical record to ensure the patient is receiving the care they need in the most appropriate environment. Regulatory compliance in some cases required final oversight of the actions of the paramedics by an emergency medicine physician.

Documentation

Given the additional team members involved in patient care, the Mobile Health Paramedic Program needed to ensure that clinical information and modifications of patient care plans were documented and accessible by all members of the treatment team. For this reason, providers use Epic (Epic Systems, Verona, WI), which is the same electronic health system as used by the rest of the medical center. This ensures consistent, accessible documentation regardless of where it occurs.

Outcomes

The Mobile Health Paramedic program at Geisinger tracked both process and outcome metrics. These metrics were used to determine the success of the program, to identify opportunities for program improvement, and to provide continuous quality assurance that the program was meeting and maintaining the desired clinical outcomes. The metrics are listed in Box 16.2.

Discussion

The Mobile Health Paramedic Program described here highlights many aspects of community paramedicine programs and some key concepts necessary to develop these programs. These concepts must be clearly understood by health system leaders, policymakers, and program developers to ensure that the programs are successfully implemented. Of importance is that these programs do the following:

1. Address a local issue identified with stakeholder involvement.
2. Have a clear structure and process, developed with stakeholder involvement.
3. Provide community paramedics with training specific to the targeted conditions.
4. Have measured outcomes to iteratively improve the program.

Local Issues Identified with Stakeholder Involvement

Successful program development usually requires involvement of key stakeholders, such as patients, advocates, hospital leadership, and clinical providers. In its development, the Mobile Health Paramedic Program was focused on the needs of the patients and on how Geisinger Health System could meet these needs. Despite being a leader in population health, Geisinger Health System found that its patients have challenges that could not be addressed by existing programs. Thus, through the formative work with stakeholder involvement, the needs of Geisinger patients helped to define the role of the Mobile Health Paramedic Program. For instance, the creation of the heart failure "pilot within a pilot" was developed because existing programs were not adequately addressing outpatient needs for this population, resulting in unnecessary ED visits and inpatient admissions.

The needs of the Geisinger Health System and its patients likely will differ from other groups with respect to distinct practice patterns, population characteristics, and existing infrastructure. However, bringing together key stakeholders is a crucial step, regardless of site, to help ensure program success.

Box 16.2 List of Process and Outcome Metrics for the Mobile Health Paramedic Program

Process Metrics

- Patient volume of service by patient type (heart failure, medical home, discharge PLUS):
  - Visit encounters
  - Phone encounters
  - Diuresis

- Service duration/turnaround time by patient type (heart failure, medical home, discharge PLUS)
  - Visit encounters
  - Phone encounters
  - Diuresis

- Daily completion of metrics

Outcome Metrics

- Avoided ED visits (captured in real time and validated by medical director)
- Avoided admissions (captured in real time and validated by medical director)
- Avoided readmissions (captured in real time and validated by medical director)
- Pre-post analysis of patients in the MHP program
  - Bed days saved
  - Patient ED length of stay
  - Patient ED boarding hours
  - Patient average length of stay
  - Patient bed days
  - Patient admissions
  - Patient ED visits
  - Patient readmissions
  - Patient days between admissions
  - Patient days between ED visits

- Patient satisfaction

Structure and Processes with Stakeholder Involvement

The Mobile Health Paramedic Program was carefully structured so that it complements existing programs (e.g., home health) and did not create role confusion or service duplication.[13] This included, at least initially, narrow inclusion criteria, limited clinical interventions, and integrated documentation to enhance communication, as well as a unique medical oversight structure to ensure adherence to EMS regulations and optimize care delivery. By positioning the Mobile Health Paramedic Program to have early successes in a limited range of focus, this helped to demonstrate early success of the program, building a solid foundation for success in other areas.

It is important to note that the Mobile Health Paramedic Program was primarily focused on medical issues (e.g., heart failure monitoring, medication reconciliation, diagnostic studies) rather than psychosocial issues (e.g., activities of daily living, home safety).

While psychosocial issues are also of great importance and may be the central focus of a program if the local needs are present, based on a local needs assessment, they were determined not to be a priority of the pilot program. However, in other settings, successful community paramedicine programs have had important psychosocial features.[8]

Training

Training is a key component of the Mobile Health Paramedic Program. Although the program did not require EMS providers to develop new skills, additional training was still necessary to ensure the use of and adherence to protocols and best clinical practices. Each program will need to carefully consider what additional training is needed. If participating EMS providers have advanced training in paramedicine (e.g., completed a community paramedic program), only targeted review may be needed. If the program is addressing a need (e.g., medication reconciliation), then further education and support may be needed on how to appropriately conduct a medication reconciliation. The heart failure pilot project is a representative example of a community paramedicine program requiring additional training. While paramedics were well trained to care for patients with acutely decompensated heart failure, the monitoring of patients with heart failure, including integrating with the cardiology team and following the individualized treatment plans, required additional knowledge and clinical skills to care for the patient rather than reflexively transporting to an ED.

Measured Outcomes to Refine the Program

Particularly while in development, it is critical to continually reevaluate these programs to determine what is working and what needs revision. These evaluations can be both quantitative and qualitative in nature, as both can provide information about the feasibility, acceptability, and effectiveness of the programs. Many programs have performed these qualitative and quantitative evaluations to optimize care delivered.[8,9,10,11] Geisinger's Mobile Health Paramedic Program carefully monitored process measures so that it could be refined to benefit patients most efficiently. The heart failure program had large numbers of participants receive both home visits and telephone calls, demonstrating feasibility and acceptability. Similarly, patients in MedStar's program were found to have lower ED use, an example of effectiveness.[10]

Challenges to Implementation

As programs like the Mobile Health Paramedic Program are developed, several common challenges have emerged. The first is, how to provide standardized training to EMS providers to deliver these medical and psychosocial services? Some formal community paramedicine training programs exist, and the Board for Critical Care Transport Paramedic Certification has announced that it will administer a "Certified Community Paramedic" examination.[14] However, given the conflicting definitions of community paramedicine and the varying roles of community paramedics, these training programs and certifications may not sufficiently prepare EMS providers to serve in these roles. Without standardized training programs, each program must develop its own educational curriculum to ensure that EMS providers have the necessary skills to deliver the needed services in their communities.

Another challenge is the regulatory environment. Each state has unique EMS statutes and regulations, and their influence on community paramedic programs needs to be clarified. Many states require that callers to 911 be taken to an acute care hospital ED, and prevent EMS programs from providing definitive treatments such as furosemide administration to heart failure patients or assisting with obtaining an outpatient clinic appointment. The EMS provider's scope of clinical practice may also be a barrier. Follow-up programs like the Mobile Health Paramedic Program use existing EMS provider skills. However, such an approach may violate state regulations, potentially putting the paramedicine program, its medical director, and the EMS provider at substantial medicolegal risk.

Payment structure is another potential issue. The Mobile Health Paramedic Program avoided this issue because the Geisinger Health System, which owns the EMS agency, indirectly benefits without direct reimbursement for the Mobile Health Paramedic Program. However, other programs (e.g., the MedStar program in Ft. Worth, Texas) may require reimbursement because they are not affiliated with a hospital system and therefore cannot collect revenue. The measurement of clinical and operational outcomes (e.g., hospital readmission) will help to overcome this challenge, as will early discussions with stakeholders.

In summary, community paramedicine is an innovation in acute and emergency care that is increasingly accepted. The role and characteristics of community paramedicine programs are rapidly evolving, but the fundamental structure of these programs, as well as the core program characteristics, are in place. A number of barriers to these programs exist, namely, regulatory and financial considerations, but considerable progress has allowed the development and implementation of these programs to ensure safe, high-quality programs that complement other healthcare services that can benefit patients.

References

1. Shah MN. An analysis of the forces affecting the formation of the emergency medical services system. *American Journal of Public Health*. 2006;96(3):414–423.

2. National Highway Traffic Safety Administration. EMS agenda for the future. Traffic Tech. 1996.

3. Garrison GH, Foltin GL, Becker LR, et al. The role of emergency medical services in primary injury prevention. *Annals of Emergency Medicine*. 1997;30(1):84–91.

4. Delbridge TR, Bailey B, Chew JL Jr, et al. EMS agenda for the future: where we are . . . where we want to be. EMS Agenda for the Future Steering Committee. *Annals of Emergency Medicine*. 1998;31(2):251–263.

5. Lerner EB, Fernandez AR, Shah MN. Do EMS providers think they should participate in disease prevention? *Prehospital Emergency Care*. 2009;13(1):64–70.

6. Shah MN, Lerner EB, Chiumento S, et al. An evaluation of paramedics' ability to screen older adults during emergency responses. *Prehospital Emergency Care*. 2004;8(3):298–308.

7. Shah MN, Karuza J, Rueckmann E, et al. Reliability and validity of prehospital case finding for depression and cognitive impairment. *Journal of the American Geriatrics Society*. 2009;57(4):697–702.

8. Shah MN, Caprio TV, Swanson P, et al. A novel emergency medical services-based program to identify and assist older adults in a rural community. *Journal of the American Geriatrics Society*. 2010;58(11):2205–2211.

9. Bigham BL, Kennedy SM, Drennan I, et al. Expanding paramedic scope of practice in the community: a systematic review of the

literature. *Prehospital Emergency Care.* 2013;17(3):361–372.

10. MedStar EMS. Mobile healthcare programs. Available at www.medstar911.org/community-health-program. Accessed August 11, 2014.

11. Tadros, AS, Castillo EM, Chan TC, et al. Effects of an emergency medical services-based resource access program on frequent users of health services. *Prehospital Emergency Care.* 2012;16(4):541–547.

12. Storrow AB, Jenkins CA, Self WH, et al. The burden of acute heart failure on U.S. emergency departments. *JACC-Heart Failure.* 2014;2(3):269–277.

13. American Nurses Association. ANA's essential principles for utilization of community paramedics. Available at www.nursingworld.org/ MainMenuCategories/ ThePracticeofProfessionalNursing/ NursingStandards/ANAPrinciples/ EssentialPrinciplies-UtilizationCommunityParamedics.pdf. Accessed August 11, 2014.

14. BCCTPC launches certified community paramedic exam. *EMS World.* Available at www.emsworld.com/news/12152172/ bcctpc-launches-certified-community-paramedic-cp-cr-exam. Accessed August 11, 2014.

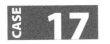

Initiating Palliative Care in the Emergency Department

Christian Jacobus and Tammie E. Quest

Introduction

Palliative care is the physical, spiritual, psychological, and social care provided to patients and families from diagnosis to death or cure of a life-threatening illness. Palliative care is practiced in an interdisciplinary team and is appropriate at any stage of illness. Core aspects of palliative care in the emergency department (ED) focus on pain and nonpain symptoms, communication skills, advance care planning, caring for patients receiving hospice services, ethical and legal issues, and support of families during the grief process after a death. Early initiation of palliative care in the ED was identified by the American College of Emergency Physicians as a quality intervention to improve end-of-life care. Patients and families benefit from a palliative care approach with increased quality of life, increased symptom control, longer life expectancy with terminal illness, increased patient and family satisfaction of care, and decreased healthcare costs.[1,2,3,4] Despite current recommendations and evidence supporting the early use of palliative care, emergency clinicians continue to struggle with implementation of palliative care in the emergency setting.[5,6] Presentation at end of life is common in the emergency setting and represents challenges regarding how to get patients high-quality care that is patient-centered and consistent with their goals. In particular, when patients present to the ED from long-term care settings (e.g., nursing homes), transfer can occur due to insecurities with nursing care, families being unprepared for the end of life, absent or inadequate advance care planning, and lack of communication and agreement within families regarding goals of care.[7] Patients are often admitted to the hospital from the ED, and palliative care consultation may be delayed by days. The following case depicts common challenges facing emergency clinicians and illustrates how an intervention can improve rates of and shorten time to palliative care consultation.

Case Study

Dr. Cynthia Adams is an emergency physician working in the ED of a large university teaching hospital. She is notified by the triage nurse of an urgent new patient being put into one of the acute care rooms. She looks over the chart on her way into the room and notes that he is a 55-year-old man with recently diagnosed metastatic lung cancer. His triage vitals include a heart rate of 132 beats per minute and a respiratory rate of 32 breaths per minute. After introducing herself she learns that his name is Bill Tucker. He tells her that he had been seeing his primary care physician for the last 3 to 4 months for a persistent cough and chest pain. After multiple rounds of antibiotics and nebulized albuterol breathing treatments his physician ordered a chest X-ray and then a computed tomography (CT) scan, which showed a right upper lobe mass with osteolytic lesions in his right humerus and multiple ribs, consistent with metastatic disease. An endobronchial biopsy confirmed non-small cell lung cancer, and a positron emission tomography scan found distant bony metastases. He has an appointment to see an oncologist at this hospital, but not until next week. His primary physician prescribed oxycodone/acetaminophen and he needs to take an average of seven tablets per day to help with his pain and shortness of breath. His dyspnea and coughing suddenly became much worse about an hour prior to arrival, prompting his presentation to the ED.

On examination Mr. Tucker is a middle-aged man sitting on the stretcher appearing in moderate respiratory distress. He looks older than his stated age of 55 years old. His cardiac monitor shows sinus tachycardia at 124 beats per minute and an oxygen saturation of 92 percent on 4 liters of oxygen via nasal cannula. Auscultation of his lungs reveals scattered wheezes and occasional coarse rhonchi but good air exchange. Dr. Adams orders a portable chest X-ray, electrocardiogram, and laboratory testing. When the chest X-ray comes back showing no change from 2 weeks ago, she orders a CT pulmonary angiogram. Multiple subsegmental pulmonary emboli are demonstrated, and she starts him on a heparin infusion. Based on his persistent tachycardia and hypoxia she decides to admit him to the intensive care unit (ICU) and pages the on-call ICU resident. The hospital's electronic medical record includes a clinical decision support rule to screen for admitted patients with a metastatic malignancy and to prompt the clinician to consider a palliative care consultation. Dr. Adams sees a pop-up window asking if consultation is appropriate based on the question "Would you be surprised if the patient died in the next 12 months?" with a negative response by the clinician triggering a palliative care consultation. It is 7 PM on a Thursday evening, and though the ED clinician orders a consult, it states that the hours of the palliative care service are Monday to Friday, 8 AM to 6 PM, and that consults initiated after these hours will be seen on the next non-weekend day. Based on this, Dr. Adams introduces the concept of palliative care as increased support to Mr. Tucker and asks whether he has an advance care plan should his condition worsen. He states that he does not, and Dr. Adams proceeds to discuss the risks and benefits of resuscitation and life-sustaining therapies. The patient states he would not want such interventions. Dr. Adams documents his advance care plan preferences in the form of a "do not resuscitate – do not intubate order."

Mr. Tucker is admitted to the ICU around midnight, and a palliative care nurse practitioner sees him the next morning. They discuss this new diagnosis of pulmonary emboli and his metastatic cancer. She helps him understand that, while the cancer is treatable, it is not curable and that he will need to be on blood thinners for the rest of his life. She recommends the addition of a glucocorticoid to help with nausea, bone pain, and fatigue as well as a long-acting opioid for more consistent pain control. They discuss his spirituality as well, and he discloses to her that he feels that God is punishing him for sins that he committed as a young man and that he will not get into heaven when he dies. She asks the palliative care chaplain to visit with him to discuss these concerns. He does not have any legal advance directive, so the palliative care social worker completes a living will and a durable power-of-attorney for healthcare with him that is consistent with his discussion with Dr. Adams. The nurse sets him up for a home palliative care visit in about 10 days to continue discussing his goals of care and to monitor his symptom management. He is discharged to home 3 days later.

Challenge #1: Identification of Patients Appropriate for Consultation

Mr. Tucker presents with an acute medical illness in the setting of a serious life-threatening and incurable condition. Areas of distress include pain and dyspnea as well as the need for advance care planning should he deteriorate, with clear focus on his goals of care. His medical care should be tailored toward that which is important to him. When patients present to the ED for an acute illness in the context of a more chronic serious illness, the emergency clinician is challenged by how much to focus on beyond acute stabilization of the medical problem.

Innovation #1: Use of Decision Support Tools to Initiate Palliative Care from the ED

Multiple studies have shown that palliative care screening in the ED can be effective. They use a variety of triggers, but there are some common elements.[8] Screens for palliative care in the ED should be simple and able to be administered within several minutes, should be able to be done by usual ED screening methods such initiation by the patient or nurse, and target high-risk such as populations for serious illness by history alone without extensive medical record review. Elements that prompt the emergency clinician to a serious illness trajectory include the "surprise question" that relies on the clinician's clinical gestalt to focus on prognostication. The "surprise" question – "Would you be surprised if the patient died within the next year?" or "Would you be surprised if the patient died on this hospitalization?" has been shown to appropriately initiate inpatient palliative care consultation.[9,10,11,12] Additional considerations that might help to identify patients appropriate for palliative care consultation from the ED include a patient chart review to identify prior hospitalizations or previous palliative care consultation, and discussions with caregivers that suggest caregiver fatigue, burden, or distress. As with the electronic medical record in Dr. Adams's hospital, potential future directions include the development and validation of a decision support rule to prompt consideration of a palliative care consultation, see Figure CS17.1. Such a decision rule could be operationalized in the context of normal clinical operations and monitored for ongoing performance. For example, such process measures could include time to palliative care consultation, time to hospice referral, or time to change in code status. Patient-centered outcomes measured can include time to pain or other symptom control, or patient/family satisfaction with care.

Challenge #2: Initiating Palliative Care in the ED until Consultation Can Be Obtained

Few hospitals have palliative care consultants who are available to come to the ED during weekend or evening hours. Workforce shortages in hospice and palliative medicine dictate that emergency clinicians initiate consultation from the ED with the expectation that the consultation may not be completed during the ED visit, as our case illustrates.[13] Dr. Adams's time is limited and she has to consider the highest yield areas of palliative care that can help the patient at that time. In an unstable or severely ill patient, discussion of goals of care and advance care planning in the ED are critical elements of primary palliative care.

Innovation #2: Advance Care Planning Discussions by Emergency Clinicians

As more education and clinical protocols focused on palliative care are implemented in EDs, more patients are likely to benefit from primary palliative care interventions. The creation of advance care plans from the ED is critical to ensure from the outset that the patient gets the end-of-life care that they wish. Mr. Tucker exhibited openness to have the discussion with Dr. Adams in the ED, which resulted in orders for life-sustaining care to be held in the event that they were needed.

Discussion

Hospice and palliative medicine is one of the newest subspecialties in medicine, focused on training a cadre of professionals with advanced skills in pain and symptom management, communication, prognostication, and transitions of care.[14] Models for tertiary palliative care integration in the ED are varied to include consultants that come to the ED in a supportive role as well as specialists who are housed within the ED.[15] While gaps in evidence exist, preliminary data suggests that when identified by emergency clinicians, the initiation of consultation of a palliative care subspecialist has been shown to be beneficial to patients with cancer, like Mr. Tucker. These patients can benefit from additional physical, spiritual, psychological, and social support. Specific benefits include improved symptom management and decreased length of stay in select patients with no evidence of harm.[16,17]

In order to effectively care for patients and families experiencing serious illness, not only do emergency clinicians need to possess primary palliative care skills for use in the ED,[18,19] but they also need to know when to call for subspecialty intervention – palliative care consultation. Particularly in patients with advanced stage cancers, earlier palliative care initiation in hospitalized patients has been linked to better outcomes, including improved symptom care, patient/family satisfaction, and decreased resource utilization.[20,21] Earlier palliative care consultation during hospital admission is associated with lower cost of hospital stay for patients admitted with an advanced cancer diagnosis.[22] However, the benefits of inpatient palliative care consultation diminish when consultations occur later in the hospital stay. If used more frequently, the implementation of palliative care in the ED could improve patient care by earlier intervention of a palliative care specialist. However, barriers to implementation exist. For example, physician-identified barriers to implementation of palliative care in the ED include lack of access to medical records and lack of availability of palliative care inpatient consultation teams. In addition, there is a lack of

Proposed Screening Tool to Identify Emergency Department Patients for Palliative Care Referral/Resources	
Proposed characterisitcs for screening tool to identify patients for specialized palliative care services (in-hospital or community)	
Time to screen	1 – 2 min
Who performs screening	ED triage nurse (preferably no additional ED resources)
Staged process	1st tier ED screen process Detailed assessment if needed conducted by other qualified personnel such as social worker or palliative care nurse
Target population	• Elderly >65 and/or • Chronic life-limiting illness (suggest each ED identify based on population served by institution; example, metastatic cancer, end stage congestive heart failure)
Prognostication	'Would you be surprised' questions
Special considerations	• Functional status of patient • Caregiver/social support • Frequent ED admits and hospitalizations (set time and definitions)

Assess outcomes of screening process	1. Completion rate of tool and number screen "positive"
	2. Referral to specialized in-hospital or community resources (palliative team, hospice care)
	3. In those who screened "positive" and are referred to specialized or community services
	    • Nature of intervention by specialized service
	    • Frequency of repeat ED visits and hospitalizations
	    • Time to disposition and discharge
	    • Adequacy of symptom control
	    • Patient and/or caregiver satisfaction

Figure CS17.1 Proposed screening tool to identify ED patients. Reprinted from the *Journal of Pain and Symptom Management*, 51:1, Naomi George et al., "Palliative care screening and assessment in the emergency department: a systematic review," pp. 108–119, copyright (2016), with permission from Elsevier.

comfort on the part of providers to initiate consultation for patients with organ failure and dementia compared with patients who have a cancer diagnosis.[23,24] Thus, while challenges to broader dissemination remain, the implementation of palliative care initiation in the ED has substantial downstream benefits for patients with serious illness.

References

1. Morrison RS, Penrod JD, Cassel JB, et al. Cost savings associated with US hospital palliative care consultation programs. *Archives of Internal Medicine*. 2008;168 (16):1783–1790.

2. Penrod J, Morrison RS, Meier DE. Studying the effectiveness of palliative care. *JAMA*. 2008;300(9):1022–1023; author reply 1023–1024.

3. Gelfman LP, Meier DE, Morrison RS. Does palliative care improve quality? A survey of bereaved family members. *Journal of Pain Symptom Management*. 2008;36(1):22–28.

4. Morrison RS, Meier DE, Fischberg D, et al. Improving the management of pain in hospitalized adults. *Archives of Internal Medicine*. 2006;166(9):1033–1039.

5. Smith AK, Fisher J, Schonberg MA, et al. Am I doing the right thing? Provider perspectives on improving palliative care in the emergency department. *Annals of Emergency Medicine*. 2009;54(1):86–93.

6. Knott DA, Hiestand BC. If not us, then who? Palliative care referral from the emergency department. *Academic Emergency Medicine*. 2015;22(2):227–228.

7. Stephens C, Halifax E, Bui N, et al. Provider perspectives on the influence of family on nursing home resident transfers to the emergency department: crises at the end of life. *Current Gerontology and Geriatrics Research*. 2015;2015:893062.

8. George N, Phillips E, Zaurova M, et al. Palliative care screening and assessment in the emergency department: a systematic review. *Journal of Pain Symptom Management*. 2016;51(1):108–119.

9. Rhee J, Clayton JM. The "surprise" question may improve the accuracy of GPs in identifying death in patients with advanced stage IV solid-cell cancer. *Evidence Based Medicine*. 2015;20(2):71.

10. Moroni M, Zocchi D, Bolognesi D, et al. The "surprise" question in advanced cancer patients: a prospective study among general practitioners. *Palliative Medicine*. 2014;28 (7):959–964.

11. Pang WF, Kwan BC, Chow KM, et al. Predicting 12-month mortality for peritoneal dialysis patients using the "surprise" question. *Peritoneal Dialysis International*. 2013;33(1):60–66.

12. Moss AH, Lunney JR, Culp S, et al. Prognostic significance of the "surprise" question in cancer patients. *Journal Palliative Medicine*. 2010;13(7):837–840.

13. Lupu D, American Academy of Hospice and Palliative Medicine Workforce Task Force. Estimate of current hospice and palliative medicine physician workforce shortage. *Journal of Pain Symptom Management*. 2010;40(6):899–911.

14. von Gunten CF, Lupu D. Development of a medical subspecialty in palliative medicine: progress report. *Journal of Palliative Medicine*. 2004;7(2):209–219.

15. Lamba S, DeSandre PL, Todd KH, et al. Integration of palliative care into emergency medicine: the improving palliative care in emergency medicine (IPAL-EM) collaboration. *Journal of Emergency Medicine*. 2014;46(2):264–270.

16. Grudzen CR, Richardson LD, Johnson PN, et al. Emergency department-initiated palliative care in advanced cancer: a randomized clinical trial. *JAMA Oncology*. 2016 Jan 14. www.ncbi.nlm.nih.gov/pubmed/26768772.

17. Wu FM, Newman JM, Lasher A, et al. Effects of initiating palliative care consultation in the emergency department on inpatient length of stay. *Journal of Palliative Medicine*. 2013;16 (11):1362–1367.

18. Quest TE, Marco CA, Derse AR. Hospice and palliative medicine: new subspecialty,

new opportunities. *Annals of Emergency Medicine*. 2009;54(1):94–102.

19. Grudzen CR, Emlet LL, Kuntz J, et al. EM talk: communication skills training for emergency medicine patients with serious illness. *BMJ Support Palliative Care*. 2016 Jun;6(2):219–224.

20. Dahlin CM, Kelley JM, Jackson VA, et al. Early palliative care for lung cancer: improving quality of life and increasing survival. *International Journal of Palliative Nursing*. 2010;16(9):420–423.

21. Temel JS, Greer JA, Muzikansky A, et al. Early palliative care for patients with metastatic non-small-cell lung cancer. *New England Journal of Medicine*. 2010;363 (8):733–742.

22. May P, Garrido MM, Cassel JB, et al. Prospective cohort study of hospital palliative care teams for inpatients with advanced cancer: earlier consultation is associated with larger cost-saving effect. *Journal of Clinical Oncology*. 2015;33 (25):2745–2752.

23. Lamba S, Nagurka R, Zielinski A, et al. Palliative care provision in the emergency department: barriers reported by emergency physicians. *Journal of Palliative Medicine*. 2013;16(2):143–147.

24. Ouchi K, Wu M, Medairos R, et al. Initiating palliative care consults for advanced dementia patients in the emergency department. *Journal of Palliative Medicine*. 2014;17(3):346–350.

18 Streamlining Patient Flow in the Emergency Department with Discrete Event Simulation

Eric J. Goldlust, T. Eugene Day, and Nathan R. Hoot

Introduction

Discrete event simulation (DES) is a method based on decades of experience in operations research and is employed to improve efficiency and reduce costs in fields such as manufacturing, air traffic control, and, more recently, healthcare delivery.[1,2] It expands on the uses of queuing theory, which has also been used to analyze waiting times and identify bottlenecks. However, DES is particularly well suited to analyze complex, nonlinear relationships between entities and resources such as those occurring in emergency department (ED) patient flow.

In 2006, the Institute of Medicine called for increased adoption of such techniques to improve emergency care, reporting that a growing body of experience suggests that using queuing theory to smooth the peaks and valleys of patient admissions can eliminate bottlenecks, reduce crowding, improve patient care, and reduce costs.[3] Similarly, in 2014, the President's Council of Advisors on Science and Technology called broadly for the healthcare industry to expand its employment of systems engineering, a broad set of methods that includes both queuing theory and DES, noting that these systems methods and tools are not yet used on a widespread basis in US healthcare.[4]

System engineering methods, in particular DES, can aid analysis of and improve patient flow in the ED. DES is well suited to model the complexities of ED patient flow, in which patients compete for departmental resources such as computed tomography scanners, physicians, or nurses. The needs of each individual patient vary according to demographics and presentation of the illness. Furthermore, arrival and departure patterns of ED patients are variable and are influenced by forces outside the control of the ED. Such competition for resources, and the variability of patient demand, tends to violate the assumptions of simpler mathematical models, thereby introducing inaccuracies and unpredictability through oversimplification. By modeling the appropriate level of complexity, DES can predict the expected effects of system changes without actually implementing them, and thus helps to guide process improvements at relatively low cost and minimal risk.

To apply DES, a modeler must first understand the processes involved in ED patient flow. These may be understood by management techniques such as process mapping and spending time in the ED itself as a direct observer of the process in situ (as is often espoused in lean management methods). Once understood, these processes can be described in terms of the five conceptual building blocks of a DES model: entities, resources and locations, events, time, and the system state. *Entities*, in DES, refer to parties or items on which work is performed – for example, the goods produced by a factory – while *resources* refer to people and equipment who perform such work. The entities of an ED might be the patients themselves, and the resources for which they compete might include physicians, nurses, laboratory technicians, or imaging equipment. Similarly, the *locations* of an ED might be physical beds, including nonstandard spaces like hallway beds or chairs. *Events* – defined here as particular moments of interest that trigger a choice, a subsequent event, or some other change – must be well defined within a DES model, and only events can modify the state of the system. *Time* moves forward in DES as in the real world – but in the model, time jumps from one event to the next, rather than capturing every tick of the clock. The time it takes for a particular type of event to occur may be a predefined constant, such as a preset on a microwave oven, or it may follow a probability distribution that can be determined empirically or approximated. Once these elements and distributions are carefully defined for the model, the sequence of events thus represents a model that continually modifies the system state. The *system state* of an ED is essentially the current "status" of the ED, similar to that represented more traditionally using a patient whiteboard, for example, describing the current patients, their assigned beds and present locations, and what has been completed (or not) as they progress through the ED.

After describing ED patient flow using these five conceptual elements of DES, a modeler can make changes to the system – for instance, by changing the available resources or modifying the demand for patient care – and use the results to make inferences about the effects on the system. This chapter will illustrate the application of DES to guide a successful intervention in emergency healthcare.[5]

Case Study

Problem

The Veterans Health Administration holds a national performance measure benchmark that no more than 10 percent of patients should spend greater than six hours in the ED from arrival to a decision to either admit, discharge, or transfer the patient.

At the Veterans Affairs (VA) St. Louis Medical Center–John Cochran Division, a Level III trauma center with 120 inpatient beds, this benchmark was exceeded in over 25 percent of its 20,000 annual ED patient visits in early 2009. The preliminary opinion of local administrators was that the inefficiency lay predominantly in the throughput processes of ED care, rather than delays in admissions (which accounted for a small percentage of patients) or an increase in patient arrivals. Thus, they sought to redesign the process of ED care in order to meet the performance standard.

Early on, ED leaders at this VA facility recognized that there were numerous potential interventions. Many such efforts to reduce ED length of stay (LOS) involve costly process interventions such as increasing staffing, modifying existing facilities, or upgrading computer or laboratory systems. Local VA physician administrators could not agree on solutions likely to achieve the desired performance improvement. Moreover, they believed that minor changes would not be a viable method for sustained process improvement. Additionally, they were concerned that any failed interventions might diminish staff morale, decreasing the likelihood of success for future process improvement efforts. As a result, this facility sought an accurate, low-cost means of testing and evaluating such interventions prior to implementation. Recognizing that DES met these criteria, administrators selected DES to explore multiple potential ED process improvements prior to finalizing their improvement strategy.

ED Processes

Characterization of ED Patient Flow

On initial presentation to the Cochran ED, some patients with less urgent requests, such as routine eye exams or medication refills, may be redirected through a process called "pretriage" to the appropriate clinic during normal business hours. Patients presenting to the ED with more urgent complaints are rapidly assigned a priority score (i.e., Emergency Severity Index [ESI]) ranging from 1 to 5 during this pretriage process. Patients with ESI 1 and 2 were directed immediately to the main ED treatment area (comprising 14 patient beds), effectively bypassing triage. Those with ESI 3 (or sometimes 4) received full triage assessments and were then directed to the main ED, while the remainder with ESI 4 and 5 were directed to the fast track area, except for a small subset of those with ESI 5, who were discharged directly from triage. The main ED area was staffed by four attending physicians during peak hours, in addition to the lone advanced practice provider (i.e., nurse practitioner or physician assistant) dedicated to the fast track area. The process of patient care within the main ED appears similar to the processes of most community EDs.

Process Mapping/Face Validation

In 2009, administrators employed a systems engineer trained in DES modeling of healthcare systems to convene with the ED team, including approximately 120 hours of observing care and existing processes. This modeler continued to observe the ED during the present study, to ensure validity of the ED process flow as characterized by administrators (above). The modeler used these observations to develop a process flow map. As part of the mapping process, the flow map was reviewed with administrators and staff of the VA St. Louis Medical Center ED and revised until all stakeholders agreed that it adequately represented the processes of care. During this review, stakeholders agreed on the appropriate level of detail needed to be represented in the model (Figure CS18.1).

Model Development

Using the patient flow map, a DES model of this ED was built using commercially available software for this purpose (AnyLogic Professional 6.4). First, the system was broken down into its constituent elements: entities on which work is performed (for this model, patients), resources that are responsible for performing that work (physicians, nurses, etc.), and the locations at which care takes place (examination rooms, triage rooms, etc.). Using these elements, events were defined to characterize the interaction of these three elements, that is, what causes entities to use resources and move between or occupy locations.

Next, the flow was mapped according to each of these elements. The statistical distributions for each process were abstracted from ED operational data reports (e.g., admission and discharge rates, ESI distributions, and daily patient arrival rates) and collected from medical records for patients presenting for care ($n = 2,194$) over a 6-week period in the fall of 2009. The average daily arrival-to-disposition time was 247 minutes (SD 39.8), with 437 (19.9 percent) visits longer than 6 hours (the primary outcome of interest). When data were not available (e.g., time spent at the bedside with each patient), mean, minimal, and maximal times were estimated from interviews with experienced staff.

Model Verification

Through a process called "verification," sometimes called "internal validation," the modeler ensured that the simulation represented a stable and well-defined representation of the actual care process. This was achieved using "audits," involving many serial runs of single patients through the simulation, and "stress tests," or single runs of massive numbers of patients. The "audits" detect anomalies in the care sequence for each simulated patient, while "stress tests" detect anomalies in the model under extreme conditions. Such errors

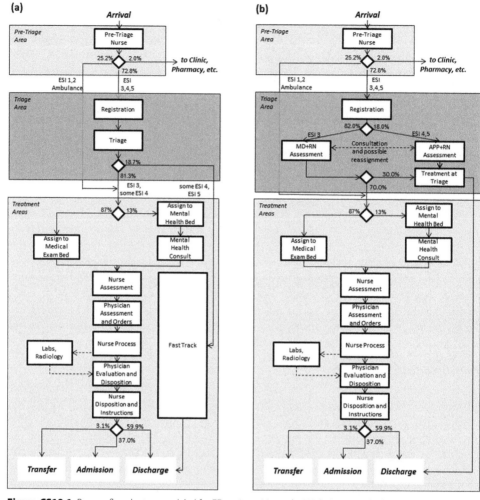

Figure CS18.1 Process flowchart as modeled for ED patient visits at the VA St. Louis Medical Center, (a) prior to intervention and (b) postintervention. Decision points are depicted as diamonds; percentages indicate the likelihood of patients assigned to each pathway, based on staff discretion or Emergency Severity Index (ESI) (in the real ED) or random assignment (in the discrete event simulation model). APP, advanced practice provider (physician assistant or nurse practitioner); MD, attending physician; RN, nurse assigned to the triage area. Adapted with permission from Reference 5.

were then corrected iteratively until no more were found. Throughout this process, the modeler continued to check "face validity," that is, consulting with ED staff to ensure that the model remained representative of reality.

External Validation of Baseline Conditions

Since events modeled in DES are randomly determined, different runs of a model can vary significantly. Therefore, the simulation was run 10 times, each for 6 simulated weeks, to match the time period for the data used to generate the model. Patient arrivals, mean LOS, and the percentage of visits greater than 6 hours were similar between observed and simulated data, further convincing stakeholders that this model represented real-world conditions and to proceed with simulated interventions.

Exploratory Analysis and Selection of Intervention

During baseline model development, stakeholders proposed process flow interventions to study based on feasibility, cost, acceptability by staff, and potential to improve the performance metrics of interest. For example, consideration was given to repurposing a physician's office into an examination room, or a nearby conference room into a holding area for admitted patients. Due to budgetary constraints, stakeholders agreed that the addition of staff was not a feasible option. Potential solutions were then modeled and validated similarly with stakeholders.

As depicted in Figure CS18.1, results suggested that the best intervention would eliminate the fast track area, moving the advanced practice provider to triage. Further, one provider was moved from the main ED to triage to evaluate and discharge some ESI 3 patients from triage, while the remainder would progress to the main ED to complete their work-up. The remainder of ED care was unchanged, with the exception that only three attending physicians were assigned to the main ED.

Analysis of the simulated results from this process change showed it to be effective in two ways. First, patients made contact with providers earlier in their visit, starting their work-ups earlier and allowing some to be discharged without taking up a bed outside of triage. This was essential in decreasing the number of visits greater than 6 hours, as it made beds available for those who needed care urgently. Alternatively, those who were less sick, with typically lower requirements for ED resources, could get all of their care without further delay for bed placement. Second, by reducing the number of patients requiring beds in the ED, this increased the availability of beds in the main ED for those who required more intensive emergency care.

The proposed change in ED care process – as simulated – reported 2,154 patient visits over a 6-week period, with a daily mean throughput time of 200 minutes (SD 19.0). Of these, 282 visits were greater than 6 hours (13.1 percent), for a relative reduction of 31.1 percent compared with the baseline simulation (Table CS18.1). Stakeholders reviewed these results and determined that this warranted implementation. Moreover, this simulation demonstrated that this could be done without adding staff, space, or other resources.

Results/External Validation

On the basis of the simulation results, hospital administration approved a 1-month real-world trial of the intervention. Staff members were educated about the changes and their new assignments. The advanced practice provider and physician stationed in the triage area were encouraged to collaborate, upgrading or downgrading acuity and reassigning patients to one another whenever appropriate.

Operational data confirmed what the simulation predicted. During the 1-month trial period, the ED saw 1,699 patient visits. Daily mean throughput time was 210 minutes (SD 16.6). There were 243 (14.3 percent) visits greater than 6 hours, and 577 patients with ESI 4 or 5 were discharged directly from triage (Table CS18.1). Notably, these results were consistent with the simulation estimates, despite a nearly 10 percent increase in mean daily patient volume.

Discussion

The experience at the St. Louis VA demonstrates how DES can be a powerful tool to understand and manage demand for emergency care. This project started with an important

Table CS18.1 Simulated versus Operational Data Results

	Simulated		p	Real-World		p
	Baseline	Postintervention		Baseline	Postintervention	
Daily LOS*	249 ±39.8 min	200±19.0 min	<0.0001	247 ±39.8 min	210±16.6 min	<0.0001
Patients with LOS >6 hours**	437/ 2,194 (19.0%)	282/2,154 (13.1%)	<0.0001	413/ 2,178 (19.9%)	243/1,699 (14.3%)	<0.0001

* Mean ± SD; p-values from Student's t tests.
** Number of patients; p-values from chi-squared tests.

foundation: understanding patient flow in the ED at the St. Louis VA, integrating knowledge from ED operations in general with direct observation at that site. This work enabled the modeler to describe patient flow in terms of the conceptual elements of DES and apply them to develop a useful simulation. The stakeholders and modeler agreed on a set of interventions that might achieve their operational goals, and the simulation was used as a means to evaluate each of the proposed interventions.

This innovation demonstrates a key strength of DES: it permits the evaluation of process improvement strategies at a lower cost, greater efficiency, and minimal risk to patient safety as compared with the trial-and-error approach. For example, changes to the physical plant of an ED or electronic health record require capital expenditure for an intervention that may not succeed. Furthermore, changes to ED processes may have unintended consequences, such as compromising patient safety or diminishing staff enthusiasm for current and future projects. Despite the cost of building a simulation model, given its potential to explore myriad process changes and focus on those with the most promise, DES yields a safe and effective approach to process improvement. Additionally, it bolsters staff morale by providing a reason to believe in the success of the planned changes.

There are numerous precedents for DES to examine patient flow in emergency medicine, dating back to 1989.[6] These studies have explored the effects of added resources (i.e., nurses, physicians, and imaging equipment) and the sources of delays contributing to ED crowding.[7,8,9,10] Interesting extensions of DES explored how operational improvement could be achieved with cost-neutral interventions, forecasting ED patient flow under various conditions, and the impact of the relationships between ED and inpatient units on admission bed availability.[11,12,13,14] DES also allows for the study and design of novel interventions, such as a study proposing the "flex track," whereby ED beds could be dynamically repurposed to accommodate high- or low-acuity patients, as indicated by patient demand.[15]

A substantial proportion of published research focuses on expanding available ED space, which is often suggested to improve throughput, despite tremendous costs. One study examined the effects of ED expansion using DES, finding that increasing bed capacity would not improve LOS, but that accelerating transfer of admitted patients to admitted units would reduce LOS by 9 percent.[16,17] Another study likewise projected that expanding ED capacity via an observation unit would not improve LOS, but that mandating transfer of boarding patients within 1 hour would improve LOS by roughly 15 percent.[18]

These findings are supported by two other studies, which did not apply DES but instead reported the effects of ED expansion that was in fact implemented. These studies found that adding bed capacity to the ED did not decrease the need for ambulance diversion or the rate of patient elopement at each site.[19,20] While differences between sites may limit generalization, at these particular institutions, ED bed capacity was not the key bottleneck in ED throughput. It is possible that less expensive alternate strategies may have improved performance. This highlights the strength of DES as a means to facilitate change, by identifying targets for improvement that are most likely to be effective, given the operational context.

Despite its practical utility, there are limitations inherent to DES. First, the reliability of simulation output is subject to the model's validity. Overly simplified or erroneous models can provide misleading results, leading stakeholders to poor decisions. This underscores the importance of model verification, as demonstrated in the intervention above. Second, some systems cannot be easily described using DES – for instance, physical or electrical systems with continuously interacting forces. Third, after DES helps guide planning, an implementation gap remains – numerous organizational and technical barriers may exist, in order for an intervention to yield the desired benefits. Because of this, modelers must consider the local culture, and incorporate stakeholders early on, which can influence the success or failure of an otherwise promising change.

In conclusion, DES is a valuable and underutilized means to address ED patient flow. While DES cannot identify a single, optimal way to operate an ED, it is quite versatile at identifying possible bottlenecks and evaluating proposed interventions. As shown here, the tools of systems engineering – in particular, DES – can help administrators identify promising interventions to facilitate change in a disciplined, careful manner that minimizes risk and lowers overall costs.

References

1. Gross D, Harris CM. *Fundamentals of Queuing Theory*, 4th ed. New York: Wiley, 2008.

2. Law AM. *Simulation Modeling and Analysis*, 4th ed. New York: McGraw-Hill, 2007.

3. Committee on the Future of Emergency Care in the United States Health System. *Hospital-Based Emergency Care: At the Breaking Point*. Washington, DC: National Academies Press, 2006.

4. President's Council of Advisors on Science and Technology. Better health care and lower costs: accelerating improvement through systems engineering. Washington, DC. 2014. Available at www.whitehouse.gov/sites/default/files/microsites/ostp/PCAST/pcast_systems_engineering_in_healthcare_-_may_2014.pdf. Accessed January 5, 2016.

5. Day TE, Al-Roubaie AR, Goldlust EJ. Decreased length of stay after addition of healthcare provider in emergency department triage: a comparison between computer-simulated and real-world interventions. *Emergency Medicine Journal*. 2013;30(2):134–138.

6. Saunders CE, Makens PK, LeBlanc LJ. Modeling emergency department operations using advanced computer simulation systems. *Annals of Emergency Medicine*. 1989;18(2):134–140.

7. Hung GR, Whitehouse SR, O'Neill C, et al. Computer modeling of patient flow in a pediatric emergency department using discrete event simulation. *Pediatric Emergency Care*. 2007;23(1):5–10.

8. Brenner S, Zeng Z, Liu Y, et al. Modeling and analysis of the emergency department at University of Kentucky Chandler Hospital using simulations. *Journal of Emergency Nursing*. 2010;36(4):303–310.

9. Paul JA, Lin L. Models for improving patient throughput and waiting at hospital emergency departments. *Journal of Emergency Medicine.* 2012;43(6):1119–1126.

10. Genuis ED, Doan Q. The effect of medical trainees on pediatric emergency department flow: a discrete event simulation modeling study. *Academic Emergency Medicine.* 2013;20 (11):1112–1120.

11. Best AM, Dixon CA, Kelton WD, et al. Using discrete event computer simulation to improve patient flow in a Ghanaian acute care hospital. *American Journal of Emergency Medicine.* 2014;32(8):917–922.

12. Hoot NR, LeBlanc LJ, Jones I, et al. Forecasting emergency department crowding: a discrete event simulation. *Annals of Emergency Medicine.* 2008;52 (2):116–125.

13. Hoot NR, Epstein SK, Allen TL, et al. Forecasting emergency department crowding: an external, multicenter evaluation. *Annals of Emergency Medicine.* 2009;54(4):514–522.

14. Levin SR, Dittus R, Aronsky D, et al. Optimizing cardiology capacity to reduce emergency department boarding: a systems engineering approach. *American Heart Journal.* 2008;156(6):1202–1209.

15. Laker LF, Froehle CM, Lindsell CJ, et al. The flex track: flexible partitioning between low- and high-acuity areas of an emergency department. *Annals of Emergency Medicine.* 2014;64(6):591–603.

16. Derlet RW, Richards JR. Overcrowding in the nation's emergency departments: complex causes and disturbing effects. *Annals of Emergency Medicine.* 2000;35 (1):63–68.

17. Khare RK, Powell ES, Reinhardt G, et al. Adding more beds to the emergency department or reducing admitted patient boarding times: which has a more significant influence on emergency department congestion? *Annals of Emergency Medicine.* 2009;53(5):575–585.

18. Hung GR, Kissoon N. Impact of an observation unit and an emergency department-admitted patient transfer mandate in decreasing overcrowding in a pediatric emergency department: a discrete event simulation exercise. *Pediatric Emergency Care.* 2009;25(3):160–163.

19. Han JH, Zhou C, France DJ, et al. The effect of emergency department expansion on emergency department overcrowding. *Academic Emergency Medicine.* 2007;14 (4):338–343.

20. Mumma BE, McCue JY, Li CS, et al. Effects of emergency department expansion on emergency department patient flow. *Academic Emergency Medicine.* 2014;21 (5):504–509.

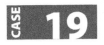

CASE 19

Using Emergency Department Community Health Workers as a Bridge to Ongoing Care for Frequent ED Users

Roberta Capp and Richard Zane

Introduction

Frequent emergency department (ED) utilizers are common, accounting for about 28–50 percent of all ED visits.[1] Decreasing ED utilization is mentioned as a goal in nearly every healthcare cost reduction initiative. Of particular scrutiny in the medical and lay press[1] have been those patients who use the ED frequently, often referred to as "high utilizers" ($\geq$4 ED visits per year). Patients insured by US public programs (e.g., Medicaid, Medicare, or both) have the highest rates of frequent ED use by far, especially Medicaid patients.[2,3] One in 12 adult US Medicaid enrollees is a frequent ED utilizer, which, by some estimates, accounts for nearly 50 percent of all ED healthcare costs.[4,5] As the Affordable Care Act has added millions of new American patients to the Medicaid rosters, this has become appropriately concerning to US policymakers and state officials nationwide.[6]

Reducing ED utilization among this group goes far beyond establishing a primary care physician relationship. Detailed studies of Medicaid-enrolled frequent ED users show that the barriers to care are myriad and complex. In fact, 60 percent of Medicaid patients have an established primary care physician yet many suffer from complex chronic diseases, have barriers to accessing timely outpatient services (which include lack of access to transportation, language, cultural, and technological resources), and major social stressors that affect their overall health (e.g., housing and food insecurity).[3,4,7] Substance abuse, homelessness, and behavioral health challenges also contribute to frequent ED use, although more notably in the small subset (1–3 percent) of "super users" ($\geq$18 times per year).[8,9,10] The trifecta of social, medical, and behavioral stressors creates the perfect storm of access and fuels repeated, potentially avoidable ED use.

Intensive, multidisciplinary, community-based care coordination has clearly been shown to decrease ED utilization in addition to achieving cost-effective, patient-centered care for these patients.[11,12,13] Several innovative programs provide primary care, health coaching, and behavioral-health home visits for extended periods (usually for 3–6 months, sometimes indefinitely) after patients leave the ED or hospital ward.[11,14,15] Patient interviews and evaluations of care coordination programs show that these programs work because they foster long-term relationships with patients – a goal best achieved by community-based care, not directly by ED or hospital staff.[16] The fundamental question remains: what is the best way to connect vulnerable, frequent ED users with existing community-based services that are proven to improve patients' health outcomes while reducing ED utilization and hospital admission?

Innovation

In 2011, several stakeholders from key organizations in Aurora, Colorado, collaborated on a community-based, multidisciplinary care coordination program for frequent ED users. The stakeholders had representation from several areas:

- Primary care: Metro Community Provider Network (MCPN), a federally qualified system of 23 community-based health centers in the Denver metro area.
- Hospital service: the University of Colorado Hospital (UCHealth) ED, a tertiary care academic center with approximately 100,000 annual ED visits, approximately 40 percent by Medicaid-insured patients.
- Mental health: Aurora Mental Health, composed of 13 clinics located throughout Aurora serving approximately 20,000 Aurora citizens.
- Community organization: Together Colorado, a nonpartisan, multiracial, multifaith community organization that empowers community members to be advocates for improving their communities.

Bridges to Care (B2C) is a multidisciplinary care coordination program that strives to achieve the triple aim of raising the quality of care, improving outcomes, and lowering costs by recruiting socially and medically complex frequent ED users. Initially funded by the Center for Medicare and Medicaid Innovation in 2012, B2C is now self-funded due in large part to its success. Most adult frequent ED users who live in Aurora are eligible for B2C services, which include up to eight home visits with a primary care provider, a health coach, care coordinator, or a behavioral health specialist, all managed by MCPN. The goal of this 3- to 6-month home visit program is to engage, educate, and provide patient-centered comprehensive services to these frequent ED users. On completing the B2C program, graduates receive their ongoing needed services at an MCPN clinic rather than at home. Engagement of frequent ED users at the right time and place was the key to a successful B2C program.

Initially, the B2C program had two full-time community health workers (CHWs), physically located at the MCPN clinic, who received a list of Aurora residents who had visited the ED the previous day. They then screened every patient to determine if he or she was a frequent ED user; if so, the CHW attempted to phone the patient to explain the B2C program and assess his or her interest in its care coordination services. We initially found that the CHWs spent most of their time in an office trying to call patients they could not reach. In 8 months, the two CHWs enrolled only 60 patients in the B2C program.

Therefore, we moved the CHWs from the MCPN office to the UCHealth ED. However, it was challenging for a CHW to conduct chart reviews on patients as they rolled into the ED to identify which ones were frequent ED users (defined as ≥ 3 ED visits/6 months). In fact, about 30 percent of all patients using the ED in any given day meet that criteria. Doing in-depth chart reviews to count the number of previous visits was too time intensive. To help CHWs use their time in the ED more effectively, we created an electronic health record (EHR) flag that allows CHWs to quickly identify frequent ED users and then do real-time recruitment for the B2C program. Within 3 months, 80 new frequent ED utilizers were referred to the program. Based on the initial positive financial impact and clinical success, the CHWs became UCHealth and MCPN shared employees. Through this shared arrangement, the CHW recruits frequent ED users for the B2C program as well as those patients with demographic characteristics consistent with patients who are at risk of becoming frequent ED utilizers and connects them with community and medical resources (e.-g., primary care providers, food pantries, etc.).

The majority of care coordination efforts by the CHWs were initiated after the patient was flagged by the EHR screening tool. The tool analyzed variables including the patient's insurance status, primary care physician status, frequent-user status, illness risk scoring, and other specific elements pertinent to care coordination. Similar to other healthcare providers, the CHWs were able to customize their view of the electronic patient tracking board to highlight patient-specific issues most relevant to their respective roles. In addition, CHWs actively engaged ED providers by making rounds with each attending emergency physician every 4 hours to review specific patient issues and to inform the care team of the capabilities of the program. After evaluating a patient, and obtaining consent, the CHW communicates what he or she learned about the patient and what services they would be able to provide. To facilitate ED provider–initiated consultation process, an electronic order set was created that automatically alerted the CHW about a new potential consultation and provided the patient's name and location in the ED.

Through the implementation of this new care coordination model, we learned that to effectively deploy this type of a program, a number of key issues needed to be addressed first: (1) the CHW must receive training on available community resources and how to do basic motivational interviewing with patients; (2) the EHR has to facilitate key pieces of information that will guide the CHWs to focus their work on high-risk patients; and (3) the CHW him- or herself has to be able to refer patients for systematic delivery of services.

Preliminary Results

Four hundred high ED utilizers were initially enrolled in the B2C program, and when compared with a nonenrolled matched control group, had an approximately 30 percent reduction in ED utilization and 50 percent reduction in hospital admissions at 6 months. For patients whose chief complaint was a mental health–related issue (e.g., depression, anxiety), there was also a 29 percent decrease in utilization at 6 months compared with a matched control group.

The B2C program impacted nonfrequent ED utilizers as well. These were patient utilizers who were still considered at risk for becoming frequent ED users (lack of a primary care physician, Medicaid enrollee, and other complex social stressors). During a 6-month period, CHWs were able to assist 228 patients to secure health insurance by referring them to a community-based financial screening location, to connect 900 patients to a new or previously assigned primary care physician, and to link 160 patients with social resources (i.e., transportation, housing, and food pantries). One full-time CHW achieved, on average, 150 to 200 successful referrals per month.

ED healthcare providers consulted the CHWs approximately 50 times per day, more than any other consultative service. Providers made comments that having the ability to provide reliable outpatient care allowed them to change management and disposition for certain patients and avoid admission. When compared with the control group, primary care visits increased 112 percent for the B2C patients. The MCPN clinic now has fixed appointment slots reserved for patients seen in the ED at UCHealth.

Discussion

Although ED utilization is often appropriate and, for a large proportion of the population, unavoidable, consistent and timely access to primary care could reduce the number of potentially avoidable ED visits by frequent ED users. Reducing ED visits could benefit three main stakeholders:

- Patients who need more effective care coordination, preventive care, and chronic disease management

- Primary care physicians, who by building relationships with patients can better manage chronic conditions, avoid duplicative testing, and reduce hospitalizations and 30-day readmissions that expose patients to hospital-acquired conditions
- Payers, who aim to reduce overall health care costs

Our innovative care coordination model achieved maximal patient outreach and significant reductions in ED utilization and hospital admissions for vulnerable populations. Most important, this model changes the patient's perspective on when to access ED and primary-care services, as patients feel empowered to be in charge of their own care. One patient gave this testimonial: "Well, my emergency department use decreased. I've only been to the ED once since I enrolled in this program. It made me more comfortable to go back to my primary care doctor and say, hey, you're my primary care doctor, you're supposed to be the one to see me and give me care. It was kind of like I didn't want to bother the primary care doctor, so let me just go to the ED. So it helped in that way."

Furthermore, we have found that although payers can offer care coordination to their members, care coordinators who work with Medicaid clients in particular report difficulty in contacting patients. This is likely because many Medicaid clients change addresses frequently, may be homeless, or may use prepaid cell phones without notifying Medicaid when their phone numbers change. Standard care coordination models typically employ a combination of nurses and social workers for this task, with approximate annual salaries of $60,000 to $100,000 per year. One employee can conduct social health screenings for 8 to 15 patients every 8 hours. A large center that treats 250 patients per day (approximately 100,000 visits annually) would need 2 to 3 care coordinators for every 8-hour shift, 24 hours per day and 7 days per week.

Novel programs have employed CHWs without formal medical training. These workers can provide individual guidance, education, care coordination, and other assistance to patients as a less expensive alternative to a nurse case manager model. For patients with diabetes, cancer, and sickle-cell disease, CHWs have been able to reduce appointment no-show rates and ED utilization, as well as increase Medicaid enrollment and patient, physician, and nurse satisfaction.[15,17,18] CHWs differ from standard hospital-based nurse case managers in that CHWs are local community members, often bilingual and bicultural, and work closely with community organizations. As the central connecters between patients and existing community programs, CHWs don't need to make duplicative follow-up phone calls for weeks or months to ensure post-ED care coordination because their role is to connect patients with already existing resources and community-based care coordination programs. In addition, most CHWs cost significantly less to employ: $25,000 to $40,000 annually, depending on their level of education and training (most have only a high school or equivalent degree).

CHWs leverage existing community-based programs by building partnerships with community organizations, educating and engaging patients about which community services to consider using, and referring patients to those services with a unique cultural competency that is patient-centered and effective. Nurses are important partners in any care coordination team, but in most innovative practices they act as leaders of the care coordination team and take on more complex cases that require medical training, such as rehabilitation placement or visiting nurse association referrals. The advantage of a blended CHW–RN model is that it is far less costly, allowing any ED to expand care coordination services to be able to touch more patients while maintaining quality.

This type of blended care coordination program has notable benefits as well as specific challenges. First, there must be a robust understanding of what the local resources are for patients who live in the community and frequent the ED. In many communities these resources will have unique characteristics, which requires local programmatic customization. Next, the blended team needs a leader. As with any blended clinical care team, previous training, knowledge of skills, and limitations need to be considered. Most program leaders are nurses with clinical training who supervise nonclinically trained CHWs. Particularly challenging is that a reasonable payment model for case management does not exist. Although some states have developed a smaller per-member per-month stipend to cover clinic-based work, there is no formal or standardized payment policy that currently recognizes the value of these services. Finally, and most important, efficient care coordination takes time and reduces utilization. In a fee-for-service environment with length of stay as a publicly reported and benchmarked pay for performance quality metric, there is a double perverse disincentive to providing adequate care coordination. New payment models will need to be instituted in order to change the current incentives and better value care coordination services.

The ED plays a pivotal role in the care for patients in need of acute, episodic, and unscheduled care beyond diagnosis and management of the acutely ill. There is also the opportunity to help patients better understand and integrate with the healthcare system by engaging community programs and existing outpatient systems. Ultimately, this will promote healthy behaviors and most assuredly result in decreased, potentially avoidable healthcare utilization and decreased overall health care costs.

References

1. Hunt KA, Weber EJ, Showstack JA, et al. Characteristics of frequent users of emergency departments. *Annals of Emergency Medicine*. 2006;48(1):1–8.

2. Foundation KF. Characteristics of frequent emergency department users. Available at www.kff.org/insurance/upload/7696.pdf. Accessed August 9, 2012.

3. Vinton DT, Capp R, Rooks SP, et al. Frequent users of US emergency departments: characteristics and opportunities for intervention. *Emergency Medicine Journal*. 2014. Epub ahead of print.

4. Capp R, Rosenthal MS, Desai MM, et al. Characteristics of Medicaid enrollees with frequent ED use. *American Journal of Emergency Medicine*. 2013;31:1333–1337.

5. Handel DA, McConnell KJ, Wallace N, et al. How much does emergency department use affect the cost of Medicaid programs? *Annals of Emergency Medicine*. 2008;51(5):614–621.

6. C. M. Targeting Medicaid super-utilizers to decrease costs and improve quality of care. 2013. Available at www.medicaid.gov/federal-policy-guidance/downloads/CIB-07–24-2013.pdf. Accessed December 16, 2013.

7. Ginde AA, Lowe RA, Wiler JL. Health insurance status change and emergency department use among US adults. *Archives of Internal Medicine*. 2012;172(8):642–647.

8. Billings J, Raven MC. Dispelling an urban legend: frequent emergency department users have substantial burden of disease. *Health Affairs* (Millwood). 2013 Dec;32 (12):2099–2108.

9. Capp R, Rosenthal MS, Desai MM, et al. Characteristics of Medicaid enrollees with frequent ED use. *American Journal of Emergency Medicine*. 2013;31(9):1333–1337.

10. Liu SW, Nagurney JT, Chang Y, et al. Frequent ED users: are most visits for mental health, alcohol, and drug-related complaints? *American Journal of Emergency Medicine*. 2013;31 (10):1512–1515.

11. Brenner J. Camden Coalition Program. 2012. Available at www.camdenhealth.org/wp-content/uploads/2011/01/Charges-Hotspots.pdf. Accessed August 9, 2012.

12. Intensive CM cuts ED visits, hospitalizations. *Hospital Case Management: The Monthly Update on Hospital-Based Care Planning and Critical Paths.* 2012;20(10):153–154.

13. Bodenmann P, Velonaki VS, Ruggeri O, et al. Case management for frequent users of the emergency department: study protocol of a randomised controlled trial. *BMC Health Services Research.* 2014 Jun 17; (14)264.

14. Kangovi S, Mitra N, Grande D, et al. Patient-centered community health worker intervention to improve posthospital outcomes: a randomized clinical trial. *JAMA Internal Medicine.* 2014;174(4):535–543.

15. Enard KR, Ganelin DM. Reducing preventable emergency department utilization and costs by using community health workers as patient navigators. *Journal of Healthcare Management.* 2013;58 (6):412–427, discussion 428.

16. Mautner DB, Pang H, Brenner JC, et al. Generating hypotheses about care needs of high utilizers: lessons from patient interviews. *Population Health Management.* 2013;16:S1:S26–S33.

17. Freeman HP. Patient navigation: a community based strategy to reduce cancer disparities. *Journal of Urban Health.* 2006;83(2):139–141.

18. Thoms E, Ryan B, Santalucia C, et al. The emerging field of patient navigation: a golden opportunity to improve healthcare. Available at http://chanet.org/TheCenterForHealthAffairs/MediaCenter/Publications/IssueBriefs/12–12_Patient-Navigation.aspx. Accessed March 20, 2016.

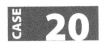

Big Data

Use of Analytics for Operations Management

Joe Guarisco and James Langabeer II

Introduction

Healthcare as an industry has a long way to go to achieve the type of efficiency and quality that provides the responsiveness and level of service quality that both providers and patients desire. Nowhere is this truer than in the emergency care setting where crowding and long wait times are common. With nearly 140 million ED visits annually, approximately one-quarter of these patients are seen in less than 15 minutes and many experience wait times greater than 1 hour, leaving ample room for improvement opportunity.[1] The Institute of Medicine's report, *The Future of Emergency Care*, outlined several key recommendations for improving the current emergency medicine crisis, including a strategy of improving hospital efficiency and patient flow using both operational management techniques and information technologies.[2]

There has been little adoption of data-driven operational techniques in the typical emergency department (ED). With the growing rate of annual ED visits in the United States combined with an increased adoption of electronic health records, there is ample information available for predictive and prescriptive decision-making.[3] What has been most effective is a process improvement approach that views data and information as essential ingredients to change.[4] Many hospitals and EDs are embracing methods such as lean or Six Sigma, which favor data and modeling of patient demands, resources available, and operating constraints to reduce variability and improve consistency of performance outcomes.[5] At their core, any process improvement project is really about understanding the underlying data – its behavior, trends, and patterns. Data offer administrators and providers the opportunity to get a clearer understanding of what is really occurring in their EDs beyond what is just observed or intuited. Analytical models can transform these data into actionable strategies and decisions to drive improvements.

The term "big data" applies to extremely large datasets that can be analyzed to reveal trends and patterns. Big data was formally defined as having three key characteristics: volume, variety, and velocity.[6,7] Applied to healthcare, *volume* represents the cumulative size of data generated about patients available from all sources. The *variety* of the sources includes the electronic health record, images, laboratory results, pharmacy prescriptions, insurance claims, and revenue cycle billing data. Finally, *velocity* represents the speed of the data generated, and how quickly it changes. Data from EDs have each of these characteristics and therefore have the potential to be "big" and to contribute to the use of analytics to make data-driven decisions that influence operations.

Retailers such as Barnes and Noble or Walmart have used analytics for more than a decade to predict sales at granular levels, such as by store and time of day. Demand predictions then drive staffing levels for clerks and cashiers, inventory orders, and even prices. For example, Walmart uses weather data to predict and subsequently increase sales. When hurricanes are forecasted in regions of the country, Walmart identified that specific items such as Pop-Tarts and alcohol dramatically increase in sales.[8] Rather than lose potential sales, Walmart can preemptively respond by increasing their availability ahead of storms, anticipating consumer demand. Another example is Amazon, which uses related item searches to suggest alternative products should a consumer not initially find a product.

Despite its potential and research already performed, implementation of analytics is low in the ED setting.[9] Given the more than 5,000 EDs in the United States and millions of ED patients subjected to delayed care, the potential is tremendous. In this chapter, we describe how one organization (the Ochsner Health System) used analytics to transform one ED into a data-driven facility with improved operational performance.

Data and Analytics Case Study: Chabert Medical Center

In 2014, the Ochsner Health System in New Orleans, Louisiana, partnered with Chabert Medical Center in Houma, Louisiana, to evaluate operations in their ED. Table CS20.1 provides a view of the performance metrics over a 3-month period for the Ochsner facility before and after the implementation of analytics. In order to address the process failures and constraints that were creating these operational issues (see Table CS20.1), robust data acquisition with an analytics focus was needed.

Although seemingly straightforward, the first step in using analytics in this ED was gaining access to the operational data. Then came the filtering, sorting, and displaying of data in ways that would reveal visual insights into Chabert's operations. The next step in moving the ED from the benchmark June 2014 performance to the July 2015 performance required a global look at Chabert's workflow, workload, and workforce while simultaneously visualizing performance through an analytic lens. With near real-time data acquisition and data management, the drivers of performance and potential solutions to Chabert's patient throughput problems were better understood.

There are many complex operational processes in an ED that can benefit from process improvement (e.g., laboratory and radiology result times), and reliance on a single performance measure ignores these processes. While those processes and the associated delays are important, room and provider availability tend to be the more critical bottlenecks from a throughput perspective. Additionally, there are standard measures (e.g., arrival-to-provider) that are available, widely understood, and easily measured and communicated during any process improvement initiative focused on operations.

It is known that best practice for "arrival-to-provider" is 15 minutes, while the national average is 40 minutes according to the ED Benchmarking Alliance. In comparison, looking at existing performance data at Chabert, arrival-to-provider was measured to be 125 minutes. In other words, patients were waiting more than 2 hours on average to initiate patient care processes. This resulted in increased waiting room congestion and downstream

Table CS20.1 Performance Metrics for Chabert Medical Center before and after Implementation of Analytics over a 3-Month Period in 2014 and a Similar Period 1 Year Later in 2015 (all times are in minutes)

	Left without being seen (%)	Arrival-to-room	Arrival-to-provider	Discharge length of stay	Admit length of stay
Before analytics	16.7	101	125	336	600
After analytics	1.8	30	43	162	372

crowding in the ED. Thus, this process improvement effort was targeted at reducing the amount of time it takes a clinical provider to engage a patient after arrival, and subsequently accelerating the remainder of the ED patient visit and decreasing patient length of stay (LOS) to an even greater degree.

In reviewing the analytics in Table CS20.1 for arrival-to-provider subprocesses, it was concluded that sufficient room capacity was the major bottleneck. Specifically, Chabert needed to create additional capacity in the form of patient rooms. Providers seeing patients promptly after room assignment, while an important issue, was a lower priority, as the room-to-provider cycle time was relatively reasonable (24 minutes) and could therefore be addressed after the room availability constraint was resolved.

Further understanding how patients were placed in a bed, the focus shifted to the two activities at Chabert that occurred prior to patient assignment to a room and placement in a bed: registration and triage. We used national operational benchmarks to evaluate the performance of our existing processes contained within the global arrival-to-provider time period. Benchmark data suggested that the initial registration cycle time (time to complete registration) should be approximately 1–2 minutes and a quick-look triage cycle time (time to complete initial nursing assessment) should be approximately 3–5 minutes. However, Chabert's global arrival-to-room was 101 minutes (Table CS20.2).

As evident in Table CS20.2, each of the processes comprising the Chabert's arrival-to-room time interval was measured; registration cycle time was found to be 7.4 minutes and the triage cycle time to be 12.6 minutes, both metrics far longer than best practices recommend. With a triage cycle time of 12.6 minutes on average, considering the impact of variation on queuing, fewer than five patients could be expected to be triaged per hour. At peak periods, arrival rates could double, surpassing Chabert's ability to triage and creating a bottleneck. When exploring potential solutions for these delays, some health systems have opted to eliminate both of these processes. The ED management team at Chabert Medical Center opted to retain them, albeit in a simplified lean form, minimizing the data requirements at registration and triage and still safely sorting the patients to the appropriate patient care area based on acuity at presentation.

Improving efficiency and shortening the cycle times of the subprocesses of registration and triage did not sufficiently impact arrival-to-provider cycle times. Looking at the patient arrival process downstream from triage, Chabert had deployed a "provider in triage." This provider, an advanced practice provider (i.e., nurse practitioner or physician assistant), initiated care immediately following triage by ordering tests before the patient was seen by a treating physician. In the end, this did not expedite care, and patients continued to wait for a room (and a physician) or subsequently left the ED before being seen. This created a potential source of liability for abnormal test results, did not help improve patient throughput, and worsened the left-without-being-seen performance measure. Ultimately, provider in triage, though attempting to improve throughput, was actually a bottleneck and was viewed as an interim process that could be eliminated.

Table CS20.2 Time Intervals for Chabert Medical Center That Comprise the Arrival-to-Room Duration (all times are in minutes)

Arrival-to-triage	Registration cycle time	Triage-to-room	Triage cycle time	Arrival-to-room
17.4	7.4	71	12.6	101

Having improved bottlenecks, room and provider availability remained as the only potential constraints. Analytics targeting room demand and supply were developed. Measurement of existing processes, comparison with benchmarks, and displaying data in an easily understood format provided good evidence that bed capacity was a major bottleneck in the ED. Using hourly census data from the third quarter of 2014 (see below, Figure CS20.2a), it was evident that ED patient census quickly outpaced room availability for the majority of the day. The percentage of patients leaving without being seen similarly increased during these times of reduced capacity.

To increase capacity, Chabert could either add additional beds, an expensive process, or build "virtual capacity." Virtual capacity allows an organization to add extra space (e.g., patient beds) without actually adding expensive physical infrastructure. Virtual capacity can be created by changing operational processes, in this case by using patient streaming in a split flow system.[10,11] Patient streaming distributes patients based on complexity and acuity into a high and a low complex stream (Figure CS20.1).

Using the retained lean processes of mini-registration and quick-look, the patients are split into less acute/less complex and more acute/more complex patient types. Acuity and complexity generally run parallel. The split flow goal is to separate patients on the basis of whether or not they can be managed in an ambulatory environment (i.e., no bed). For example, a patient with heart failure exacerbation or severe abdominal pain would be a high complexity patient, requiring laboratory work, radiology, and a decision whether to admit the patient. Most important, these patients need a bed. On the other hand, low complexity patients, for example, those with pharyngitis or low back pain, whorepresent 65 percent of all ED patients, could have quick decisions about their care.[10] These patients can be managed in an ambulatory fashion and do not need a bed. Deploying split flow thus creates "virtual capacity." However, addressing bed capacity was not enough – sufficient staffing levels were necessary to provide care once a patient arrived. Managing the supply demand for these resources is a challenge for a busy ED and requires simple but effective analytics tools. To determine the number of rooms and providers, Chabert used optimization tools from Intrigma to efficiently match patient demand with room and provider capacity. To meet peak demand for rooms, as the Chabert experience showed, the hourly census at 2 PM (31 patients) would require a near doubling of the existing 17 ED beds to meet patient demand. Using split flow work

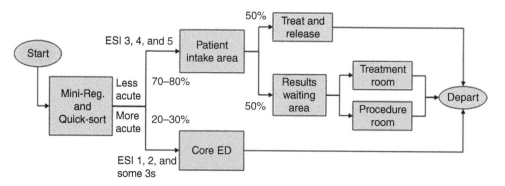

Figure CS20.1 Split flow system patient flow diagram. ESI, Emergency Severity Index.

processes, low complexity patients either were immediately discharged after seeing a provider or went to a results waiting area to await further test results and minor treatments. This results waiting area could accommodate a far larger number of patients than a traditional ED bed, freeing up a real ED bed for patients with a higher complexity illness. As a result, Chabert not only reduced ED LOS for discharged and admitted patients, as shown in Table CS20.1, but also reduced the peak number of patients in the ED by over 16 percent, from 31 to 26.

Additionally, again relying on analytics, Chabert focused on provider productivity (i.e., LOS for admitted and discharged patients). These data revealed a significant variability in LOS when filtered by provider, and these results were shared with the clinicians. Unblinding the data gave providers insight related to their practice patterns and enabled ED management to tailor provider education. Arrival-to-admission cycle time was further broken down into the following time periods for admitted patients: arrival-to-disposition decision, and admit-decision-to-departure. Again, simply producing and unblinding this type of data resulted in effective practice pattern behavioral changes and enabled management to target process improvement efforts toward individual provider performance.

The resultant improvement in capacity from the process improvement work as described above reduced LOS and in turn decreased the maximum number of patients in the ED from an average of 31 to 26 at peak census periods. Further, the patient census was decreased for 21 of 24 hours of the day (Figure 20.2a), and the reduction in LOS not only decreased for all patient categories but was sustained more than 1 year later (Figure CS20.2b).

The same analytics approach that was deployed to improve and efficiently match bed demand to bed supply was applied to provider staffing. This would complete the arrival-to-provider cycle time improvement project. The lower acuity/less complex patient stream is staffed by advanced practice clinicians (physician assistants and nurse practitioners) with emergency physician oversight, and the higher acuity/high complex patient stream is staffed by board-certified emergency physicians. To determine the appropriate number of providers for each stream, the optimization tool Intrigma was deployed once again. This software allowed Chabert to create a staffing model that could effectively manage patient demand and its inherent variability, providing for high probability that a provider would be available at patient arrival. Intrigma uses patient demand data (arrivals per hour) adjusted for hourly variation, interactivity between different levels of providers, including scribes, and further adjusted for the specific provider productivity profiles.

The front-end process changes described earlier created room availability, and optimization using predictive analytics increased the probability that a bed and a provider would be reasonably available, thereby improving the "arrival-to-provider" time.

This multifaceted, data-driven approach using analytics resulted in substantial and sustained results in a relatively short period of time for this ED (Figure 20.2b). Though the improvement after 1 year for the project was not at the goal of 30 minutes for arrival-to-provider time, the target of 2 percent left without being seen was achieved and the reduction in arrival-to-provider time from 120 minutes to 45 minutes was dramatic (Figure CS20.3).

At the 18-month time mark in February 2016, Chabert achieved a 25-minute arrival-to-provider time and 0.5 percent left-without-being-seen as a result of continued process improvement.

(a)

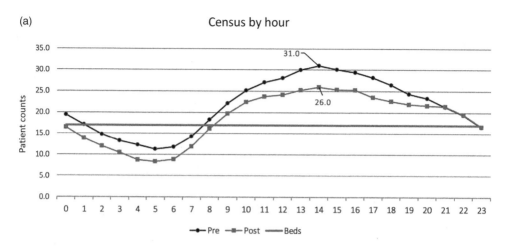

(b)

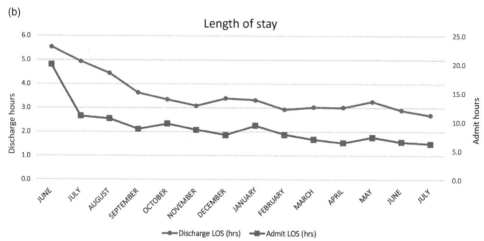

Figure CS20.2 (a) Bed occupancy versus bed availability by hour of day. (b) Discharge and admit cycle times by month.

Discussion

The innovations described in this case study demonstrate how one healthcare system used analytics with existing ED data to identify and implement changes to clinical ED operations. This aligns with a commonly used approach employed by most hospitals, the "Plan-Do-Study-Act" process improvement methodology. As demonstrated here, these data helped to identify and prioritize process improvement opportunities by performing the following steps:

1. Visually displaying operational data to identify trends and patterns for patient demand, census, and performance over time.
2. Understanding performance and identifying outliers by provider or time of day.
3. Identifying variability and tendencies in existing processes.

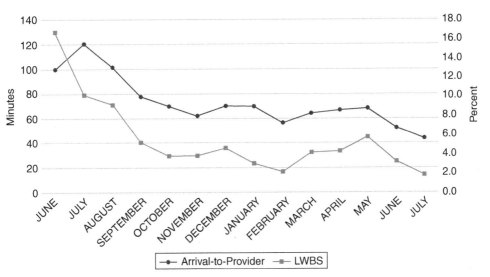

Figure CS20.3 Arrival-to-provider versus left-without-being-seen.

4. Using these data to develop staffing models that are better matched with patient demand, leading to better ED performance.
5. Incorporating these multidimensional process improvement efforts into a comprehensive process improvement project that was successful in accomplishing its original goal of making the ED more responsive to patient needs.

The widespread implementation of electronic health records makes large operational datasets ubiquitous.[3] This reduces barriers to use and facilitates application of analytics to the ED and other clinical settings. Others have documented similar improvements in EDs, such as for personnel scheduling and resource allocation or to identify high-utilizers that impede care coordination and bottleneck the ED.[12,13] The *Annals of Emergency Medicine* published an article to help explain the big data concept and provide instruction for how to utilize it appropriately.[14] Clearly, big data and analytical models not only are here to stay but will be used with increasing frequency and sophistication. Future applications could allow EDs to increase an ED's flexible capacity in response to current and predicted conditions. There is a potential for incorporating frequency of infectious diseases, such as pneumonia and influenza, along with recent ED volume, weather, and public events to predict patient volume for the day. Dynamic changes in bed capacity and staffing could make not only the ED but the hospital more responsive to ever-changing conditions.

The use of analytics holds great promise and can enable EDs to achieve improved operational performance through faster throughput, with a reduction in errors and unnecessary costs. Lessons can be learned from other EDs that have revolutionized their processes through data and process improvement to nearly eliminate all waste and waiting.[15] Streamlining processes and eliminating the waste in many EDs will be possible only by making data-driven decisions. Never before has so much data been available.

However, obstacles lie in this path and challenges exist with using tools for pattern identification and in determining what to do with these data. Ensuring that the data resources are accessible to practitioners is a major hurdle; and then if they are available there are often problems with data integrity and quality. Ensuring the data are complete and accurate often involves substantial effort. Having access to technology analysts and information technology staff who can help to run reports and assist in this project are vital, but they are often resource constrained. Finding alternative paths around these obstacles will take leadership. The challenges can be overcome, and those who take this journey to master their systems and data will be best prepared to succeed.

References

1. Centers for Disease Control and Prevention. Emergency department fast facts. Available at www.cdc.gov/nchs/fastats/emergency-department.htm. Accessed January 2, 2016.

2. Institute of Medicine. *The Future of Emergency Care: Key Findings and Recommendations*. Washington, DC: National Academy of Sciences, 2006.

3. Centers for Disease Control and Prevention. Progress with electronic health record adoption among emergency and outpatient departments: United States, 2006–2011. Available at www.cdc.gov/nchs/data/databriefs/db187.pdf. Accessed March 27, 2016.

4. Langabeer J, Helton J. *Health Care Operations Management: A Systems Perspective*, 2nd ed. Boston: Jones and Bartlett.

5. Deblois S, Lepanto L. Lean and six sigma in acute care: a systematic review of reviews. *International Journal of Healthcare and Quality Assurance.* 2016;29(2):192–208.

6. McAfee A, Brynjolfsson E. Big data: the management revolution. Available at https://hbr.org/2012/10/big-data-the-management-revolution/ar. Accessed March 27, 2016.

7. Ghosh R. Healthcare and big data: hype or unevenly distributed future? Available at www.analytics-magazine.org/november-december-2015/1465-healthcare-analytics-healthcare-and-big-data-hype-or-unevenly-distributed-future. Accessed January 2, 2016.

8. Hays C. *What Wal-Mart knows about customers' habits. New York Times*, November 14, 2004. Available at www.nytimes.com/2004/11/14/business/yourmoney/what-walmart-knows-about-customers-habits.html?_r=0. Accessed January 2, 2016.

9. Saghafian S, Austin G, Traub S. Operations research/management contributions to emergency department patient flow optimization: review and research prospects. Available at http://papers.ssrn.com/sol3/papers.cfm?abstract_id=2420163. Accessed March 27, 2016.

10. Agency for Healthcare Research and Quality. Door-to-doc patient safety toolkit. Available at https://innovations.ahrq.gov/qualitytools/door-doc-patient-safety-toolkit. Accessed March 2, 2016.

11. Saghafian S, Hopp WJ, Van Oyen MP, et al. Patient streaming as a mechanism for improving responsiveness in emergency departments. *Operations Research*. 2012;60 (5):1080–1097.

12. Cerrito P, Pecoraro D, Browning S. Visits to the emergency department as transactional data. *Journal of Healthcare Management.* 2005;50(6):389–395.

13. Bates DW, Saria S, Ohno-Machado L, et al. Big data in health care: using analytics to identify and manage high-risk and high-cost patients. *Health Affairs.* 2014;33(7):1123–1131.

14. Janke AT, Overbeek DL, Kocher KE. Exploring the potential of predictive analytics and big data in emergency care. *Annals of Emergency Medicine.* 2016;67 (2):227–236.

15. Goralnick E, Walls R, Kosowsky. How we revolutionized our emergency department. *Harvard Business Review*. Available at https://hbr.org/2013/09/how-we-revolutionized-our-emergency-department. Accessed March 2, 2016.

Index